Psychology Revivals

Fifty Years of the Tavistock Clinic

Originally published in 1970 this title commemorates the men and ideas that started, inspired and established a pioneer institution in British psychiatry. Based on the impetus of Freudian and related innovations after the First World War, the Tavistock Clinic offered treatment, training and research facilities in the field of neurosis, child guidance and later on group relations.

Dr Dicks, who had been associated for nearly forty years with the work and personalities that helped to develop the Tavistock venture, describes the struggles and capacity for survival of the clinic. He shows how, belonging neither to the older classical psychiatry nor to orthodox psychoanalysis, and suspect to both, the Clinic nevertheless became increasingly used by the rest of the profession as a psychotherapeutic resource. Dr Dicks describes the influence of the Tavistock on the medical, psychological and social work scene both before and after the Second World War, and assesses its achievements as a centre of psycho- and socio-dynamic thinking.

The Tavistock is shown as a pioneer *sui generis*, launching psychosomatic research and initiating the exciting ventures in social psychiatry associated with the Army in the Second World War. As the Tavistock was the outcome of work with shell-shock victims in the first war, so its offspring, the Institute of Human Relations, was the natural continuation of the military effort in man-management, morale and group dynamic studies. The book includes an account of the inter-relationship between the Clinic, now part of the National Health Service, and the Institute, a private corporation. Still going strong as part of the Tavistock and Portman NHS Foundation Trust today this is an opportunity to revisit its early history.

Fifty Years of the Tavistock Clinic

H.V. Dicks

Routledge
Taylor & Francis Group
LONDON AND NEW YORK

First published in 1970
by Routledge & Kegan Paul Ltd

This edition first published in 2015 by Routledge
27 Church Road, Hove BN3 2FA

and by Routledge
711 Third Avenue, New York, NY 10017

Routledge is an imprint of the Taylor & Francis Group, an informa business

Publisher's Note

The publisher has gone to great lengths to ensure the quality of this reprint but points out that some imperfections in the original copies may be apparent.

Disclaimer

The publisher has made every effort to trace copyright holders and welcomes correspondence from those they have been unable to contact.

A Library of Congress record exists under ISBN: 0710068468

ISBN: 978-1-138-82194-1 (hbk)
ISBN: 978-1-315-74302-8 (ebk)
ISBN: 978-1-138-82195-8 (pbk)

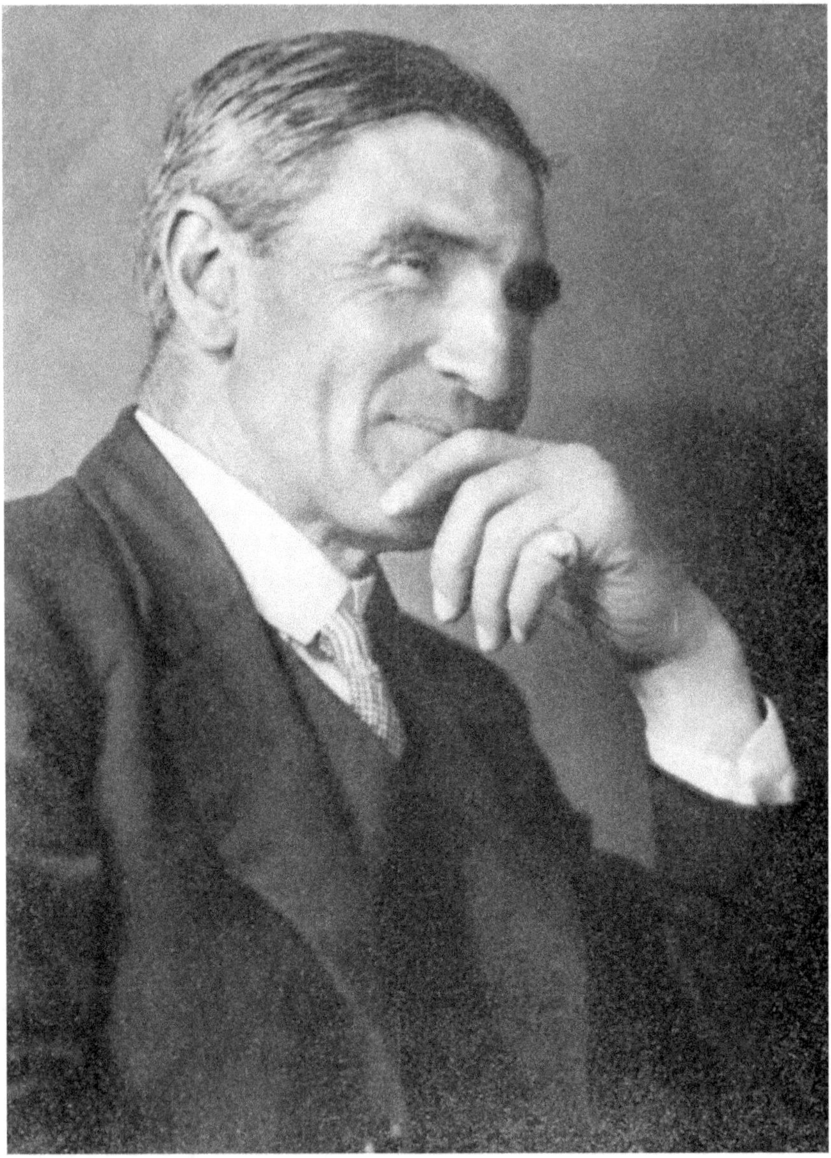

H. Crichton-Miller, M.D., F.R.C.P.
Medical Director 1920-1933

Fifty Years of the Tavistock Clinic

H. V. DICKS

with a foreword by Sir Leslie Farrer, K.C.V.O.

London

Routledge & Kegan Paul

First published in 1970
by Routledge & Kegan Paul Limited
Broadway House, 68–74 Carter Lane
London E.C.4
Printed in Great Britain by
Ebenezer Baylis & Son Limited
The Trinity Press
Worcester, and London
Set in 11 on 12 pt Baskerville

ISBN 0 7100 6846 8

Contents

List of Illustrations

Foreword

I have been asked to write a Foreword to this book; mine not to reason why, but, given both the subject and the author, it should not be too difficult.

By the end of the First World War the importance of psychological stresses had become clear, but the close study of the subject was not one that appealed to many doctors. A small group, however, imbued with the conviction that these stresses were the source of much suffering, under the leadership of Dr Hugh Crichton-Miller, created the Tavistock Clinic as a centre where this work could be furthered and taught. As so often for those breaking new ground, financial worries were constant; nevertheless, as also happens, dedicated persistence and good work began to bring their rewards. The small band of pioneers soon attracted others who wished to pursue this daunting yet fascinating subject, and by the mid-thirties the Tavistock Clinic was becoming known throughout the world.

From the start there was a breadth of vision which readily allowed these doctors to realize the importance of what was going on in the social groups in which the individual lived as well as the factors that his own development had formed inside himself. As a result, training was soon extended beyond doctors to the new professions of the psychiatric social worker and the clinical psychologist—an invaluable innovation for those attracted to the possibilities in these fields.

When the late Dr J. R. Rees, the Medical Director of the Clinic, became the psychiatric adviser to the British Army, this dual perspective on the individual and the society in which he had to function enabled the 'Tavistock Group', as they came to be known, to make many major innovations in handling the urgent social psychological tasks of the Army in the Second World War. After the war the Council of the Clinic agreed with the plans put forward by the staff—now augmented by many new members who had shared their experience in the Army—for a new sister body to complement the work on the clinical side. The Clinic was to enter the National Health Service, and the new body, the Tavistock Institute of Human Relations, was established in 1946. In the next two decades both Clinic and Institute made the name of the Tavistock renowned amongst those concerned with mental health and with social science. Despite the administrative separation of the two bodies, the combination of the viewpoints, the forces internal to the individual and those in his social milieu, persisted. It was an inspiring recognition of the work of both bodies after twenty years in extremely restricted premises, when the Minister of Health, Mr Kenneth Robinson, agreed to provide magnificent new premises, and the staffs are permanently indebted to his encouragement. In the spring of 1967 the late Princess Marina opened the new building. Her Royal Highness had succeeded her husband, the Duke of Kent, after his tragic death in 1942, as the Patron of the Tavistock, and her keen and informed interest, expressed in several informal visits as well as on more formal occasions, was a constant source of satisfaction to the Councils and to the staffs. The Tavistock is very happy that the daughter of its first two patrons should now have accepted the office.

It is, however, unnecessary for me to try to write the history of the Tavistock myself. As the fiftieth anniversary approached, the Council of the Tavistock Institute of Medical Psychology, the original Council, which had remained in being, considered the project of getting a history written to mark the occasion. Little thought was needed as to who should do it. Dr Henry Dicks was the obvious choice. He was one of the early distinguished members of the Clinic staff and had been at the centre of its affairs for over thirty years. The Council was delighted when he undertook this task, an arduous one, but, I believe, for him, who had the welfare of the whole Tavistock so much at heart throughout this period, a labour of love. His book admirably conveys his deep identification over this long period with all that was going on.

The history of an institution is naturally of interest primarily to those who have been connected with it. Nevertheless, the history of the Tavistock should have a wider appeal. For, along with their professional work, the staffs of both bodies devoted a great deal of effort to making their own organizations function as satisfyingly as possible for their own members and for their governing bodies. Staff participation in the management of their affairs is a widespread and urgent concern today. How the Tavistock did this is a most important feature of their work, and many institutions will find much of interest in the way the staff created its own democratic organization with a clear structure of responsibility attached to the various leadership roles, both in their relationships internally and to their external authorities.

As one who has been connected with the Tavistock in one capacity or another for thirty years or more I find this book extremely interesting and hope that it may be widely read.

Leslie Farrer

Author's Preface

The Council of the Tavistock Institute of Medical Psychology has honoured me in asking me to prepare this jubilee volume on the history and vicissitudes of the Tavistock Clinic during its first fifty years. In some ways I am, I suppose, the most obvious person, since I have lived through some thirty-eight of those years as a member of its medical staff—a sort of latter-day Talleyrand who survived all régimes until my retirement from the active staff in 1965.

I am aware that this book has perhaps become too long, with some tendency to repetition. Undue and rigorous compression and strict logic might, however, have made it too formal and abstract. I have aimed to avoid the narrowness of a mere parish chronicle, but rather to afford the 'outside' reader some notion of the place of the Tavistock Clinic in the history of British psychological medicine, while, also paying, in some instances all too brief, tribute to those men and women, professional or administrative, who in my view have made the greatest contributions to the growth and good name of this rather unusual institution in their several roles. I hope that those colleagues and helpers, past and present, whose share in carrying the responsibilities of clinical work, education, research or administration has been just as essential, though not named by me, will forgive my subjective emphases.

I was fortunate in having, at an early stage, the help of our greatly loved Dr J. R. Rees, C.B.E., recently deceased, whose tape-recorded account of the origins and first few years is the main source material for 1920–7. It tallies with his own brief account in *Reflections* (1968). As some readers will know, after 1945 the original Tavistock Clinic budded off a new institution —the Institute of Human Relations. It would have been impossible, on the one hand, to write the post-1945 history of the

Clinic itself without constant references to its vigorous twin. On the other hand, it was also beyond the scope and intentions of this present volume to include a detailed account of the complex development of the Institute, very much a flourishing body, corporate in its own right. I therefore, on my sole responsibility, invited the Institute's own Secretary, Mr Sidney G. Gray, to contribute a chapter covering in outline the main events and developments from the Institute's standpoint, which he has, I think, done admirably. It was the best practical solution I could think of. To Mr Gray, therefore, as well as to the late Dr J. R. Rees, I want here to express my gratitude for their part in this volume. To Miss Marjorie Harborough I owe thanks for her transcription of tape-recordings and help with the secretarial side, including some appendices, and to Mrs Mollie Tupholme (herself a former staff member) for her excellent and patient preparation of several versions of the manuscript. Mrs Maureen Wright and Miss Veronica Nicholson have kindly helped with the appendices.

I am greatly indebted to Dr J. D. Sutherland, John Bowlby, A. T. M. Wilson and Professor E. L. Trist for valuable suggestions and correction of inaccuracies in the text, which Mr Gray has also improved.

To Sir Leslie Farrer, K.C.V.O., in his role as Chairman of the Council of the Tavistock Institute of Medical Psychology, I am grateful for his kind Foreword to this book, which has only been made possible through the generous encouragement of that Council, the direct heirs of the original Tavistock's governing body. I wish to add, however, that for the views and orientations expressed in what follows I assume sole responsibility.

Lastly, I wish to thank the Crichton-Miller Trust for permission to quote passages from the memoir, *Hugh Crichton-Miller, 1877–1959* (privately printed), in which I have drawn on the contributions by Mrs Leith-Ross and Mr Donald Crichton-Miller.

H.V.D.

I

Introductory Outline

The Tavistock Clinic was established in 1920 as one of the first out-patient clinics in Great Britain to provide systematic major psychotherapy on the basis of concepts inspired by psychoanalytic theory for out-patients suffering from psychoneurosis and allied disorders who were unable to afford private fees. The clinic owes its foundation to the vision and energy of the late Hugh Crichton-Miller, M.D., F.R.C.P. (Founding Medical Director), who had worked with a group of doctors of academic standing on what was then called 'shell-shock' (battle neurosis) in the First World War. He wished to carry into the civilian sphere their fruitful military experience of gaining understanding and power to help neurotic sufferers by adapting Freud's theory of neurosis to treating these shell-shocked soldiers. This origin of the Tavistock Clinic in psychodynamic thought is stressed from the outset of this book because it has imparted a lasting orientation to the Clinic's structure and staffing, despite departures from strict psychoanalysis, and because it has provided a special image of the Clinic both to its staff and to the British medical scene.

The focus that is characteristic of the Tavistock is the emphasis on the until then ignored or misinterpreted sphere of the neuroses and personality disorders now illuminated by the 'New Psychology' originating in Vienna and Zürich. This distinctive 'mix' was in the fourfold aim of *understanding and treatment*, the furthering of *research* into causation in the hope of finding rational means of *prevention* in mental hygiene, and on *teaching* the emerging concepts and skills to future specialists as well as to all those, medical and non-medical, concerned with mental health and human relations.

On the basis of this orientation, it was logical that there should be emphasis on understanding the patient as the product of his environment and of his own history. This led to the Clinic being organized in two parts; the Adult Department and the Children's Department, conceived as a unity although differentiated in roles, where the aim was to understand the child as the father of the man and the parents as conditioning the new generation of children. It also led from the first to the notion of the multi-disciplinary team to cover all aspects of personality study: the psychiatrist, the psychologist and the social worker. The first patient ever seen in 1920 was a child; this was some years before the first 'official' Child Guidance Clinic opened in London. The Clinic from the first had a curiously independent, indeed isolated, position somewhere between official psychiatry and medicine on the one hand and 'orthodox' psychoanalysis on the other. Both of these were in development, and the Tavistock was, in a sense, part of this forward movement.

The Clinic's revenues were derived from sympathetic guarantors and donors with impeccable credentials, who provided social support at high levels; from public subscriptions as the result of appeals and charity functions; and to some extent from such small fees as the patients could afford. With few exceptions, the medical staff gave their services free or for nominal honoraria, as in other voluntary hospitals of that time.

While psychodynamic, the Clinic's doctrine beyond this general orientation was to 'have no doctrine', but only aims: to help, to understand more and to teach its work. As such it was the meeting-ground of psychotherapists of several schools or of none, making for a certain vagueness and lack of theoretical homogeneity, but also for flexibility and a wide variety of techniques and viewpoints. These were from the beginning debated at monthly meetings of the compact, small staff. The Clinic's existence as a medical institution, not wholly committed to the then still much-feared and suspect psychoanalytic school (to whom none the less the Tavistock staff group owed most of its conceptual basis), made this new approach to psychoneurosis more acceptable and 'respectable' to British medicine in the 1920s. Its image was always that of an open forum, of a synoptic viewpoint and ethically above reproach.

Contrary to Crichton-Miller's hopes, other clinics were slow in being established. Crichton-Miller had conceived the Tavistock as a model, as we should now call it, which he expected would be copied by the teaching-hospital psychiatric departments and by out-patient centres elsewhere based on mental hospitals; but this development was slow and halting. Consequently, this little pioneer centre in a decrepit building in Bloomsbury was before long swamped with immense demands for both clinical services and for training facilities, to which the staff responded to the best of its ability. By 1932 it was already necessary to make a move to a larger home than the original dwelling-house in Tavistock Square (from which the Clinic derived its name). This move was made possible by the good husbandry and the generosity of the voluntary help from Treasurers and Finance Officers who were able to secure a lease of some disused mews in Malet Place, by University College, where a reconstruction was carried out. Here we had premises suitable for instituting systematic training in psychotherapy, in child guidance, in psychiatric social work and in the then existing elements of clinical or educational psychology. Some of these courses were later sponsored and recognized by London University.

Shortly after this move, which was still under the direction and inspiration of Crichton-Miller, events occurred which led to Dr Crichton-Miller's resignation, when the direction passed to his Deputy Director, J. R. Rees, in 1934. The phase from 1932 to 1939 represented the period of greatest expansion in treatment, training, external lecture courses and in numbers of staff and trainees. Many former students of both sexes and from many countries who received their training at this time came to occupy leading positions in psychiatry and child guidance and in related fields in Britain and overseas. Two closely-related centres were founded by members of the Tavistock Clinic in association with others during this period, and may be said to be 'daughter colonies'. The first of these was the Davidson Clinic in Edinburgh; the second was the Portman Clinic, as it was later called, originally the Institute for the Scientific Treatment of Delinquency, opened in 1931.

Research as a major activity in the Tavistock Clinic was a

relative latecomer, due largely to economic conditions. The medical staff, as mentioned, were all working part-time, mostly unpaid, and burdened with big case loads. Such 'academic' time as they had was devoted to teaching their skills to the younger generation while having to earn their livelihood in private practice. It is also fair to add that the psychotherapist is not often a rigorous research methodologist by nature. However, the volume of publications of papers and books flowing from the Clinic was quite considerable, and individual members of the Tavistock staff achieved eminence for their contributions to the growing mental-health field and to psychopathology. By the mid-1930s we were fortunate in securing two research fellowships endowed by the generosity and belief in our work of the Rockefeller Foundation and of the Sir Halley Stewart Trust respectively. By the onset of the Second World War a number of original contributions of more rigorous research design and content had appeared. These were chiefly along the lines of the then novel psychosomatic method of enquiry. The two holders of these fellowships, Dr A. T. M. Wilson and Dr Eric Wittkower, made a considerable impact on the younger generation of teaching hospital physicians by pointing to this link between psychological and somatic aspects of sickness. Their work answered to some extent what had been justifiable criticism of the Tavistock Clinic's tardiness in research.

In these first twenty years of its development the Tavistock Clinic thus came to be a national school for the skills and approaches required for the treatment and understanding of neurotic illness and many similar conditions. It consequently was able through its various staff members to play a considerable part in the diffusion of the concepts and practice of a somewhat eclectic dynamic psychology, not only in its everyday work with children and adults and in its intra-mural teaching, but also by the great demands made upon it for extra-mural activities covering the country: the British Mental Hygiene movement, the fostering of interest in the problems of neurosis in provincial centres, by lectures and discussions to divisions of the British Medical Association, participation in scientific societies, notably the British Psychological Society's medical section, etc., which were to a surprising extent Tavistock-linked.

This activity was to have resulted in a move to a larger permanent home planned by our Governing Council. A site had been bought and was to be developed in close proximity to the new London University curtilage. However, this project was not implemented because the outbreak of the Second World War brought an abrupt change as well as great new opportunities to members of the Tavistock staff. The destruction of our Malet Place building by bombs was perhaps the least of these.

The Influence of the Second World War

The premises of the Tavistock Clinic were, fortunately, together with most of its clinical records and a large part of its library evacuated to temporary wartime premises in Hampstead, where a core staff of those not mobilized for the armed services carried on an uninterrupted service. The appointment of the Clinic's Medical Director, J. R. Rees, as head of the Army's psychiatric services during the war was not only a well-deserved tribute to the man, but a mark of confidence on the part of the Army medical authorities in the approach which he and the Clinic had consistently upheld. The greater part of the Clinic's professional staff joined the armed services as psychiatric specialists, mostly the R.A.M.C. under J. R. Rees's active leadership. This experience with massive human-relations problems under stress and dislocation has strongly influenced the second post-war era of the Clinic's life and thought, as will be seen in subsequent pages. The problems thrown up in Army psychiatry were perceived by the group around J. R. Rees to be largely those of social psychology, of interpersonal relations. We were not concerned ourselves so much with treatment of war casualties, of which during long stretches of the war there were few. The focus of interest was on the questions of morale-building, as exemplified in man-management problems between officers and other ranks, hence on selection methods for such leadership; on re-adapting the displaced and the traumatized, especially of those who had long been prisoners-of-war (civil resettlement); on the proper allocation of skills for the various roles of the soldier in military life, including the use to which the dull and backward soldier might be put; on the study of the mentality of enemy nations, with its feedback into social and political psychology, and many more.

It was within this group drawn from among staff members of the pre-war Tavistock and from psychologists, psychoanalysts and psychiatrists from other centres that a new trend of thinking grew which they were as eager to apply to peacetime problems, as Crichton-Miller and his colleagues a generation earlier had been to transfer their new insights and skills to civilian life. These concepts came to be based on clinical psychiatry and dynamic psychology, on psychoanalysis and on recent work, especially from the United States, on the frontiers of psychoanalysis and cultural anthropology, on the social psychology and the group dynamic studies of the field theorists among the *Gestalt* school, and also on some sociometric techniques. This preoccupation with social, large-scale group phenomena in the Forces dominated the interests of this very closely-knit Army group. Thus it came about that we made scarcely any major new contribution to the treatment of traumatic neuroses, which were largely 'farmed out' to the emergency medical services run by the Ministry of Health. It inevitably also resulted in something of a gap between the Army group and those who had not been called up, but had carried on gallantly the hitherto customary services of the Tavistock Clinic in its wartime premises.

1945–8

In the years immediately following the Second World War, and indeed before it ended, the new trends became embodied in the policy and structure of the Clinic. A planning committee with wide powers had been *elected by the whole staff* in order to implement them. It was already apparent that a National Health Service was on the way. That the Clinic should play its full part in the psychiatric area of that Service was generally accepted with considerable enthusiasm, because we had become accustomed to working without the need to consider the voluntary hospital financial difficulties or the claims of private practice during our war service. So once again war was the stimulus of the 'second birth' of the Tavistock Clinic into its more or less present-day guise. However, it was only for three years that the old Tavistock Clinic emerged as a new entity which we called the Tavistock Institute of Human Relations, embodying the multi-disciplinary and integrative approach to the behavioural sciences listed a moment ago. Once more the Rockefeller Foundation generously came to help us with the start of this momentous new development. There were also other substantial grants from anonymous donors. In this new Institute it was hoped to integrate the study of personality development and its vicissitudes with medical sociology and with group dynamics. The work retained its clinical base in the therapeutic and training activities of the 'old' Clinic rejuvenated by the infusion of new staff members, among them a much higher proportion of doctors and psychologists appointed for whole-time or near whole-time service. Some of the older staff members who could not visualize themselves working happily in the changed conditions withdrew. The group of those who started the new venture had been close collaborators in the Army and developed a common viewpoint on their future problems and on the theoretical basis for approaching them.

In this new setting, in a house procured by the sale of the old Bloomsbury site on which the pre-war Tavistock was to be re-erected, there could be a promise of continuity of teamwork and a concentration on teaching and research as well as on improved skills in dealing with clinical psychotherapy. It was perhaps because of the inherent sociological interest no less than for their clinical importance that the staff of the whole Institution began its development of group methods (of study and of therapy) with which the Tavistock Clinic was now to become largely if inaccurately identified at home and abroad. The theoretical framework characteristic of the Tavistock Clinic's approach to group therapy had been laid down by W. R. Bion and the late John Rickman originally for purposes of economy in manpower, as well as for leadership studies in the Army. Now the therapeutic group became the main link connecting personality study, the endeavour to change personality disorder and the study of group dynamics or interaction psychology.

The staff group during this time spent much effort in debates on the decisions to be taken about our role in the National Health Service and the plans for it. In view of the likely preoccupation of that Service with clinical work in the strict sense rather than with developments in what was likely to be viewed as the 'para-medical field', it was to be assumed that only the clinical departments would easily fit into the National Health Service. That part of our new structure concerned with social psychology and group dynamics of institutions – e.g. industry – was more likely to succeed in its pioneer function if it retained its independence. In consequence, the Tavistock Institute of Human Relations was separately incorporated before the Health Service took effect. There remained in legal being also the old Council of the pre-war Tavistock under the name of the 'Tavistock Institute of Medical Psychology'. This continued to contribute to developments from what resources it had and was legally entitled to accept legacies and donations helping the Health Service body with free moneys. This is the body which is making possible the publication of this present volume.

It was inevitable also that there should be considerable conflicts of orientation. It was as the result of such difficulties that a second crisis in leadership structure resulted in the resignation of J. R. Rees from the directorship of the Clinic, to be replaced by Dr J. D. Sutherland, the third Medical Director, in 1947. Limiting ourselves for the moment to the organization of the Clinic, the division into departments for adults and for children was preserved because of the necessarily different skills and approaches required. Dr Sutherland also acted as head of the Adult Department, while Dr John Bowlby, another of the post-second-war recruits to our staff, was appointed head of the Department for Children and Parents and Deputy Director of the Clinic. In their day-to-day work the departments remained largely autonomous, but the unity of the whole was preserved by a Professional Committee drawn from staff members of all disciplines of both departments and by frequent joint meetings and seminars.

Medical responsibility for the treatment and disposal of every patient accepted by the Clinic has always rested, from the beginning of the Clinic, with psychiatric consultants, though the actual work of therapy and of certain diagnostic procedures is shared by non-consultant members of the medical, or by non-medical staffs.

The National Health Service

On 5 July 1945, then, in common with nearly all other voluntary hospitals of the country, the Clinic became part of the National Health Service. Administered for some seven years by the Central Middlesex Group Hospital Management Committee of the North-west Metropolitan Regional Hospital Board, it changed in 1956 to the Paddington Group Hospital Management Committee for geographical and administrative reasons. Whilst thereby the necessity for having a Governing Council for the Clinic was done away with, the now separately incorporated Institute of Human Relations came under the administration of a new Council, partly recruited from members of the Tavistock Clinic's pre-war Council and partly from new professional circles with the relevant interests. Until 1959 the Clinic and Institute occupied parts of the same building at No 2 Beaumont Street, W.1, but with the growth of both organizations additional accommodation became an urgent necessity. A large house at No 3 Devonshire Street, in the vicinity of the Clinic, was acquired by the Institute in that year, and by arrangement with the Health Service authorities this building also was shared by both Institutions. These two bodies continued to have close working ties, with some overlap in staff. Senior members of both staffs constituted a joint Staff Board. The Institute was able to raise considerable funds from private foundations and from grants by public authorities to finance training and research based on the Clinic. These funds are now administered by the Institute through a special Sub-Council for Family Psychiatry and Community Mental Health. From 1949 the Clinic developed a new unit devoted to the study and treatment of marital conflicts. In 1957 the Institute took over the administration of another marital casework centre, the Family Discussion Bureau, founded originally within the Family Welfare Association. Both these units have substantially added to the resources for treatment of family and marital problems. The Clinic also developed, in 1959, a new unit devoted to problems of adolescents, who often do not fit readily into a department organized either for adults or for younger children. This unit is developing into a full new department.

To summarize: the structure of the total Institution as it now stands is that, *qua* Tavistock Clinic (with which my history is largely concerned), it is a special centre not designated as a teaching hospital, for the diagnosis and treatment of neurotic and personality disorders. This is financed by the State. *Qua* teaching institution and research centre, it largely relies on its twin sister, the Tavistock Institute of Human Relations, which, as a private corporation, is able to accept donations and grants to organize teaching and to finance and administer major research work. This dichotomy arises from N.H.S. policy and structure, which limit these latter functions to designated teaching hospitals. Many of the developments of the post-war era sponsored by the Clinic and the Institute have been generously supported by grants to the Institute from the Ford Foundation, the International Children's Centre, the Josiah Macy Junior Foundation, the Foundations Fund for Research in Psychiatry, the Old Dominion Foundation, the Grant Foundation and the Field Foundation in the United States of America, by the Sir Halley Stewart Trust, the Carnegie United Kingdom Trust, the Gulbenkian Foundation, the Home Office, the Joseph Rowntree Memorial Trust, the Mental Health Research Fund and the Mellanby and Southfield Trust in Great Britain, and by the Regional Office for Europe of the World Health Organization.

In 1956 the Clinic and Institute were invited to submit plans for future development to the Regional Hospital Board which were worked out in a liaison committee with the Institute's Council. After consideration of the programme, the Ministry of Health approved the plans for our new building in Belsize Lane at Fitzjohns Avenue, which we now occupy. The new premises are a much more fitting home for the work of treatment, teaching and research for which we have become known. In October 1965 our former Medical Director, J. R. Rees, was able to lay the foundation-stone, suitably inscribed. Our present building, about three times larger in floor space than our previous one in Beaumont Street, was taken over at Easter 1967 and opened officially by our Royal Patron, the late Princess Marina, Duchess of Kent, on 4 May in the presence of a large and distinguished company. At this point its history merges into the present.

II

Origins

All sources that we have been able to consult are united in describing the inception of the Tavistock Clinic as something which originated in Dr Crichton-Miller's[1] mind. Thus in a private biography of H.C.M., Mrs Leith-Ross, who was our first and voluntary Secretary, refers to his 'vision' of founding a clinic. The same kind of statement is made by Dr J. R. Rees.[2] This 'vision' H.C.M. expressed in words in his first Tavistock Clinic report, which will be cited later in this chapter. On the level of action, the Tavistock Clinic may be said to have been launched at a meeting which took place some time in 1919 in the drawing-room of Lady Margaret Nicholson in Pont Street, Chelsea. Lord Wolmer (now the Earl of Selborne) was in the chair, Dr Farquhar Buzzard (later Sir Farquhar), then a physician at St Thomas's Hospital, the Reverend Lionel Ford, Headmaster of Harrow School, and H.C.M. himself spoke. There was a promise of £300 and the Tavistock project was now a reality. This was to be, as stated in ch. i, a clinic where psychotherapy would be offered to people of modest means, in order to continue what had been achieved in the Army with cases of war neurosis or shell-shock. At this meeting, also attended by a medical member of the Army, Lieut. Colonel H. Gordon Mackenzie, D.S.O., it was pointed out that 'the treatment of functional nervous disorders had received a great stimulus as the result of war experience . . . that much had been

[1] We shall mostly refer to Dr Crichton-Miller by his well-known initials, 'H.C.M.', by which he was nearly always addressed by his friends and even by his juniors.

[2] We shall often refer to Dr J. R. Rees, second Medical Director, by his habitually used initials of 'J.R.' in the Tavistock. In his W.F.M.H. contacts he appeared to prefer 'Jack'.

done for the war neurotics and much was being done for pensioners, but little, if anything, was being done for civilians'. It was also suggested that 'many of the younger medical men who had had war experience might be given an opportunity of working at a clinic with such [i.e. neurotic] civilians'. It was expected that the larger hospitals would soon establish psychotherapeutic clinics. It was therefore agreed to start a clinic on an experimental basis of three years' duration, with the understanding that it should be closed if and when the hospitals could meet the need.

As mentioned above, subscriptions and donations were given or promised that assured an income of £300 a year for three years. A committee was formed and an honorary medical director appointed. The latter was, of course, H.C.M. himself. The Committee should here be named. It consisted of J. Douglas C. White, M.A., M.D., who became the first Chairman; the famous Dean of St Paul's, the Very Reverend W. R. Inge, Sir Lindon Macassey, K.B.E., K.C., the Hon. Mrs Edmund Pery,[1] Mr Owen Hugh Smith (Chairman of Hay's Wharf) and Sir F. J. Willis, K.B.E., C.B., the Chairman of the Board of Control, which at this period of history looked after the welfare of mental patients with direct responsibility to the Privy Council. In addition there were in attendance the officers of the Executive Committee. These were the Honorary Medical Director, Mr Dougal O. Malcolm (later Sir Dougal), our first Honorary Treasurer, and Mrs Leith-Ross who, as mentioned, was the first Honorary Secretary, a position which she occupied for some six years.

Progress

The hunt for suitable premises which were central and easily accessible from the Harley Street area (in the expectation that doctors would give what time they could from their private practice to this new venture) proved difficult, not only because after the First World War the housing problem was as acute as it was after the Second World War, but also because it was difficult to secure permission from ground landlords for what they

[1] Later the Countess of Limerick on the succession of her husband to the title.

feared might turn out to be a clinic for wildly disturbed lunatics! At last, however, a house was secured in Bloomsbury at No 51 Tavistock Square, W.C.1. This had been run as a 'Victory Club' (a veterans' hostel) after the war but had failed, and the lease was very cheap. It had a number of small rooms and one considerable drawing-room which could be used for meetings and lectures. As all of us who worked there knew, it was a depressing, gloomy, tall old house, but it was situated close to the centre of things, and it looked out over the trees of Tavistock Square. Furniture and furnishings were supplied by Mrs Leith-Ross and her personal friends and the friends of the early staff members; these fittings were both sparse and ramshackle. No one wanted a high-sounding title, so the new venture simply came to be called the 'Tavistock Square Clinic for Functional Nervous Disorders', and quickly became 'Tavi' to all its friends.[1] It was here on 27 September 1920 that the first case was seen, and H.C.M. said, 'My dream has come true'. The first case seen was a child; the second case seen was an adult.

Owing to the loss of pre-1939 records due to bombing, the earliest details are in some cases not very reliable. Thus it was stated that the original staff consisted of seven persons, but in fact nine are listed as having been appointed in September 1920. Here are the names, with such details as can be found: H.C.M. himself as Honorary Director, J. R. Rees (to be made Deputy Director in 1926), Dr Mary Hemingway, who was soon to become Mrs J. R. Rees; Dr J. A. Hadfield, Dr E. A. Hamilton Pearson, Dr D. Leslie Tucker. But there is also the name of Dr Neill Hobhouse, who was to be the neurologist and general physician in order to keep an eye on the physical state of every patient who applied. There also occurs the name of Dr W. A. Potts, whose work lay in Birmingham, but who became honorary head of the children's service of the early Tavistock. Then there was a lady doctor, Dr Evelyn Saywell; and Dr David Yellowlees (brother of Dr Henry Yellowlees) was attached to the Tavistock for a few months before moving to

[1] J. R. Rees suggests that the original name was the 'Tavistock Clinic', but that, owing to many complaints by the G.P.O., who were always sending letters to Tavistock in Devonshire, the name was changed and the word 'Square' inserted between 'Tavistock' and 'Clinic'.

Glasgow, where he became one of the earliest exponents of psychotherapy.

Dr W. A. Potts was a Medical Officer with Birmingham City Corporation, in care of mental deficiency and a psychological expert to the Birmingham Justices. He published a good deal on the subject of subnormality and entered child psychiatry through the mental-deficiency field. He was also a Jungian.

Dr Leslie Tucker was a recently qualified man who had just done house jobs and then went to Bowden House (H.C.M.'s private nursing-home) as a resident medical officer, and was brought in by H.C.M. to help at the Tavistock.

Dr Hamilton Pearson qualified in 1912 and with his adventurous temperament became a surgeon in the Chilean Navy after leaving the R.A.M.C. He then came into psychiatry via a resident post at the Lawn at Lincoln, then a private mental hospital for paying patients. He served the Tavistock Clinic as Director of the Children's Department until the outbreak of the Second World War, when he went back to his love of the sea and volunteered, no longer a young man, to be a medical officer on board the ships that were taking child evacuees to overseas countries just before the Blitz. Thereafter he served in the Children's Branch of the Home Office as a senior medical officer, until his death some few years ago.

Two other near-original members of staff should be mentioned here. Dr P. F. Barton, who qualified in 1890, was a senior and experienced general practitioner with strong talents for psychotherapy who served the Clinic well until his retirement around 1929. Similarly, Dr Eleanor Montgomery, a venerable mother-figure and also a retired general practitioner, did, according to J.R., very good work in the earliest days, using the Crichton-Millerian psychosomatic or 'double-barrelled' approach to the neuroses.

Before going on to describe the kind of clinical life that was lived in this austere building, we should perhaps note that, however sketchily the physical base of the Tavistock was organized and financed, there was no lack of influential community and medical support for H.C.M.'s new Clinic. Thus, one is impressed with the list of Vice-presidents, varying from marquesses and marchionesses to the two First World War

Commanders-in-Chief of our two services, Earls Beatty and Haig; academic support in the persons of William McDougall (at this time already gone from Oxford to Harvard) and Sir Henry Newbolt; Dame Katherine Furse of the Red Cross. No less impressive was the earliest Medical Advisory Board, which contained many of the most distinguished physicians of the London teaching hospitals, including the already mentioned Sir E. Farquhar Buzzard (of St Thomas's and the National Hospitals), who later became Regius Professor at Oxford; Dr Walter Langdon-Brown (later Sir Walter) of St Bart's. Hospital, later to be Regius Professor of Physics at Cambridge; Dr Adolphe Abrahams (later Sir Adolphe), the Dean of Westminster Hospital, Mr Wilfred Trotter, F.R.S.,[1] and many more. It was interesting that Queen Square and organic neurology were well represented. A particularly valuable supporter was Dr C. W. Kimmins, the Chief Medical Officer of the London County Council Education Department. A word should perhaps be said about our first Chairman of Executive, Dr J. Douglas White, who was not a psychiatrist, but a Harrow doctor who was greatly concerned with the then nascent interest in social factors in health, and in health education. In addition to chairing the Executive of the new Tavistock Clinic, he was also the originator of the Council for Health Education, of which he later became the first Executive Officer.

As without doubt the Tavistock was very much the creation of that remarkable man, H.C.M., his general orientation and attitude towards the treatment of neurotic and personality disorders should be placed on record. This is not only in order to praise him, but also to emphasize the continuity through all these years in the ideas and values which the Tavistock has consistently represented, and which remain very much closer to his original vision than he himself at a certain point in the history of the Clinic was willing to believe. The principle on which H.C.M. wanted the Clinic to develop was one of freedom from administrative and institutional bureaucracy, a place where a patient could come with a sense of privacy and confidence; a place where each person was seen punctually by

[1] A pioneer of neuro-surgery and famous also for his book on *The Instincts of the Herd in Peace and War* – an early essay in group psychology.

appointment and always by the same doctor, in which there were no forms to fill in and no awkward details to be given in cold blood, so different from the dreaded long hours of waiting in the hospital out-patient departments, never knowing which doctor you might see. It is true that many patients and many referring doctors were at first nonplussed by this great difference from any then-existing medical institution. Only bare rooms with tables and chairs and an occasional couch; no apparatus, no dispensary, no medicine to take away, no white coats or syringes, except in one room!

H.C.M. had gathered a small band of early enthusiasts around him who belonged to all manner of orientations in psychotherapy and who had varying academic or clinical backgrounds and standing. Having himself begun as a most successful general practitioner with experience of the rich and idle on the Riviera and also in Aviemore, he knew the prejudices of the medical world against neurotics as the people of imaginary illness who were under-employed and lacked purpose in life. H.C.M. was most anxious to dispel this image of neurotics as either the *malades imaginaires* of the 'useless Society woman type' or else as 'dregs of society', idle, unemployable and malingering. In fact, from the first he visualized the Tavistock as a place where people who were still struggling to hold on to work and to being useful members of society could find comfort and support. One knew that his sympathy and focus of interest lay with these middle sort of people whom he called 'the educated poor': the students, the clerks, the overworked housewives of the middle class and similar sections of the population, who had slender means and a maximum of social stress in the post-war world. Strangely enough, this kind of clientele has also remained the majority of the existing patient load, probably because it was this class of person who had both the intelligence and the insight to understand, in the light of their reading, the essentials of the nature of psychoneurotic problems and symptoms, and who were not content to be fobbed off with bottles of medicine or with various magical techniques which they had had before and which they knew did not touch the core of their difficulties. H.C.M., an aristocrat in temperament, was none the less a man of deep compassion and patience and continually stressed the importance of respect due to even the most foolish of patients. He also propounded the doctor's own need for self-examination and humility, which naturally led to his advocacy of personal insight derived from a training analysis. He was keen to preserve what he used to call binocular vision – that is to say, paying attention both to physical and to mental factors of the given illness. He felt that the private consulting-room, the 'Harley Street' atmosphere, was more suitable to the treatment of such disorders than the institutional atmosphere. Despite his strong views and values, Crichton-Miller tried not to be an autocrat. He left everybody free to use their best endeavours to produce results. I will quote some of the words he wrote in his first report to the Council of Administration. He said:

> The medical profession suffers from a tacit convention that its business is to cure a diseased condition of the body. *Our* avowed aim is to investigate, and if possible to remedy, disabilities of the personality as a whole. If a man contemplates suicide it is of little use to assure him that he is 'free from organic disease'. He has found that life is not worth living; it is our business to find out why, and if possible to make him feel that life *is* worth living. If a woman complains of numerous and vague pains which have driven her to the out-patient departments of half the hospitals in London, it is not enough to assure her that her pains are all imaginary. An imaginary disease is a disease of the imagination, and as such it may be just as disabling as a disease of the heart or lungs. It is our business to find out why her imagination continues to generate such unpleasant and crippling sensations. Similarly if a child of 12 is referred to us by the headmaster of his school for persistent pilfering, it is futile to say, 'Stealing is an anti-social act; he must learn the consequences of his actions; let him have a good caning or be handed over to the police; that will teach him a lesson he will not forget.' But will it? Our attitude is that a reason must be found to explain why this particular boy should need such drastic penal treatment. What is it in his personality that makes him incapable of assimilating the usual lessons of honesty? If we can find out

> the answer to that question we may possibly save the community from having on its hands in years to come one more incorrigible criminal.

The report continues:

> Now in these three cases we see personalities that are unharmonized or maladjusted and as such of little or no value to society. The ideal of mental hygiene is incompatible with such social waste. It demands that the healer's function should be interpreted in the broadest way and that consideration be given not only to the body but to the mind, not only to the patient, but if necessary to his environment. Thus it comes about that in his work of salvaging maladjusted personalities, we found ourselves confronting all sorts of problems, applying all manner of remedies and meeting with very varied results.

H.C.M., in a few pungent words, gives us an insight into the catholicity and breadth of his therapeutic outlook. He continues:

> It took but twenty minutes to recognize that the man who was contemplating suicide required thyroid treatment. The woman with the 'imaginary' aches had to undergo a lengthy analysis before she obtained freedom from the results of a forgotten sex incident which occurred at the age of five. Six interviews were needed to straighten out the 12-year-old thief, and two of these were devoted to the unconscious cause of his misdeeds, to wit, his new stepmother. Therefore, when the captious critic hints that people who complain of 'nerves' are not worth treatment we reply that there is work to be done – the work of creating harmony in the unharmonized, adjustment in the maladjusted, independence in the dependent, and social worth in the socially worthless: and when we speak of the 'socially worthless' we are thinking of our average patient not as he is but as he may become if he is allowed to drift.

H.C.M. was also keenly aware of the epidemiological distribution of mental inefficiency and suffering. He listed the minority of patients chronically confined in the mental hospital, an intermediate group who may be allowed to alternate between mental hospital and the community, and, thirdly those who are what he calls

> Men and women by the hundreds who will never enter an asylum but are as good as inside in so far as their value to the community is concerned. These are 'nervous breakdowns' less popularly described as minor mental disorders, that represent a very appreciable proportion of the lost working time in all but manual occupations. In fact it would be a conservative guess to say that at any given moment there are for every certified lunatic at least ten workers not certified but disabled by psychoneurosis or a mild psychosis.

With the help of a table analysing the composition of the case load of the moment (1927) at the Tavistock Clinic, H.C.M. showed that something like three-quarters of the patients were at work and none the less thought it worth while to carry on with their treatment, because he says:

> Without such out-patient psychotherapeutic help they would either be out of work or drifting to the inevitable breakdown . . . hence the economic importance of early out-patient treatment is a logical corollary of the acceptance by the community of the principle of supporting the worker during disability.

H.C.M. next went on to demonstrate by an analysis of occupations of the patients attending that nervous disorders were by no means a prerogative of either 'the idle rich' or of the weak-minded, self-indulgent or hysterical. He says: 'A considerable number of our patients are of outstanding force of character and some of unusual intelligence', after which he proceeds to show the composition of the patient group of teachers, social workers, clergy, artists and students, as well as clerks, artisans, small traders and many housewives. He continues: 'If then we contemplate this vast array of those who are inefficient from mental causes it behoves us to ask ourselves how far so great an evil is unavoidable and how far we are called to endure it'. He then proceeds to plead the essential curability of mental disorders:

> Public opinion is not sufficiently enlightened to realize that in many asylum cases we can recognize no brain changes, and that many a neurosis is a potential psychosis, just as many a cold is potential tuberculosis. Such hard-and-fast differentiations between sane and insane do not belong to life nor yet to science; they belong to social exigencies and are based upon behaviour rather than the origin or presumed course of any given case of mental disorder. Enlightened opinion realizes today that some asylum cases are curable, that many uncertified cases of mental breakdown can be saved and that a very great proportion of both might be prevented.

H.C.M. concluded this part of his first report with a plea for ample funds so that the Tavistock Clinic could continue not only to apply measures for alleviation of maladjustment, etc., already known, but mainly to try to do research into causes with the aim of obviating avoidable mental inefficiency. He expressed his belief that the work of the Clinic, regarded in this light, had a definite economic value to the community. He, moreover, also showed that, owing to lack of whole-time workers, fellowships and proper schemes of training, the mental health professions were being starved of progress in which even in 1920 the United States had shown themselves to be much in advance.

H.C.M. wrote all this some years before the Mental Treatment Act of 1930, which is commonly held to have ushered in a new era in British psychiatry. Here we see not only an appreciation of the economic and epidemiological aspects of the so-called minor mental disorders, but also a very considerable depth of insight into the continuity and possible overlap between the categories of the neuroses and the so-called 'insanities' still called 'lunacy' in 1920, as well as a kind of blue-print for much of what would nowadays be called 'preventive psychiatry'. Thus the three small case vignettes that he chose showed at once that he regarded mental aetiology as between the suicidal depressive with his low thyroid function, the anxiety-hysterical housewife with her unconscious sexual problem and the stealing child as in some way all tied together by a set of common factors for which he uses the word 'unconscious'. With this broad vision of the scope which the Clinic was to cover, it behoves us to try to examine the sources of our Founder's attitudes and scientific orientation.

It would be wrong to assume that H.C.M. learnt his ideas from his work as an Army medical officer in what would nowadays be called a 'neurosis unit', to the possible influence of which I shall return. We read in his son's brief biographical perspective of his father that

> In 1910 the new psychology was very new indeed; a virgin field lay open to a young man whose imagination had been fired by the writing of Freud and who knew intuitively and by experiments he had made in hypnotism and the treatment of 'nervous' cases that he was peculiarly fitted to exploit the weapons now available to medical psychology. In a flash he saw what could be done to save people from mental depression, from the asylums, from suicide.[1]

It would seem, then, that H.C.M. was already a psychotherapist when the war came, and in fact he implemented this new vision of his by starting in 1911 a new-style nursing-home for psychoneuroses and early or mild psychoses in the famous Bowden House at Harrow-on-the-Hill of which he was the Director and moving spirit for some forty years. While it is true that H.C.M. was already a psychotherapist, it seems to be fairly certain that before the First World War he drew his concepts and methods from the French School deriving from Charcot and represented by Déjérine and Janet. His later, more psychoanalytic orientation was probably enhanced by work with the war-time Army unit that treated cases of shell-shock by the 'new psychology' in the not yet inaugurated buildings of the Maudsley Hospital. In 1912, for example, he published a book called *Hypnotism and Disease*, whereas soon after the war he edited a very different book called *Functional Nervous Disease*. William McDougall, one of the group who took part in the war-time applications of Freud's original doctrines, lists H.C.M. among the school he called British or 'integral'. Among them he pays particular tribute to W. H. R. Rivers, and also lists Drs William Brown,

[1] *Hugh Crichton-Miller, 1877-1959*, A personal memoir by his friends and family (1961), privately published and printed by Longmans (Dorchester) Ltd., pp. 6–7.

Millais Culpin, J. A. Hadfield, Bernard Hart, T. W. Mitchell and some others. Among those men William Brown, Millais Culpin, J. A. Hadfield and Bernard Hart, as well as the Editor of the then *British Journal of Medical Psychology*, T. W. Mitchell, were intimate collaborators with H.C.M. during the war and later supported the work of the Tavistock Clinic. Rivers died in 1922. The characteristics of this group were that whilst they accepted Freud's basic propositions concerning the unconscious and conflict and the various mechanisms, they had rather individual approaches, some leaning towards more eclectic and others towards more McDougallian interpretations of the dynamics of behaviour and neurosis. In some cases Jung's ideas also found representation, notably so in H.C.M. himself. Hadfield, a former pupil and assistant of McDougall's during his Oxford days, was a member of the staff from the beginning. Culpin, Bernard Hart and others were at various times members of the Medical Advisory Board and regularly lectured in the Clinic courses. Another influence on the ideas found in the Tavistock at its inception were those of a British pupil of Jung's named Maurice Nicol, who had a hand in analysing several of the early staff members. Others had training analyses by the late James Glover, the brother of Dr Edward Glover, himself a well-known psychoanalyst who died young.

The picture, then, emerges of H.C.M. as the indubitable leader both as regards administration and public relations and as regards the stock of theoretical concepts brought to bear on the practice of the Tavistock. J. R. Rees, who has helped me with the preparation especially of this chapter, recorded his view that H.C.M.'s mind was quite open about Freudian, Jungian, Adlerian and many other ideas, including the French School deriving from the Suggestionists. In addition, he was also very alive to the developing sciences of biochemistry and endocrinology and to the focal sepsis theory, which was just then a fashion in British medicine. It is also fair to call H.C.M. a follower and admirer of the psychobiology of Adolf Meyer of the Phipps Clinic, Baltimore. This is shown in his view of man as developing from the vicissitudes of childhood through human relationships on the basis of inherited traits and instinctual organization which reacts with the environment. Hence his emphasis on having a Children's as well as an Adult Department in which the staff should gain experience of the whole range of ages – and hence, perhaps his best-known and most important mental hygiene books called *The New Psychology and the Parent*, and *The New Psychology and the Teacher*.

It would, however, be an incomplete picture of H.C.M. were we to confine ourselves to his medical and psychopathological orientation. He was above all a deeply religious person. This was shown not so much by the fact that he became an Elder of the Scottish Presbyterian Church of St Columba's, London, as by his quite open emphasis on the force of Christian moral ideas as bearing upon human conduct, and especially on the development of individuals' moral responsibility for their actions. Among his cherished ideas were those contained in Kipling's 'If', which, if one knew the man, one did not find ridiculous in those early days, because he lived this kind of strenuous, dedicated life. It was not generally known that, hard pressed though he was with a large family to educate, he made up deficits of the Clinic's earliest budgets from his own pocket, i.e. the profits of Bowden House, which he regarded as a way of 'soaking the rich in order to help pay for the poor'.

With this background we may begin to construct something of a picture of the early days at the Tavistock Clinic, its practice and its education work. It would seem that the 'public relations' aspect of the Clinic was from the beginning based on personal links which H.C.M. and J.R. developed with some of the personalities that have been mentioned, and many others. Among these were consultants who advised on the somatic aspects of H.C.M.'s private patients at Bowden House and in Harley Street, those colleagues with whom he came into relationship through his membership of the Medical Section of the British Psychological Society and the many Society people who formed his clientele in Scotland and on the Riviera. In addition, J.R. has told us that one of the first things that was done was to distribute circulars to the profession giving briefly the aims of the Tavistock and its purpose in being founded, and appealing for support in both senses, professional by referral of patients and financial by donations and subscriptions. It certainly is an imposing list of institutions that sent patients in the very first years of the Clinic's life. Evidently in 1920 there was already some recognition that psychotherapy was a valid treatment even though highly suspect, and, secondly, that there was a woeful lack of facilities for it elsewhere in London. It would be wearisome to list all these bodies, but, as already mentioned, they included such citadels of orthodox medicine as the National Hospital, Queen Square and the major teaching hospitals of London.

H.C.M.'s philosophy and aims seem to have been shared by the small staff. Essentially they continued to regard themselves first and foremost as doctors with the binocular approach to the body as well as the mind of the patient. From the first a pathologist, Dr Gloyne, was employed to help with the necessary investigations; while, as mentioned, Dr Neill Hobhouse acted as the consultant physician and neurologist covering our responsibility for somatic factors. Social enquiry, in the absence as yet of a psychiatric social work profession, was carried out by one or two volunteers whose qualifications it is now impossible to ascertain. The name of the first honorary 'social service worker', as she was styled, was Miss N. K. Satow, who was later joined by Miss Doris Robinson. Other early voluntary social service workers were Miss Angela Trotter, later the Hon. Mrs Pery (now the Countess of Limerick), and Miss Sellar, who functioned both as a social worker and as the Librarian. H.C.M. had a wonderful way of inspiring devotion and effort on behalf of his causes in both men and women because he never spared himself and was clearly perceived as a charismatic personality. Miss Robinson became one of the first batch of social workers to be sent to the United States to train as psychiatric social workers and bring the new skills and techniques to this country. She stayed with us as Chief P.S.W. for a number of years. The first few years show no record of any professional psychologist having been appointed to the staff. However, of two of our staff members, Dr J. A. Hadfield was first and foremost a psychologist by training, whilst on the children's side we had Dr W. A. Potts, who was expert with the then prevailing test procedures. Likewise, Dr Hamilton Pearson, who actually saw the very first patient in the Clinic, was well versed in techniques of psychological testing and the ascertainment of intelligence quotients, which was just about all that the psychological services were supposed to provide in those days.

In so far as H.C.M. recruited Tavistock doctors from the Bowden House staff (that is to say Dr Leslie Tucker, J.R. and Dr Mary Hemingway, later Mrs J. R. Rees), they were taught by H.C.M. himself. In the case of J.R., this was on demobilization from an exciting period in the R.A.M.C. in the First World War. The method of teaching was by case conferences and by discussions on diagnostic and theoretical psychopathological lines. H.C.M. had apparently always used this method of joint discussion in his private practice with any doctor who came to see him about his patient or with his junior staff, whom he would make go through the history of the case. This was the method of supervising and instructing which he introduced into the Tavistock and used as his way of keeping contact with his then small staff, both for verifying diagnosis and for watching treatment progress. The whole staff would attend once a week and report what they were doing with their patients and how the patients were doing. In this way the conference learnt from each others' concepts, techniques and habits and were also confronted with their own blind spots and mistakes. It would seem that H.C.M. was more of a chairman than a dictator during these meetings, but, as J.R. says, he was very dynamic, a person who did not have to *try* to impose his views. 'It was not a leaderless group exactly, one cannot imagine that with H.C.M. there, but they were enormously inspiring. H.C.M. has never got his full credit for what he did, and the Tavi is his monument.'

It is true that the group round Crichton-Miller, including himself, were not psychiatrists in the old sense of the term; few had done long spells of service in mental hospitals. They did, however, supplement this lack by attending seminars and ward rounds in various mental hospitals. For example, J. R. Rees went to Bethlem Royal Hospital in Lambeth, which was then the main teaching hospital in London. Here J. A. Hadfield had an honorary appointment as a teacher in psychopathology, while the staff, Dr Porter-Phillips, Dr Thomas Beaton and others, did the instruction in clinical psychiatry. This deficiency in institutional experience has been very much held against the

Tavistock from the beginning of its life. The stereotype persists to this day. The exceptions were those mental hospital psychiatrists who themselves were able to incorporate 'the new psychology' into their aetiological thinking. Some of such early supporters should be mentioned. Dr H. W. B. Stoddart, a former Superintendent of Bethlem Hospital, became not only interested, but a fully qualified analyst. Dr Bernard Hart's writings are classics on the application of Freudian viewpoints to the theory of mental disease. Another such who served with Dr Stoddart was Dr (later Sir) Maurice Craig, whose inspiration not only helped the mental hygiene movement in Great Britain, but also to found our sister institution, the Cassel Hospital at Penshurst. Its first Medical Director, T. A. Ross, was also always a good friend and the best of rivals with the Tavistock Clinic. Another closely related group was the psychiatric team which had gathered in the West End Hospital for Nervous Diseases, with whom there was some overlap and interchange of staff in the first few years of the Tavistock's life. This group was the forerunner of the St Marylebone Hospital for Psychiatry and Child Guidance, now the Paddington Clinic and Day Hospital.

Early in my own attachment to the Tavistock I had the impression that H.C.M. seemed glad to receive any recruits and asked little in the way of training or experience in psychiatry. But J.R. informs me that from the very first days of the Clinic there were many applicants who for various reasons wanted to work at the Tavistock. In so far as they were not people whom H.C.M. knew well and trusted, he apparently exercised a fairly stringent selection on grounds of personality, and he turned down more than he accepted. He often sat with two assessors – a selection board – for this purpose, of whom Dr T. W. Mitchell was one. Among applicants, strangely enough, there were many Americans. It would seem that people were soon beginning to be aware of this novel institution and came over specially to see what the Clinic did, became interested and reported back, spreading our renown. At this time there were no places comparable to the Tavistock in the United States (or anywhere). It has remained a fact that the Tavistock as a carrier of certain ideas and methods has interested the Americans more than our own people from the earliest years to the present.

While on the subject of the United States, it should be mentioned that very early in the Tavistock's life contact was made with the new 'mental hygiene' movement begun by the American pioneer, Clifford Beers, who had founded in 1908 the Connecticut Mental Health Society. This link was effected through the old National Committee for Mental Hygiene, in which the moving spirits were then Dr Helen Boyle, Dr Doris Odlum and Sir Maurice Craig, as the result of Dr Boyle going to see Clifford Beers in the United States. It should also be mentioned that Dr Helen Boyle was the founder of an even earlier venture in psychotherapy, the Lady Chichester Hospital at Hove, which to this day maintains its excellent reputation as a treatment centre for neurotic and minor psychotic disorders and is now, like ourselves, in the National Health Service. It was Dr Helen Boyle who brought back the news of what the new American mental hygiene movement was doing. She interested Sir Maurice Craig, who was soon to become President of a new National Committee for Mental Hygiene. This, of course, is one of the parent bodies of the present National Association for Mental Health after its amalgamation with the Child Guidance Council and the Association for Mental Welfare. As early as 1923 J.R. went to the U.S. to attend the first international congress for mental health, in which the Tavistock experiment and aims were further presented to an international professional gathering.

We learn that in 1920–1 the supply of patients hung fire, but that it soon increased. As expected, they came chiefly from among the educated poor whom H.C.M. was most anxious to help. Soon there was a waiting list, but with a certain amount of juggling and the general co-operation of staff it was seldom more than a few weeks before a patient could be taken on. The time at which patients could be seen depended on the free hours of the doctor concerned. As now, so all that long time ago, the evening hours were always the fullest because our patients came after work. From the beginning the time allotted to every patient was a full hour, no doubt based on the Freudian model. After diagnostic sessions H.C.M. would scrutinize the records and order whatever additional investigation might be necessary.

The physical examination was generally thorough, and such things as dental examinations and the hunt for focal sepsis were carried out in nearly every case. It has been said that there were no administrative facilities. It is true that even when I arrived at the Tavistock in 1927 the card index of people's names and addresses and who was treating them, etc., was still kept in old shoe-boxes. None the less, proper case sheets had already been printed, at first copied from those in use at Bowden House, and from the beginning also there was adequate provision for the confidentiality of all the documentation appertaining to every patient. The only piece of equipment freshly bought was a fine lockable steel filing cabinet.

The kind of therapy given depended, firstly, on the needs of the case; secondly, on the predilections and training of the doctor in question. Most of the little rooms had couches of a sort (some were camp-beds!) and cushions or pillows, so that the analytic procedure could be carried out under conditions resembling the orthodox method; indeed, some patients received full analytic therapy from those who themselves had been analysed. Others received treatment more nearly resembling the Jungian technique, or the kind of therapy which can be summed up as analytic counselling with liberal doses of suggestion or persuasion. No one indulged in the more spectacular forms of Faradic stimulation or other magical practices derived from the French schools of suggestion and hypnotism. On the children's side, with which I personally have never had very close contact, J.R. assures me that the practice was not at all unlike what goes on in a contemporary child guidance clinic. Dr Potts, though nominally the head of the Children's Service at the Tavistock, had to commute from Birmingham, and he used his skills mostly for supervision and for testing. The effective head of the Children's Department was Dr Hamilton Pearson, soon joined by Dr Alice Hutchison and Dr C. L. C. Burns. It is noteworthy that, even in the first year or two of the Tavistock Clinic's life, H.C.M. thought it essential for the children's psychiatrists also to interview and deal with the parents and to investigate home and family conditions through the agency of the volunteer social workers. Staff members were supposed to give a minimum of six hours per week. This frequently meant that they saw two patients three times a week or three patients twice a week, but they were free to use their time in whatever way they thought they could help in a fairly intense form of reductive insight therapy. They were, of course, welcome to give more than the minimum time to the Clinic.

Teaching and lecturing to medical and other professional audiences began almost as soon as the Clinic had opened. Whilst it is not necessary to outline all the lecture activities, it might be worthwhile mentioning some of the titles. For example, in the autumn of 1920 H.C.M. gave ten lectures on elementary psychotherapy and J. A. Hadfield ten lectures on psychology and ethics. In 1921 Potts lectured on mental deficiency, H.C.M. again on elementary psychotherapy and also gave a further eight lectures on the 'New Psychology and Its Bearing on Education'. Dr Maurice Nicol, mentioned earlier, gave five lectures on analytical psychology (meaning the Jungian system) and Mary Hemingway six on the psychological aspects of nursing. H.C.M.'s course was repeated three times that year. During the course of the first seven years a total number of 389 lectures were given, and the average attendance per lecture worked out at seventy persons. Of these courses some were reserved for the medical profession and medical students, others, as can be gathered, had wider audiences, such as teachers, social workers and at times the clergy. Very soon the scope of these lectures was widened to include Sir Walter Langdon-Brown on endocrinology and the children's physicians, Potts, Hamilton Pearson and Alice Hutchison (from 1923), on the psychology and the abnormalities of childhood. There were also lectures from Dr George Riddoch, a leading neurologist at Queen Square Hospital, and Dr John Freeman, an expert on allergy. In addition to this activity and on top of their clinical work, the staff, so few in number, managed to give very many addresses to medical and similar audiences in most of the large provincial cities. I myself heard of the Tavistock Clinic as a second-year undergraduate in 1922 when H.C.M. addressed a student audience at Cambridge chaired by Dr Joseph Needham.

In the first seven years the staff grew from seven members to nineteen. Some of these were younger people intending to specialize; others were rather senior or even retired general practitioners whose training was largely on the job by supervision and seminars by H.C.M. himself. None the less, the case attendances did not show a corresponding increase, except in one direction. Whereas there were 247 new patients seen in the first twelve months, in 1926–7 there were 489, less than double. Attendances in the first year were 2,200, and these grew to only 3,800 six years later. Thus a very high proportion of cases were either seen once or only a few times. But the total of patients under treatment grew from 247 to 690. It should be added also that, like Dr Potts, some staff members mostly took part in teaching and lecturing and did very little clinical work. Among these was J. A. Hadfield, who had never been a very active clinician inside the Tavistock, whereas he influenced the theoretical orientation and teaching to a considerable extent.

Summing up the origins of the Tavistock, here was a very precariously financed new model of a mental health institution devoted almost entirely to the psychodynamic diagnosis and treatment of cases of neurosis and stress, including psychosomatic disorders and the behaviour disorders of children. It utilized the discoveries and general hypotheses of the schools deriving from Freud with much empiricism and much dilution, but possibly more clinical realism for mass-therapy purposes. In addition it was a venue for eclectic or non-orthodox therapists who wanted to learn or apply their skills to the relief of neurotic suffering; it was a centre where, moreover, through H.C.M.'s breadth of vision, a new dimension could be added also to the treatment of psychosomatic or even superficially somatic disorders. The position of the Clinic then was, as it still remains, one between standard organic medicine as practised in 1920, the older mental hospital world and orthodox psychoanalysis. Both the latter regarded it with scant respect: the one because of the lack of prolonged training (such as it was) and experience in the psychoses, and the other because of the strong influence of Freud's warnings to keep its doctrines and practices unalloyed and undiluted. This strange position, however, made the Clinic perhaps more readily acceptable to many of the more enterprising and progressive physicians and general practitioners who either had themselves experienced the impact of war neuroses or had otherwise become interested in the new psychology. What was perhaps more remarkable was that from the beginning Crichton-Miller and his staff not only saw the continuity between the child and the adult and had implemented this in the structure of the Clinic, but had also demonstrated that, at least in principle, psychotherapy was a multidisciplined affair, particularly in the children's field, where both child and parents would receive treatment. Moreover, there was also the early endeavour to go out into the community and to regard the activity of psychotherapy and the dissemination of aetiological knowledge to doctors as part of the prevention of more serious deterioration of patients as social beings, with an envisaged possibility that psychotic breakdown might be a result of non-intervention. H.C.M. and J. R. Rees were already that long time ago stressing the economic loss which neurosis represented to the community. On these grounds they confidently expected that this new model would quickly be copied by other hospitals, and that similar departments would within a short space of time be established in the teaching hospitals and other medical centres throughout the country, and that the Tavistock as such would then become superfluous. In fact, it has taken many years before anything like it happened. Even to this day the Tavistock presents a highly idiosyncratic institution, at least on the British scene, essentially with the same aspirations and indeed very similar methods of going to work as originally, but refined and more sophisticated. At no time did the people who founded Tavistock attempt to compete with the then existing two major psychiatric post-graduate institutions, the Bethlem Royal Hospital and the newer Maudsley Hospital. The focus was always on the holistic approach to people suffering from a certain range of disorders and on the effort to forestall deterioration by attention to the aetiological factors, whether social, somatic or psychodynamic. It is questionable whether this position outside the three major orthodoxies mentioned was a weakness or a strength. Some of what follows in subsequent chapters may help us to answer this question, and whether the Tavistock might have done better if from the beginning it had established itself as a neurosis hospital with in-patient facilities like those of the Lady Chichester at Hove and later on the Cassel Hospital, or even as a new kind of psychiatric hospital with a psychodynamic orientation. What is easier to show in the remainder of this book is how, almost without knowing it, the successive generations of the Tavistock have remained essentially faithful to H.C.M.'s original conception of its scope and purpose.

III

Consolidation (1923 - 32)

We have seen that H.C.M. had scarcely anticipated or provided for the Tavistock experiment to be more than the setting-up of a model which he thought would be taken up and improved upon by other hospitals and institutions with larger resources. This provisional existence, in fact, went on until the 5 August 1929, when it had become evident that the Tavistock was there to stay because it obviously met a felt need not catered for elsewhere, both for therapy and also as a training school for psychotherapy in a somewhat broader sense than the small and esoteric classical psychoanalytic movement of those days provided. On that date in 1929 the Tavistock Clinic was formally incorporated as a non-profit-making, charitable body and acquired the requisite legal existence. This sense of permanence was brought about by the growing demand on its services and by the Clinic's response to these demands by recruiting more staff and by gradually, despite H.C.M.'s dislike, 'institutionalizing' its structure.

The appointments to the staff were now made chiefly from those who had decided to devote themselves to psychotherapy or psychological medicine as their way of life. These had usually been people who had served apprenticeships in mental hospitals, or, in some cases, at Bowden House, where they were trained by H.C.M. himself and also encouraged to undergo training analyses, although seldom in the terms required for qualification by the Freudian school. Among this category should be mentioned Leonard F. Browne, who was destined to become a pillar of the Institution, although not primarily in clinical work. More will be said about his role in later chapters. Another such man was E. A. Bennet, M.C., a staff member from

1923 until the outbreak of the Second World War, who became well known in psychiatric circles outside the Tavistock. Another early recruit was E. Graham Howe, who came from residences at Bethlem and Bowden House, which had opened an offshoot for psychotics at Oxhey Grove. There was myself, ex-Bethlem, and a little later Mary C. Luff, with higher qualifications in psychiatry, and Ian and Jane Suttie, husband and wife. Others in this group were Dr Grace Nicolle, who throughout her career at the Tavistock was resident medical officer at Bowden House, and Basil Crowhurst Archer, who worked in the Children's Department.

The second kind of recruit has been already mentioned in connection with the names of P. F. Barton and Eleanor Montgomery in the preceding chapter. An only slightly later recruit was Dr Edwin Clegg, who also came from general practice. There was thus quite early on a rudimentary division, not in internal status, but in actual or potential expertise between a younger 'consultant' and a somewhat older 'S.H.M.O.'[1] group. This division was not accurate in regard to the Children's Department, where Dr C. L. C. Burns, destined to become the Director of Child Guidance for Birmingham Corporation some years later, was recruited from general practice. On the whole, this class tended to fade out fairly soon. Dr Alice M. Hutchison, who joined us in 1922 from paediatrics, was a full-time children's psychiatrist from the beginning. Some Diplomates in Psychological Medicine began to appear among a staff list which in the period around 1927 to 1929 numbered nineteen permanent staff with something like consultant status. But apart from this core staff of the first seven or so years there was a constant flow of post-graduate students already representing, not only the United Kingdom, but also, as mentioned, the United States, New Zealand, Australia, Malta, Ceylon and the colonial medical services. The same period saw the beginnings, not only of consultant appointments to our staff for the more recondite specialities, such as oto-laryngology, ophthal-

[1] For the benefit of readers unfamiliar with the terminology of the National Health Service, S.H.M.O. is short for Senior Hospital Medical Officer, a rank below that of Consultant, which carries permanence of tenure. Lately it has become 'Medical Assistant', but will doubtless be further changed.

mology, dentistry and radiology, but also around 1928 of the eminent physician and writer F. G. Crookshank as so-called 'diagnostic physician'. These were to have special charge of the physical investigation side as a way of overcoming the problem of the analytic relation with our patients. The same period saw the establishment of a pathological laboratory in which the simpler tests could be performed without calling upon external services. The first pathologist, Dr Roodhouse Gloyne, was followed by Dr Hilda Cunnington. She was succeeded by another lady, Dr Isabel G. H. Wilson, who also did psychotherapy. Later she joined the Board of Control and – from 1948 – she was one of the two senior psychiatrists at the Ministry of Health. She was the first woman to be elected President of the R.M.P.A. at the end of her distinguished career. Among birds of passage who came to sample us and perhaps stay as clinical assistants or post-graduate students for a year or two may be mentioned a number of well-known members of our profession, such as C. P. Blacker, subsequently consultant at the Maudsley and an eminent geneticist and eugenist; the late Dr Noel Harris, later the Medical Superintendent of Springfield Hospital, whence he was appointed Consultant in Psychological Medicine at the Middlesex Hospital (President of the R.M.P.A. in 1954–5); the late Dr Henry Wilson, who, starting at Bowden House and remaining on our staff for some eleven years, went to the York Retreat, and then returned to be the first full Physician in Psychological Medicine at the London Hospital until his retirement. Then there was the late Dr Kathleen Todd, who came and went from New Zealand, and who for a time during the Second World War was acting Director of the Child Guidance Training Centre evacuated from Canonbury to Oxford; and Dr Angus McRae, who had worked in the National Institute of Industrial Psychology and left us to become the Secretary of the British Medical Association a little later. For an even shorter period we had Dr Desmond Curran and Dr Walter Maclay, who made brilliant careers in spite rather than because of their sojourn among us.

It would be tedious to repeat the description of the general conceptual orientation of this rather empirical and non-doctrinaire group which was presided over by H.C.M., at this stage with much less contribution from J. A. Hadfield, with his own somewhat original approach based on McDougall plus psychoanalysis. This was a group of pioneers who consciously wanted to differentiate themselves from the rigid orthodoxies of the early Freudians, at the same time, however, acknowledging the debt they owed to Freud, Jung, Adler and others in the field of dynamic psychiatry and the broad analytic or reductive approach to problems of neurosis. We certainly recognized the techniques of free association and interpretation, dream-analysis and the then not very well understood phenomena of the transference and of resistance, which were freely used concepts in the Clinic. An eclectic and enquiring spirit was fostered by H.C.M., who, as already mentioned, not only encouraged and took seminars and discussion groups, but held regular staff meetings at which views were freely aired and debated. Through the generosity of the late Dr T. W. Mitchell, at one time a practising Freudian analyst and for many years Editor of the *British Journal of Medical Psychology*, and of two other benefactors, a Miss Green and a Miss Reynolds (details not available), a library came into being, both of books and of back numbers of many specialist journals of the day. In general, the quite extraordinary enthusiasm and sense of drive and common enterprise which prevailed made both medical and lay staff, still largely voluntary, co-operate in making the Tavistock an exciting place to work in, despite its physical discomforts in extremely cramped premises and its shoe-string finance.

Perhaps the success and consolidation of the Tavistock was due to its independent position and to H.C.M., and increasingly also J.R., managing to enlist the constant and enthusiastic support of the kind of representatives of the community who carried weight and were also regarded as guarantors of the Clinic's own respectability and integrity. The three-tiered supporting edifice of Vice-Presidents, Executive Committee (or Council) and Medical Advisory Board contained persons who were not merely ornaments of their time and Society, but were also exceedingly active. Some of these have already been mentioned, but it does not follow that those not named might not have done more for the Tavi behind the scenes. For this reason, a complete list appears in Appendix I. It was certainly by the efforts and personal contributions of such eminent sanctioning and supporting personalities that public interest was quickened and the growing momentum of donations and subscriptions reached a point at which legal incorporation as a charitable institution became possible. By 1927 and 1928 some modest honoraria for junior and often very impecunious medical staff became possible (*7s. 6d.* an hour!), and a professional secretary and one or two shorthand typists could be employed. There was now also assessment of means for the charging of modest fees, and cost accountancy of overheads and budgeting, which gave the financial side of the Clinic a more businesslike look. Doubtless there was also a feedback in the shape of small subscriptions and donations from the mainly middle-class clientele and their friends, and from the gradual public recognition that our handling of neuroses and related mental disorders was more effective and rewarding than the other methods for treating 'functional nervous disorders' of those days.

Thus the general public and the general medical profession, including high permanent officers of the B.M.A., were much more favourably disposed towards the treatment of psychoneurosis by the new psychology in general, and the Tavistock in particular, than the prevailing type of mental hospital psychiatrist. This fact was borne in on me as a one-time resident in Bethlem Royal Hospital, where its then Physician Superintendent spoke in no uncertain terms of disdain and suspicion about H.C.M. and all he stood for. Only worse than the Tavistock for him was, needless to say, the psychoanalytic movement proper. Intimations of similar hostility also reached one in one's young days from the then newly established Maudsley Hospital under Edward Mapother. This neurological and Kraepelinian orientation had already made it difficult for the wartime psychotherapists to work on the traumatic neuroses, as the official doctrine had it that shell-shock was an organic state due to punctate haemorrhages in the brain. The then emerging 'neuro-psychiatry', however, somehow did not commend itself by any means to all of the top neurologists of the day. I have already mentioned that many of them saw in the new psychotherapeutic method a useful complement to their own skills in the difficult elucidation of organic nervous diseases. But just as fierce in hostility against us was the psychoanalytic movement, itself very much on the defensive within the medical fold and under the very considerable influence of Freud's paper on 'Wild Psychoanalysis'. They feared dilution and the loss of inner cohesion and professional discipline if their members accepted posts or even mixed too freely with the unqualified or half-qualified. It was a phenomenon comparable to Lenin's anathema on the Mensheviks. It should be added that H.C.M. and J.R., and Hadfield in lesser measure, returned the sentiments of the official Freudian group, whom they regarded as a sectarian, inturned coterie with whom reasonable scientific intercourse was impossible. But the Clinic provided a field of activity and a haven for those who, though analysed by Freudians and in some instances even accepted for training, did not desire or were not given their formal qualification. They were able to practise more flexibly in the permissive atmosphere of the Tavistock. Among two notable men in this category should be mentioned Dr Charles Berg, whose two books subsequently attracted considerable interest, and Dr Maurice Wright, O.B.E., who became one of the stalwarts of the consulting team at the Tavistock for many years, much loved and respected, a wise, sceptical teacher as well as a marvellous therapist. Dr T. W. Mitchell, who has already been mentioned, was also an analyst a little bit away from the Psychoanalytic Society. He was consistently friendly and generous and could see the need for a more 'popular' or diluted form of psychotherapy still based on dynamic if not rigidly Freudian methods.

In the consolidation of the Clinic's activities a number of notable events took place in the period up to 1931. Thus in 1928 we were fortunate in securing the part-time services of Miss Constance Simmins, a member of the staff of Professor (later Sir Cyril) Burt's department at University College, London, as our Clinical Psychologist. She served in this capacity until her retirement in 1952 and over these years she devised and led the training of a large number of clinical psychologists, about which more will be said later. There was also established a speech-therapy unit under the direction of Miss Elspeth McLeod, who was later assisted by one or two junior speech therapists. This unit functioned at first mainly in the Children's Department.

Miss D. F. Robinson returned to us after her full training as a psychiatric social worker to head the P.S.W. team. We also appointed a Registrar in the old sense of that term – namely, a medical officer concerned exclusively with clinical records, statistics and follow-ups, in which she rendered admirable service. This was Dr Marjorie Garrod, the daughter of Dr Bedford Pierce. Her father was for a short time, before joining the Board of Control, the chairman of our Executive Council, having been for many years head of The Retreat at York.

In his annual reports the Medical Director published not only analyses of the patients falling into each classificatory category within the spectrum of cases taken on, but also the graphs of attendances, the sources of new patients, the length of time taken for treatment and some estimate of the results. In a subsequent chapter I shall make allusion to a large follow-up study by Dr Marjorie Garrod and Dr Mary Luff. Ian Suttie and his wife, Jane, began their joint work of revising psychopathology, resulting in the volume, *Origins of Love and Hate*, a notable contribution to dynamic psychiatry. Ian was a lively spirit who soon organized private discussion meetings in which Tavistock staff were engaged in most amicable but also quite rigorous doctrinal discussions with their psychoanalytic 'opponents'. His premature death was much mourned by us.

In 1929 we could afford to secure another ramshackle Bloomsbury house close to the Clinic. Here was opened a hostel for patients who either could not live at home for reasons of stress or else lived too far for regular attendance. The hostel was under the medical supervision of E. A. Bennet and was run by Miss Muriel Payne with the help of a resident Matron. There were fourteen patients resident at any given time, and in the first year thirty-four patients were admitted. This was an early experiment in creating a 'therapeutic community' at minimum cost for the patients. Patients needing special nursing or supervision were not admitted. All the work of the hostel was done by themselves, including the organization of social and recreational life. Their psychotherapy was given in the adjoining Clinic.

The hostel was not the only activity looked after by Miss Payne, another of those dynamic and unpaid helpers who responded to our work and philosophy. She was also the Secretary of the so-called Extension Fund. This development was a direct consequence of J.R.'s official appointment in 1926 as H.C.M.'s Deputy Director at a small honorarium and devoting much more time to the affairs of the Clinic. Already at this time J.R. was conceiving of the Tavistock as a developing school for psychotherapy and related mental-health disciplines. It was characteristic of his mind and energy that the Council's effort towards securing larger premises became for J.R. the vision of a new institution to which increasingly, and for a time formally, the name of Institute of Medical Psychology began to be applied. Miss Payne's first report on the Extension Plan stated that it was not only 'needed for the relief of suffering, but also for research into causation, thus contributing to the progress of civilization and medicine'. One should perhaps have expected to see added to it, 'teaching and education of the medical and allied professions', but this was by then clearly taken for granted. In 1929 a special appeal setting out the programme of the extension was launched over the signatures of ten prominent persons, including the Archibshop of York, Mrs Stanley Baldwin, the wife of the then Prime Minister, and Sir Humphrey Rolleston, President of the Royal College of Physicians. The appeal aimed at £160,000 (when money was worth so much more), necessary for the establishment and partial endowment of the proposed Institute of Medical Psychology. The hostel itself was conceived as a small early instalment of this plan, although it was never contemplated that we should have an extensive bedded psychiatric hospital.

In this activity an important early link was formed with the National Council for Mental Hygiene in the shape of a special committee known as the Joint Committee of the National Council for Mental Hygiene and the Tavistock Square Clinic. The object of this committee was not only to promote the scheme for an Institute of Medical Psychology, but also other matters relating to mental health which might appear to assist in forwarding the movement. Not only did this Joint Committee actively promote fund-raising in various ways, but it also organized in the autumn of 1929 what was probably the first Mental Health Conference in Britain at the Central Hall,

Westminster, having run a two months' Press propaganda campaign in preparation for it. At this Conference, where the newly formed Child Guidance Council was also represented, there were delegates from countries of the European Mental Hygiene Movement; messages were received from the Minister of Health (Mr Arthur Greenwood) and Mr Lloyd George. The topics were: sex education, the working of juvenile courts, problems of delinquency, the personal equation in industry, and public health work in relation to mental health. It seems that the themes of that early Conference were already those which remain the staple of mental health conferences everywhere! It was perhaps a pity that this Joint Committee was dissolved early in the following year for reasons not given, except that the report states 'the Joint Committee feeling that interest in the promotion of the Institute of Medical Psychology had been well established, dissolved'. There was now formed an 'extension committee' for the Tavistock Clinic alone, but two members of the National Council for Mental Hygiene joined it, our old friend, Dr Doris Odlum, prominent for many years in the British National Association for Mental Health and the European League for Mental Hygiene, and Lieut.-Colonel J. R. Lord, the Physician Superintendent of Long Grove Mental Hospital and subsequently a Senior Commissioner of the Board of Control. Dr Lord edited the report of that first Conference on mental health.

Educational activity now took a more organized form. In addition to the usual short, intensive courses of lectures for general practitioners and for the other audiences already mentioned, there was held for the first time an advanced course for recognized social workers in the field of mental health and psychotherapy. A beginning was also made with more formal seminars for post-graduates, taking some weight off H.C.M.'s own shoulders, by the appointment of two clinical tutors. The first incumbents of these new posts were Isabel Wilson and H. V. Dicks. On the resignation of Isabel Wilson when she joined the Board of Control, Graham Howe was appointed as the second tutor. These seminars were essentially weekly discussion groups on a given subject treated systematically.

We now began to have distinguished speakers from abroad.

The first of them was Dr Ira S. Wile of Mount Sinai Hospital, New York, who in 1928 gave a full week of lectures and demonstrations on his diagnostic and counselling techniques with children and their parents, perhaps the earliest teaching in the Tavistock on joint-interview techniques. In 1929 we had several lectures from Alfred Adler of Vienna and from Dr William Healy, Director of the Judge Baker Foundation of Boston, who spoke about his studies in delinquency. Apart from such renowned guests, the senior staff, who now numbered twenty-six, were taking a much greater part in the lecturing, and less reliance had to be placed on audience-appeal of outside speakers. In all, in 1929 the medical staff gave seventy-seven lectures to the medical profession and to social workers, and Dr Isabel Wilson also lectured to nurses on problems of mental health.

It may be of interest to note H.C.M.'s policy of giving beginners cases which were either easy and rewarding, producing good results (with or without the help of the seminars) in a relatively short time for symptomatic relief or the actual remission of the neurosis, or else cast-iron chronics, such as stable obsessionals or cases of impotence of twenty years' standing, from which one could learn a lot and where at least it seemed one could do no great harm. In connection with the early years of training, I should like to pay tribute to a lady who from the earliest days of the Tavistock was an indefatigable voluntary helper as well as generous benefactor – Miss W. E. Hollingsworth. In her exacting and unpaid role of organizer of the lecture courses, she did all the backroom work by way of publicity, registration and documentation for these activities in the Clinic over many years, and all this in addition to helping in the Secretary's office.

Turning now to the administration, our first Chairman had been replaced by Dr Bedford Pierce, who resigned on becoming a Commissioner of the Board of Control. He was in his turn replaced by Dr H. H. Brackenbury (subsequently Sir Henry), who was then the Chairman of the B.M.A.'s Council and a distinguished medical figure. It was around this time also that our first professional full-time Secretary/Administrator was appointed in the person of Miss Dorothy Poole (later Mrs

Harold Mattinson), who transformed the efficiency of our administrative work – and not before time. The Clinic was now (in 1930) treating some 900 patients, with a total of 7,500 attendances per annum. A waiting list had already come into being, a feature which we were never to be rid of again. It was calculated in 1930 that the cost per patient-attendance was 9*s.* 6*d.*, whereas patients' contributions amounted to between 2*s.* 6*d.* and 3*s.* 6*d.* The difference had to be collected by donations and subscriptions and various charitable entertainments and drives, in which our Council and our Vice-Presidents played a most active role. Total expenditure in 1931 ran at £5,040, the hostel in addition costing £1,500, but was more or less self-supporting. The Extension Fund for the Institute of Medical Psychology stood then at nearly £7,000 in a separate account not to be touched for current or routine expenditure. It was also at this time that we acquired a new Treasurer. Sir Dougal Malcolm resigned, although he stayed on the Council, and his place was taken by Mr Walter Roch. Mr Roch was never a very active Treasurer, but delegated much work to another voluntary helper, who took good care of our finances. This was Mr Richard A. Howden, a member of Lloyd's, who remained a personal friend of many of us long after his voluntary job ceased. A cultivated man with a flair for psychodynamics, he published two useful popular books on medical psychology in the 1930s.

We now find in H.C.M.'s reports an increasing impatience with the slowness of the progress towards better premises; that, in the face of waiting patients and with more and more doctors trying to join us in order to be trained, we had to turn down urgent cases and to close the waiting list, so that the quality of work should not unduly suffer. Quality was always a very important consideration for H.C.M.

The year 1931 was particularly full of change. A second honorary psychologist, Mrs Hocart, was appointed, Dr Crookshank was lost to us, but we gained Dr Eric Blake-Pritchard, who joined Dr John Barrie-Murray as a diagnostic physician. Blake-Pritchard later became a distinguished neurologist on the staff of University College Hospital. There also arrived a new psychiatric social worker who was to become one of our mainstays before the war, Mrs Phyllis Hamlyn whose husband later joined our Council. 1931 saw lecture courses by George Groddeck and by McFie Campbell of the Boston Psychopathic Hospital on schizophrenia. The Children's Department underwent notable expansion both in the number of cases taken on and in the recognition given to it by the various public bodies it served. This was a pay-off of the long-standing association of especially the London County's Chief Medical Officer, Dr C. W. Kimmins, with our work, as already stated. Thus the growing interest in delinquency led to the Children's Department being asked to give evidence before the Home Office Committee on Persistent Offenders and to supply regular advisory attendance at the children's courts. Partly as a result of her experience with us, Miss Muriel Payne, mentioned earlier, left us to become the Secretary of the Home and School Council, a body of considerable influence in the 1920s and 1930s and which, it is interesting to note, was reconstituted in 1967.

By 1931 our total attendances were nearing the 11,000 mark. The only persons we could still give priority to were juveniles under seventeen, those who came from far away to stay at the hostel, and those on whom police court action was pending and for whom reports were needed. It was around this time that negotiations began with the psychoanalysts for the creation of the Institute for the Scientific Treatment of Delinquency (as it was originally called). From our side the leading personalities were Hadfield, Crowhurst Archer and Emmanuel Miller, and from the psychoanalytic side Edward Glover and Dennis Carroll, who was to achieve international renown in this sphere. A modest beginning had been made in our treatment, not only of neurosis, but also of behaviour disorders, including some criminals. Among the more sensational events of the week for some months was the arrival three times weekly of a prisoner serving a sentence for homosexual offences, with two uniformed warders, to one of whom he was always handcuffed. In the course of these visits the handcuffs came to be left off. The gradual increase in criminals seen at the Tavistock led to the explorations by H.C.M. and a Dr Jensen into how and with what conceptual base a separate institute for the study of delinquency should be formed. The Tavistock was beginning to get complaints from 'law-abiding' patients, who were not unnaturally disturbed to arrive in the waiting-room to find scenes such as the one just described!

The Move to Malet Place

By the end of 1931 the Extension Committee and the supporting Friends of the Institute of Medical Psychology group under the dynamic leadership of J.R. and of Muriel Payne had done their work well. We now actually acquired premises in what used to be Shoolbred Stables,[1] at the corner of Torrington Place and Malet Place, W.C.1. These were planned and adapted for our use by Mr (now Sir) Graham Dawbarn, a rising architect with considerable interest in our work. Much of the tasteful re-equipment and *décor* were planned by the indefatigable Miss Hollingsworth, and by a new arrival, Mr Harry Downes, a lovable man who was to give us several years of devoted service both as a Council member and later in the now arduous post of honorary Lecture Secretary. We moved in 1932. The staff felt renewed and immensely stimulated by being at last in premises which seemed spacious and pleasant to work in. We now had not only an adequate number of fair-sized consulting-rooms in the attractively contemporary taste of those days, but also a library where we could read quietly or where we could hold small seminars and committee meetings. We had a large lecture hall seating several hundreds, with movable partitions and a stage/platform – by no means a negligible feature in view of our constant need to raise money by various entertainments. This was a long, low building of only two floors, of which the ground floor was set aside mainly for the Children's Department and held the lecture-room, while the upper floor housed the adult waiting and treatment rooms and central offices, which now assumed recognizably modern shape. Even better for our collegiate life was the provision of a cosy canteen, also comprising a separate refreshment bar for patients. The social possibilities of the refectory were at once

[1] Shoolbred's was a department store which was beginning its demise during this period.

utilized by our instituting monthly dinner discussion meetings (in addition to the other more clinical occasions), at which a staff member or some guest would present a paper after dinner, which would then be discussed for a long time in comfortable surroundings. The playroom on the ground floor for the Children's Department had at one time been Shoolbred's Undertakers' Department Mortuary and had a forbidding Gothic doorway to the outside world which however, we never used! In it was installed a primitive one-way screen for students to observe children's behaviour.

With this new move the attendance figures for 1932 leapt by several thousands. In particular, the number of new cases we were able to see increased from some 500 to well over 700, despite the dislocation and temporary closure of the Clinic for some weeks during the move. The staff were not slow to begin projects until then impossible. Not only were the seminar events and supervisions intensified, but the Children's Department at once appointed a research assistant, Dr Augusta Bonnard, who was later to become a well-known psychoanalyst. The Clinic was now in the very heart of the University of London, with University College and University College Hospital as its very near neighbours, with the central buildings of the University in Malet Street nearing completion, and the School of Tropical Medicine and Hygiene nearby, where one of our best friends, Millais Culpin, held the Chair in Industrial Mental Health. There was no doubt that in some ways we now considered ourselves to have 'arrived'. This was emphasized by two eminent psychiatric teachers, D. K. Henderson (later Sir David) of Edinburgh and Moorhead of Dublin, joining our Medical Advisory Board and Professor Cyril Burt joining our Council.[1] The library had grown steadily: we had by this time some 400 volumes and subscribed to a number of journals. It was always available to our staff and students and was supervised by an honorary Librarian, the Rev. Harold Mattinson, who played an active part in stimulating the intellectual self-education of our staffs. He also promptly proceeded to

[1] Sir Cyril Burt, head of the Department of Psychology at University College, was famous not only for his contribution to psychometrics but also for his pioneering book, *The Young Delinquent.*

marry our first professional Secretary, Miss Dorothy Poole. Upon her resignation for this happy purpose, there was appointed another no less effective and admirable General Secretary to the Clinic and to the Council in the person of Miss V. Joan Howard, who was to remain with us until her marriage in 1939. Much of the excellent organization and cheerful *élan* in the administration was due to her energy and liveliness, which all of us came greatly to value.

The Children's Department seemed to benefit almost more than the Adult Department by the expansion. Not only were extra medical staff appointed, but our desideratum of a truly interprofessional team could be implemented by increasing the psychological and social work staffs and adding extra speech therapists and a number of play therapists, at this period a new and untested development.

We now started 'exports', always an ambivalent reward to an institution aspiring to teach. Perhaps the most notable such loss was Birmingham's gain in the appointment of Charles Burns to the position of Director of Child Guidance for the city of Birmingham. Another weighty export was the appointment of Miss D. L. Robinson, our first psychiatric social worker, to the newly-established Child Guidance Unit of the West End Hospital for Nervous Diseases. The Adult Department now numbered twenty-two senior staff members with a number of clinical assistants or trainees. Some of these went back to their own countries as teachers. The Children's Department staff numbered three consultants and three more permanent clinical assistants, who might in present terminology have been called senior registrars. The children's work was always at a much lower numerical level than the Adult Department, partly because the needs of treating young children were not yet so generally recognized as the acute breakdowns and neurotic difficulties of adults. Moreover, the Commonwealth Fund had set up a new Child Guidance Training Centre in North London ('The Canonbury Clinic') with Dr William Moodie (ex-deputy to Professor Mapother) as its Director. This was taking both clinical and training loads off the Tavistock by the early 1930s.

A notable acquisition to our Council was the young Earl of Feversham, a trained probation officer, who made mental health his main concern in his full life of service to the community. In due course he became the Chairman of the so-called Feversham Committee on the co-ordination of mental health work. It published its famous report in 1939. The document was shelved owing to the war, but became the blueprint for later developments that led to the unification of three hitherto separate bodies, the Child Guidance Council, the Central Association for Mental Welfare and the national Council for Mental Hygiene in the National Association for Mental Health.

In those years the Tavistock Clinic, the Cassel Hospital, the West End Hospital, and a little later the Child Guidance Training Centre and the I.S.T.D. were the main clinical bases from which the three voluntary movements concerned with public education in mental health drew technical advice and backing.

IV

The Search for a New Institutional Structure

In H.C.M.'s report as Medical Director for 1932 there was a remarkable lack of enthusiasm for the changes which resulted from the move into our new home which had so much inspired many staff members. An explanation came soon enough. The third paragraph cryptically recorded: 'A committee of the medical staff has been in existence for a year. It has planned all the lecture and training courses and *has made itself responsible* [my italics – H.V.D.] for other professional activities.'

This brief statement expresses what in the light of history proved to be his negative attitude to a rising demand among the senior staff for a greater share in the running of the Clinic. There were by this time some twenty-five 'full physicians', as well as some psychologists and social workers. There was also a fairly large number of post-graduate students in training, some of them with considerable experience. A fair proportion of senior staff had served their proper psychiatric apprenticeships elsewhere and held the Diploma in Psychological Medicine or M.D.s in Psychiatry. The ferment began in the old premises. It can bear some description, because it was to recur again in the 1940s in somewhat different circumstances, and may therefore be typical of certain stages in the maturing of social organizations. The régime of benevolent autocracy or monarchy tends to be assailed by the needs of the oncoming generation for a real stake in the institution; or a certain power group has outlived its creativeness.

H.C.M. himself in the 1932 report had lamented the fact that, owing to lack of funds, there could not be any paid part-time appointments made. The only consultant at that time in receipt of a nominal salary (£50 *p.a.*) was J. R. Rees in his capacity as very nearly full-time Deputy Director. J.R. never spared himself for the Tavistock, and one always felt he was neglecting his private practice in favour of institutional development. He was always about the place and was the *de facto* chief, seen by all. Time has somewhat blurred the memory of the events and attitudes that produced the drive towards forming a Medical Staff Committee to take responsibility and interest in the growth of the institution in its clinical, teaching and research aspects. There are no documents saved from the Blitz. I was certainly among those favouring the replacement of the monarchy by a constitutional medical government. Some time around the turn of 1930 I recall a long meeting with J.R. at his home, in which he and I discussed ways and means of broadening the responsibility and involvement of staff in the Clinic. This amounted to an elected staff committee. As far as I now recall, J.R. proposed the matter to H.C.M., who did not overtly oppose it. Consequently, the first Medical Committee was elected by secret ballot by the senior staff in 1931. It consisted of H.C.M. as Chairman, J. R. Rees, Edward Bennet, Leonard Browne, Mary Luff and H. V. Dicks from the Adult Department, and Hamilton Pearson and possibly Charles Burns (before he was translated to Birmingham) or Crowhurst Archer from the Children's Department.[1] The Medical Committee was concerned first with working out its own terms of reference, which included the right to make recommendations to H.C.M. for transmission to Council as well as to comment on his policy plans. H.C.M. cannot be remembered to have openly objected to or opposed the formation or transactions of this Medical Committee, who for their part had no sense of disloyalty or parricidal intent. It is not easy to put in proper perspective the inner experience which must have been H.C.M.'s in relation to this change. This appeared to amount to feeling 'put on the shelf' and rejected by the staff. The nearest to what might have gone on in his mind is contained in the affectionate and insightful paragraph of the private biography, already mentioned, by Mr Donald Crichton-Miller, his eldest son, shortly after H.C.M.'s death. I quote certain passages:

[1] A year or two later Alan Maberly and Emanuel Miller represented the Children's Department.

> My father, desperately pressed with his own work, was unhappy about it. The Clinic was his 'baby', but this aspect of its growth worried him. He could not give the time to supervision himself and he was scrupulously fair about not interfering with those who took on the responsibilities. Gradually he relinquished control and finally resigned (p. 11).

His resignation took place some time in the year 1933, shortly after what should have been a great sense of achievement for him. The possible reasons why he should have been so cast down by the growth of the Clinic and maturing of his senior staff are perhaps best stated in the words of his son:

> In the beginning the clinic was the home of a small band which he led with enthusiasm. He had in turn loyal and eager disciples. Gloyne [not a psychiatrist, but a clinical pathologist – H.V.D.], Bennet, Rees, Howe and others were in every way the men he sought. But they did not multiply nor were they joined by younger people ready to learn. Instead there was an influx of people who considered they had learned better elsewhere and, though anxious to forward their knowledge by experiment and discussion, were more often critical than appreciative of the work done by their more experienced colleagues (p. 11).

In trying to find the explanation for this highly significant passage, it should be said that among the twenty-five or so people there was now only a minority of those quoted as having been largely trained by and closely identified with the values of Crichton-Miller himself. There were others in the new group of senior staff who had had Freudian analyses, just as there were quite a number who had had analytic training by J. A. Hadfield and had done a fair amount of psychiatry before coming to the Tavistock, rather than being, as it were, 'brought up' by H.C.M. via Bowden House, etc. It is my belief that the passage in which Donald Crichton-Miller refers to 'the influx of people who considered they had learned better elsewhere' refers to these people who did not fully share H.C.M.'s philosophy of medicine, and in particular, perhaps, his doctrine of psychophysical parallelism, with the great emphasis he put on the then fashionable doctrine of focal sepsis and his slightly naïve endocrinological faith. This indeed was perhaps a pity, since a holistic view of the interaction of body and mind was then, as it has always remained, one of the great planks of medical psychology denied only at the physician's peril. However, what the Hadfield-trained people, who were a fairly influential and by now successful group, did not realize was that between Hadfield and Crichton-Miller there was some kind of private feud or coolness not obvious to outsiders. With hindsight, one could have seen this as the reason why Hadfield's name merely appeared on a list of staff and as an occasional lecturer for the Tavistock, but why he seldom came near it. Bennet, Leonard Browne, Wilfred Bion (who had by now joined us), Archer, myself and some others were in this group. Others again, like Charles Berg and Mary Luff, came with good qualifications from elsewhere after training analyses, M.D.s in psychiatry and D.P.M.s, with backgrounds owing little to H.C.M. Yet it was he himself who had been the arbiter of staff appointments by promotion of clinical assistants selected by himself, the Council merely confirming the appointments on his recommendation. Commenting on this point, Mr Donald Crichton-Miller continues as follows:

> At first sight this [development of criticism – H.V.D.] would seem to be a natural development and so it was. But there were features which made it hard for my father to bear. In the first place he had by nature an idea of discipleship which was outraged by this [i.e. people differing from him – H.V.D.]. It is easy for me to say that his teaching was not pedantic; I believe that to be true. I also claim that he never thrust his leadership on anyone. In the circumstances he wistfully withdrew from the teaching as he had done from the administration of the Clinic (p. 11).

Mr Donald Crichton-Miller continues with an atrocity story which perhaps reveals his father's outrage at the 'arrogance' and independence of the newer staff members. The story concerns a woman patient whom H.C.M. himself had been treating with little success. He then thought he detected a physical deficiency for which he prescribed endocrine extracts [in the early years of the century not very effective – H.V.D.]. Donald Crichton-Miller says: 'This idea was ridiculed in quarters where it was held that diseases were either the sort that the mind controlled, like asthma, or purely coincidental, like a cut finger. In any case, if there was interaction it could only be tackled from the mental end as it were.' This is, of course, a layman's travesty of the controversy which is still raging within psychiatry. The point of the story is that H.C.M. transferred this patient to a younger colleague. When after some weeks he asked how the case was going, the colleague is said to have replied, 'Not very well, but at any rate we got her off your rat poison pretty quickly'. Donald Crichton-Miller continues: 'The Founder of the Tavistock Clinic "couldn't take" this. He was silent but he was deeply hurt.'

J. R. Rees had perhaps most insight into the reasons for H.C.M.'s sense of rejection and abrupt withdrawal from the active leadership, since he had worked with him daily for some thirteen years. He had little doubt that H.C.M. was somewhat jealous of Hadfield's more systematic teaching based on solid academic training, didactic analyses and a consequently bigger following. J.R. fairly seriously put some of the blame on myself, who, unaware of the tensions between Crichton-Miller and Hadfield, argued that with the intensified teaching activities in the new premises we should have a well-known medical psychologist with academic connections, such as Hadfield had with King's College, London University, in charge. I had formally proposed in the Medical Committee that Hadfield should be made Director of Studies at the Institute of Medical Psychology, as we were now called. J. R. Rees further recalls, although he cannot quote exact incidents, that H.C.M. had felt in a fairly irrational way hurt and diminished by proposals such as this, and during this period was blocking our Committee's proposals systematically at Council level rather than in the Medical Committee. J. R. Rees, in my recorded talks with him, said: 'I was Deputy Director, and I don't know what he was opposing, something about the educational scheme, and he was just blocking it and being quite unco-operative,' and he didn't like the proposals, and he resigned the next day after a very considerable row with J.R. in which harsh things were said. J.R. felt that H.C.M., as the person who had started the Clinic, wanted to keep complete control, felt that he had got all the right kind of ideas for the growth of the Clinic and could not bear that new people with bright ideas were, as it were, shaping the future not according to H.C.M.'s idealized blueprint. When I asked J.R. how this was so, since J.R. was certainly not a new person, but the oldest collaborator, J.R. said, 'I did not have any new ideas because I had been with him since 1920,' but that H.C.M. did resent as gross disloyalty the fact that J.R. sponsored ideas emanating from the Medical Committee and from the newer members, of whom I was one of the youngest at that time. All records except copies of annual reports having been destroyed during the Second World War, there is no very good additional evidence to show what really took place in either the Council or in H.C.M.'s mind, but it does seem as if he found difficulty in handing over more responsibility to others and in having his own vision assailed by different, even if on the whole closely related, ideas and projects. It has to be said that H.C.M.'s resignation produced in some staff members a very considerable 'sense of liberation'. This was reaffirmed to me in 1967 by a retired colleague in those very words. It is hard to say why there should have been this effect, because H.C.M. was certainly not an ideological tyrant who obviously demanded conformity. Throughout his active directorship there had been people working in whose training he had had no hand and who represented all kinds of points of view, some almost ludicrous. One whom I recall with amusement, even thirty-five years later, was a clinical assistant who shall be nameless, who called his system of therapy 'neuro-induction'. One saw him always in the passage, where he waited, pipe in hand, while two patients in separate darkened cubicles were lying, supposedly meditating on sentences he had given them. He then passed from one to the other doing what must have been some form of suggestion. We had also fully fledged and enthusiastic followers of Adler, notably James Young and A. R. Redfern; and we had Alan Maberly (ex Bethlem), fresh from a training analysis with Stekel. But it seems that somehow H.C.M. must have had a difficulty in squaring such broad tolerance with his belief in leadership and the 'right way'. It was perhaps easy to be permissive with lesser people than himself. But now men and women joined our staff who, let us face it, had a much sounder and more thorough grounding than H.C.M. in general psychiatry, in some instances in general medicine as well, *and* had been through training analyses in one or other of the schools or with prominent psychoanalysts. It was perhaps this threat of people with the right to criticize and dispute his ideas and methods which may have created his insecurity. He remained very much in the background, much to my personal disappointment, since I have always had unconcealed admiration for this creative charismatic personality whose faults were all obvious and who was so much a child of his generation and his background.

The New Régime

Towards the end of the year 1933 the change was formalized by the Council, who invited J. R. Rees to become the Medical Director. They appointed H.C.M. Honorary Senior Physician, in which role they hoped he would still co-operate in whatever way he preferred. In this, however, we were disappointed. As one of the by no means hostile protagonists of the change, I had visualized H.C.M. remaining the Director, but handing much of the detailed planning of the content of the now great volume of teaching, such as seminars, case supervisions, formal lectures, staff meetings, case conferences, acquisition of books and journals and the rest of it to another eminent senior man, functioning as a kind of embryonic Dean of the Institute, while H.C.M. retained the overall clinical and policy-making directorship and represented us at Council. However, this was not to be, and in the upshot the new structure emerged with the responsibility on J. R. Rees. He recommended that there should be two Assistant Medical Directors to help him: one of them, myself, to be responsible for clinical work and its standards, and Mary C. Luff to be responsible for the efficiency of the medical administration. This directorate functioned as the executive of the Medical Committee.

In H.C.M.'s last report as Medical Director he comments

with apparent satisfaction on the immense growth of the institution: 248 new cases in 1920 and 893 new cases in 1933, and from 2,300 hours treatment to 14,500 in 1933. He makes no allusion to J.R.'s taking over, but comments that the passing of the Clinic from humble beginnings to full institutional status involved the sacrifice of certain informalities and elasticities that made for personal rather than structured organization. He adds, however, that patients would, if they were asked, still maintain that the personal atmosphere associated with the early days had been conserved as far as possible under the new conditions.

During the year 1933, despite these sad and probably inevitable concomitants of change and growth, which could so easily be seen as the 'expulsion of the old leader', there was nevertheless also a very considerable accession of new strength. For the first time there appears in the list of the physicians to the Children's Department the name of Emanuel Miller. Among the Adult staff Ian Suttie and his wife and Maurice Wright have already been mentioned. Wilfred Bion is promoted to the senior staff. Hadfield appears again among the 'physicians'. The work in the Children's Department grew in proportion to that of the Adult Department; we now had three qualified P.S.W.s, two psychologists and two play-group workers, headed by Miss Theodora Alcock, who was to remain with us in her other role as an international authority on Rorschach techniques until comparatively recently. She is still working for the Institute of Human Relations as a consultant and lecturer on projective techniques.

New types of ancillary treatment in addition to psychotherapy were instituted: as well as play-group therapy for children there was occupational therapy for adults, mainly in various arts and crafts, for which the lecture-room was used by day. Speech therapy was extended to adult stammerers and other speech defects. There was also greater concentration on remedial teaching for children. All of these were made possible by the enlarged premises and were to be the feature of the next few years until the outbreak of the war. But possibly the greatest innovation was the recognition, made explicit in the departmental report, that children's conditions almost inevitably called for treatment of the parents' difficulties, from which they 'could rarely be distinguished as individual illness'. Thus the Tavistock Children's Department under the leadership of Dr Emanuel Miller was probably among the first in Great Britain to include something like the whole family in the treatment. The concept of family therapy, of regarding the family as a unity and the patient's difficulties in no small measure related to the interpersonal nexus with the parents, runs with great continuity through the theoretical base on which the Tavistock Clinic and the later Institute of Human Relations was developing. This was far from being a method in orthodox psychoanalysis of those days (despite the emerging hypotheses on introjected objects), which isolated the therapeutic relation on the practical level from the patient's relatives. Freud had discovered Oedipus, but Laos and Iocasta were not allowed in.

The change of atmosphere after J. R. Rees took over was certainly very great. J.R. was in most ways H.C.M.'s opposite. J.R. is a much more familiar figure to many people outside Tavistock circles, at the time of writing still happily amongst us, now in his late seventies, and will be remembered both by his Army work and by his great contribution to mental hygiene through the World Federation of Mental Health, which he founded in 1948. In 1933 he was reaching the height of his powers. Always rotund and always genial, he was in most ways an excellent complement to H.C.M. during their joint direction of the Tavistock Clinic. Now his more creative and, in the best sense of the word, 'promoting' qualities had full scope. J.R. was a man to whom all geese began as swans and who enjoyed the sense of good relations and co-operation with his 'team', as he would think of them, and with the Council. He was affectionate, warm and outgoing, and highly supportive of the younger generation. He was immensely tolerant, and under him it was possible for individuals to develop their own lines with genuine encouragement. Some may have felt that this was due to a certain lack of intellectually systematized concepts in psychological medicine, and this he would have been the first to admit – indeed, almost boast about! He regarded himself as psychiatrically ill-educated, having gained nearly all his experience in practice under the tutelage of H.C.M., whom he joined after First World War Army service without formal previous training. J.R., however, underwent a didactic analysis at the hands of Maurice Nicol, who has already been mentioned earlier. Many of his ideas he shared with H.C.M.; and he also held strong Christian values, being like H.C.M., a son of the Manse, but in his case of a Methodist minister. He had moved about the country every few years, and got to know many people in many kinds of living conditions. It is no disrespect to make the analogy that if H.C.M. was a Don Quixote with a very high aim, J. R. Rees was the necessary complement as his Sancho Panza, the much more down-to-earth, practical, organizing and executive personality who actually made the Tavistock Clinic function as a living institution. He had the great gift of 'roping in' and imparting his infective enthusiasm to all he met. He was always alert to ways of tirelessly promoting the development of the supporting bases for psychological medicine: in the National Council for Mental Hygiene, the Home and School Council, at various conferences and get-togethers, always on the platform. He was early in the counsels of the international mental hygiene movement, attending the first International Congress for Mental Health in the United States, making countless friends. In many ways his was an 'American personality', and he was very naturally at home with the less stuffy, less status-conscious and less conservative American psychiatrists and medical psychologists whose help and goodwill to the Tavistock was to become of crucial importance in our subsequent history.

One of the differences between J.R. and H.C.M. was that J.R. was a much more natural democrat, with more insight into his own mind and attitudes. He was thus able himself to joke about his 'ignorance' and lack of psychological sophistication, which he humorously accused some of us younger people as believing of him and whom in return he christened 'the psychopathological snobs'. It was characteristic of J.R. that he readily supported the movement for a Medical Committee, and that it was in fact popularly elected by the suffrage of all the medical staff members and not appointed from above by the Council. This democratic structure, rare in medical institutions, has been retained as a feature of the Tavistock's inner life throughout all subsequent years. But perhaps the chief characteristic of J.R. was his almost missionary zeal to promote not only the particular baby – namely, the Tavistock of which he was now in charge – but the whole subject in the wider field of medicine. I think it was J.R. who was the virtuoso at enlisting important personalities in the *élite* of the community to help run the Tavistock and make them spend money and effort for it. Thus he managed to recruit to the Council not only the Earl of Feversham, but also Mr P. K. Hodgson, C.M.G., C.V.O., who was the Private Secretary to the then Duke of York, subsequently King George VI. He was tirelessly at work also to get the best people for the Medical Advisory Board, which, as stated, ranged from as far afield as Professor D. K. Henderson of Edinburgh to the Regius Professors of Medicine at Oxford and Cambridge and Sir John Weir of the London Homoeopathic Hospital, then already a Royal Physician. For a brief spell he even managed to interest Professor Edward Mapother, then the only professor of psychiatry south of the Border, with his newly created chair at the Maudsley Hospital,[1] whose co-operation he was most anxious to secure. Mapother in that position of academic power was, of course, the 'gatekeeper' to University recognition, which it was from the first J.R.'s aim to secure, if not initially for the Tavistock as a post-graduate institution, then at least for some of its staff members as recognized teachers in the University. In 1933 J.R. wrote on behalf of the Chairman of the Council (whose report was largely drafted by the Medical Director) the following sentences:

> We give the warmest welcome to every sound new venture in this field of psychiatry. Many of the old-established hospitals have now started psychotherapeutic departments. Independent Child Guidance Clinics have come into being, more are projected. The Maudsley Hospital, with its splendid backing from the London County Council, provides a steadily increasing service and in its therapeutic and educational work embraces a wider group of mental and nervous disorders than this Institute has ever aimed at touching. No rivalries, save those that are friendly, will ever be allowed to spoil work that is so much needed and so far-reaching

[1] Opened in 1923 – three years after the Tavistock.

> Co-operation might, in any case, almost be said to be the 'watchword' of psychology.

These remarks were clearly intended to disclaim any wish for outdoing or competing destructively with the new Maudsley, which, as we recall, also sponsored the setting up of the so-called Child Guidance Training Centre with Commonwealth funds, which was headed initially by Dr William Moodie, at one time Deputy Superintendent of the Maudsley Hospital, who was sent for training in the United States and then returned to take up the new position.

J.R. was, however, always aware of the great insecurity and resentment felt by Mapother, and some of the figures round him, towards the Tavistock; in fact, J. R. Rees was told by Mapother that he would sooner see another 'Maudsley' set up on the north side of the Thames than that the Tavistock with its conceptual framework should flourish. We know from Mapother's writings how energetically he rejected psychodynamic psychology in psychiatry. It was all the more interesting that he did in fact create a psychotherapeutic department in the Maudsley. Indeed, his Clerk of Works came to our new premises in Malet Place in order to see how psychotherapeutic rooms should be laid out and furnished. But if he made this concession to fashion, as he might have called it, he certainly was no friend to the Tavistock, and as Professor of Psychiatry blocked all attempts by the Tavistock to secure University recognition as a specialized post-graduate institute, though we were turning out trained psychotherapists in increasing numbers. This disdain and dislike of what the Tavistock stood for and what we did perpetuated by Mapother in his teaching and in University counsels has in no small measure contributed to the quite unnecessary division between so-called 'organic psychiatry' of the psychoses in which the Maudsley had special competence and the Tavistock's contribution to the therapy and aetiology of the psychoneuroses based essentially on psychoanalytic principles, but leavened with contributions from other schools of thought.[1] J.R. knew and often discussed with

[1] This statement is not weakened by a recent Mapother Memorial Lecture by his successor, Sir A. Lewis.

Mapother the latter's unreasoning opposition to our getting University recognition, which he was able to rationalize on many grounds familiar to all those who are aware of both intellectual and, more importantly, unconscious resistance to the acceptance of medical psychology and psychoanalytic ideas into the body of medicine. J.R. always kept up friendly personal relations with his ideological opponent. It is a poignant fact that when J.R. visited him during his last illness, Mapother confessed and apologized 'as a good Catholic' that he had opposed us and that he now regretted this opposition. Knowing him well personally, J.R. had no difficulty in recognizing that Mapother, another 'principled' introvert, had felt lacking in medical support and was deeply envious of the numbers of post-graduates and various overseas visitors that flocked to see the Tavistock at work and to join training courses.

Perhaps, like H.C.M. on our side, Mapother was also something of a monopolist. It is in my personal recollection that H.C.M. not only spoke with dislike of Mapother, but even with greater disdain of, for example, Porter-Phillips of Bethlem Hospital and of Ernest Jones of the British Psychoanalytic Society. Somehow with H.C.M. one felt that he always had the notion that 'they were all out of step'. Rees was a genuine unifier, to whom co-operation and pulling in the same direction were a real need and value in his personality. He clearly went a long way to disarm the opposition by what in modern ethology would be called postures of non-aggression; the mechanisms of denial and idealization played a part in this. Somewhat later in our history it will appear that London University Post-graduate Federation, which was then beginning to take shape, had already been quite seriously prejudiced against the Tavistock, whom Mapother had at various times called 'the Parson's Clinic' or compared unfavourably with those who followed Adolf Meyer's psychobiology, then the ruling doctrine or dogma of the Maudsley Hospital. This went for anyone who tried to use the new psychology in the treatment of neurosis, save when they worked under his control. It was mentioned earlier that this battle began, strangely enough, within the very walls of the Maudsley Hospital before it was ever opened, when it was a military neurosis unit for shell-shocked soldiers, by the men of the 'new psychology' against the 'organicist' views of Sir Frederick Mott and Dr Gordon Holmes over theories of shell-shock. Although Mott later came down on the side of psychogenesis, none the less this early and bitter cleavage seems to have had quite lasting consequences and repercussions on the *genius loci* of that building and on British psychiatry in general, and particularly therefore on the position of the economically weak voluntary Tavistock Clinic, which lacked formal University, Government or local authority backing. To this extent it was no part of 'established institutions', but an upstart, a cuckoo in the nest. It was by its respectable clinical results and the good informal relations with doctors and teachers of the community, generated by the enthusiasm of the staff and J.R. in particular, that the Tavistock in fact survived, expanded and became well known. This itself was by its critics regarded as a piece of vulgar promotion, rather than that its claims to making a serious contribution to medical psychology and to psychiatry were recognized as valid. I do not doubt that our having no beds and no large pile of bricks and mortar played its part in this irrational process.

Yet our claim was increasingly obvious, not only by the quality of work and the results of psychotherapy which were evident to the practitioners and other agencies referring cases but also by the painstaking search for and exclusion of organic disorder by our diagnostic procedures. There was also the growing contribution to the literature and by lectures and so forth which now flowed out of the Tavistock, moulding the medical climate of the era. Also this was the beginning of the 'export' of trained therapists from the Tavistock to other centres, as already mentioned. All these contributions in men and ideas are contained in the lists in the Appendices to this volume.

If J.R. Rees was not a giant in original contribution to theoretical psychopathology, he was certainly a man keenly and generously interested in applying the results of other people's work to the notion of prevention and to the epidemiology of mental disorder within the range of conditions with which we dealt. He became instrumental through Mary Luff in organizing the kind of case records which could be easily abstracted into follow-up material. She initiated what is perhaps the best pre-Second World War follow-up study of the effects of treatment on neurotic disorders, which will be referred to in more detail below. J.R. was, as mentioned, a hard driver, and a great deal of work had to be done for him. It was almost impossible to plead private preoccupation or a family anniversary as an excuse for not attending the weekly directorial meetings, or any other Tavistock function. He genuinely could never understand why anyone should wish to go to the theatre or have a party when the great work was there waiting to be done.

V

The Period of Expansion

In this chapter I shall present an overall picture rather than a stroke-by-stroke chronicle of all the major events up to the Second World War. The subject matter can conveniently, if somewhat artificially, be divided under various sub-headings: Clinical Work; Educational Activities; Research; Position of the Tavistock in the Community; Scarcity Economics; Aspirations for the Future.

Clinical Work

In general the pattern of this work has already largely been described. Between 1933 and the coming of the Second World War it developed perhaps in quality and intensity rather than in form. It is difficult to separate it from the internal training activities, since a good deal of the clinical work, especially of therapy, was done by our trainee staff as part of a new two-year course in psychotherapy. For the directorate this meant constant attention to the regularity of supervisions, case allocation, checking up on due and useful communication with referring doctors and social agencies, perhaps even more important in the Children's than in the Adult Department, but regarded by us in any case as a most important feed-back to the profession and the community. In this respect the Director and the two Assistant Directors regarded themselves as the planners and executives on behalf of the Medical Committee, having been democratically confirmed by it in our roles. This made our due and responsible authority much easier, especially as, unlike other institutions of the period, there was scarcely any of the authoritarian 'medical superintendent and deputy superintendent' feeling about our jobs or about our relations with all levels of staff. Such a stance would have been quite out of place in a group among whom the trainees were often our equals, both in seniority and distinction in other branches of psychiatry or previous medical experience, and were with us mainly for learning additional skills. These were not 'medical apprentices' who might be senior house officers elsewhere. In only one respect was it necessary to 'chase' people: that was in the keeping of adequate records which, before the advent of tape-recorders and sufficient clerical staff, was a matter of handwriting. It constituted a valuable training experience and a guarantee of the records being usable for later reports, follow-up or research work.

There was a steady rise in attendance figures between 1933 and the first half of 1939, from about 15,000 attendances in the Adult Department to about 26,500, with parallel rises at a lower level in the Children's Department. In 1938 the figure for new patients was about 1,200, with 341 children. It should be pointed out again that these attendances were always of at least from fifty to sixty minutes' duration – mostly longer for diagnostic interviews. The latter were nearly always done by a senior staff member, and physical investigation with all necessary tests was carried out in our own diagnostic unit and laboratory under a skilled pathologist before any treatment decisions were made.

The work of the in-patient department or hostel ceased in 1937 because the lease of its premises came to an end, and we did not think it wise to renew it. We could not really offer to treat the whole nation as presented by provincial referrals in any case; we also felt that the hostel community demanded better structural arrangements and had best wait until we were able to implement our further 'permanent' extension plans, about which more will be said later on.

The shape of work and the methods tended to become a little more uniform, perhaps inevitably when the powerful personality of J. A. Hadfield dominated training and when several of the senior staff had been trained by him. Most of us were convinced that for out-patient therapy with a long waiting list rigorous full analyses were seldom justified. While individual 'styles' of psychotherapy were encouraged and fostered in discussion and supervision, Hadfieldian 'reductive analysis' (his term) had a great vogue in the inter-war years and is still practised by a number of people originally coming under the Hadfield/McDougall influence. There were many advantages in its somewhat more flexible views. Hadfield had anticipated Freud by some years in postulating an independent instinct of aggression. Hadfield had stressed that there was at least a triad of instincts – namely, the sexual libido, aggression or self-assertion, and dependence, with its need for attachment behaviour, which he regarded as the source of tenderness and infantile self-preservation. He could not bring every kind of affective manifestation under the libidinal or sexual hat. This conceptual scheme made it possible without loss of inner consistency to use, for example, Adlerian hypotheses, with their stress on the need to dominate or compensate for a sense of insecurity or weakness or over-dependence, or, again, to use a much more friendly approach to the patient rather than the extremely rigorous and conceptually motivated impersonality of the classical Freudian technique. The aim of treatment was to discover the dynamic links between the symptom and its causes in the past. The search was by free association and dream analysis for what Hadfield termed 'nuclear incidents'. These need not necessarily be grossly traumatic, but were crises or turning-points in the inner life of the child, as recollected on the couch. The patient relived and realized a repression of one attitude – for example, dependence – by adopting a new attitude – for example, defiance – and a splitting off of his need for love, etc. In practice this method frequently worked quite well. The criticism made of it by the more discerning of Hadfield's trainees was his deliberate and reasoned rejection of the significance of the transference. Not that he failed to observe it; but he did not evaluate it in the same way as the psycho-analysts. To him it was a transient phenomenon in the uncovering of infantile behaviour and material. This is no doubt fair enough, but what he tried in practice was to push it as soon as possible away from himself, believing that he was only a peg on which such transference feelings were hung. In treatment he tried to relate them back to the early incident with which the psychotherapeutic analytic search was there and then concerned. He was always working on 'an incident'. This lent a certain unreality and artificiality to the procedure best described by the notion of 'forced fantasy'. Several of his pupils in due course rebelled and sought further training. From this 'rebel' group then forming in the senior and middle ranks of the Tavistock staff of the later 1930s have come quite a number of eminent psychoanalysts. The first was Dr Augusta Bonnard, who, though not strictly a pupil of Hadfield's, felt our concepts wanting and sought psychoanalytic qualification. She herself and I recall that at this stage she was regarded by a good number of Tavistock people as a bit of a renegade and apostate who went 'supping with the Devil'. Among later converts who obtained their regular training at the Institute of Psychoanalysis were W. R. Bion, Geoffrey Thompson, Lois Munro, Margaret Little, A. T. M. Wilson, and a number of others stretching into the post-war era. I also went for further training analysis in the mid-1930s, without the intention of joining the organization.

It seems to me that the Hadfieldian inter-war analytical psychotherapy was a bit too tidy and intellectually remote, and scarcely paid enough respect to the interchanges at the patient's and the doctor's irrational levels of the unconscious. It was apt to make the therapist stay too much outside the patient's subjective experience, play the role of an outside, detached observer rather than participant. Neither the transference nor the therapist's counter-transference were used creatively. But it would be a mistake to regard the Tavistock as in any way a monolithic school in which everybody marched in step and used only this one method. It remained always an eclectic, ideologically free place where people could both try new techniques or use pharmacological aids as well as the venerable tools of earlier years; thus we had on the staff at least one 'cast-iron' hypnotist, as well as those who had in their own development as psychiatrists used suggestion and hypnosis. In the middle 1930s Mary Luff and I were already investigating the clinical value of the then novel intravenous barbiturates for 'chemical' hypno-analysis, at this stage mostly for diagnostic confirmatory purposes. We found it diagnostically of some help, but therapeutically useless. The wilder, or fringe kind of techniques, never prominent, now disappeared. Even in hypnosis the aim was more the facilitation of abreaction or the uncovering of depth material for analytic purposes than the forced 'brain-washing' by suggestion techniques of the pre-Freudian era.

In 1934 J.R. and I were appointed by the Home Office to examine and assess the qualifications of the many German and Austrian psychotherapists who came to this country. We invited some of them to work with us as clinical assistants. The 'vetting' work in respect of general psychiatry and for qualified German and Austrian psychoanalysts was done by others. In 1938, when the rape of Austria brought another wave of refugees, we were joined by Dr Leopold Stein, who reorganized our speech services on a truly psychodynamic basis and who was soon to become the leading exponent of speech therapy and the psychopathology of speech in this country.

(i) *Follow-up Studies*

It will be recalled that both H.C.M. and J.R. had always felt a need to try to validate the work of the Tavistock. Now, with greater resources in manpower and space and the appointment of Marjorie Garrod as Registrar with the sole duties of follow-up work, we were able to implement these hopes. By 1935 Mary Luff and Marjorie Garrod had published what was then a pioneer survey to assess the results of our treatment three years after discharge. It may be of some interest to give an abridged account of this study, the full text of which appeared in the *British Medical Journal* on 13 July 1935 under their joint authorship. After describing our range of treatments, the authors divided the 500 patients on whom this follow-up was possible (out of 1,000 questionnaires sent out), by diagnoses, as set out in the following table:

Anxiety states	44%	Paranoid states	4%
Hysteria	15%	Delinquencies	4%
Obsessional states	12%	Schizoid states	3%
Depressive states	6%	Backwardness	3%
Sexual difficulties	4%	Epileptics, alcoholics, migraine, together	2%

In the main these were severe and long-standing cases – the Tavistock was chiefly a 'last resort'.

The results at discharge were compared with the results after three years under four headings:

(a) *Much improved:* which meant that the patients were free from symptoms, leading normal lives, usefully employed and able to meet difficulties with self-confidence without lapse into neurosis.
(b) *Improved:* this category indicated that patients had been much benefited, had become self-supporting members of the community and able to withstand ordinary stresses, but were liable to show some return of symptoms under particularly difficult situations such as bereavement or unemployment, and whilst not relapsing into a 'break-down', needed to return to the Clinic for one or more interviews to assist readjustment.
(c) *Slightly Improved:* those who had had some benefit but had never become free from symptoms and were liable to break down again under strain.
(d) *Not improved.*

For purposes of the follow-up the 'Much Improved' and 'Improved' groups together were called 'Relieved'. In this way the figures showed that on discharge the 'Relieved' were 65·6%, which after three years had dropped to 55%. The largest group, the *anxiety states*, showed an 80% improvement rate on discharge, which remained at 64% after three years. Interestingly enough the stablest benefit (73%) was in *sexual difficulties*. These included not the deviations, but *impotence* and *frigidity* and similar dysfunction. Once 'relieved', they remained at the same figure of 73% after three years.

Comparison in length of treatment showed that 50% of cases had under twenty interviews, and 58% of these remained relieved after three years; a further 39% had from twenty to sixty interviews, and of these 51·2% remained relieved after three years; lastly, 11% of cases had over sixty interviews, and of these 54·5% remained relieved. An interesting point in the sample was the ratio of women at 61% as against 39% of men. The authors made the point that the discrepancy might be accounted for not so much by the fact of sexual differences in liability to psychoneurotic illness as by the fact that it was often easier for women to find the time for courses of regular treatment at a time when employers would not give men time off.

By and large our women patients did rather better than men: women with anxiety states remained relieved to nearly 70% after three years, whereas the men with anxiety states showed only 55% relief after this period. It was argued that the greater difficulty for men patients to stay well might be connected with the then prevailing economic stresses, such as unemployment.

A separate follow-up was also done in the Children's Department, and here the sex ratio was almost reversed. Of 500 consecutive cases, 304 were boys and 196 were girls. The preponderance of boys was attributed to the fact that their symptoms tended to take a more obvious acting-out form than those of girls, so that parents or other agencies were more likely to feel the need for referring boys for treatment. The authors commented that with our culture values it was easier for boys passing through neurotic phases to adjust through better outlets as they grew up, whereas girls with latent or unrecognized neurotic tendencies developed more definite symptoms in later life, having fewer social and work outlets in those years, and so swelled the adult female patient quota.

There was also a breakdown into occupations which showed that, as now, so in 1934–5, the Tavistock was a clinic for the middle and lower middle classes. These classes, assumed to contain the people with better intelligence, as indicated by their professional status, showed a higher percentage of 'relieved' than manual workers (66·7% professional groups as compared with 51·8% non-professional groups). The results of the lowest three occupational groups, unskilled workmen, factory hands and unemployed working class, were considerably below the average for the group as a whole.[1]

The last point Luff and Garrod made was the relationship between psychopathic heredity and adverse early environment, a subject still to the fore at the present time. Psychopathic

[1] This seems to point to the conclusion that analytic methods are perhaps best suited to the intelligence groups above the median. H.V.D.

heredity in gross form was scored as present when a history of psychosis, mental deficiency, epilepsy or severe neurotic symptoms in one or more first-degree relatives was recorded. The authors said 'the incidence of this factor was therefore under- rather an over-estimated'. Among the early environmental factors Luff and Garrod included cruelty or drunkenness in the parents, illegitimacy, orphanage upbringing, divorce, separation or serious quarrelling among parents, and conditions of severe poverty. Psychopathic heredity as above defined was recorded in 36·6% of the 500 cases. In this group the proportion 'relieved' three years after discharge was 52·2%, suggesting that such a factor was not as serious a handicap to successful treatment as is sometimes thought. The number of patients giving a history of adverse early environment (naturally, with some overlap from the psychopathic heredity group) was 59·4%. Among these 47% remained relieved, a lower figure than the average for all patients. The point was made here that where early adverse environment and psychopathic inheritance coincided, the results of psychotherapy were probably least good.

The second piece of follow-up work done by the Registrar's Department appeared in 1937 and concerned 500 cases received and treated in the Children's Department between 1921 and 1934. The main findings of this follow-up were that approximately 70% of the cases recorded were in a satisfactory condition at the time of the follow-up, which might be anywhere from three to ten years after their discharge. A particular point was made of following 53 available patients originally seen in the Children's Department during the earliest years, 1921 to 1927, which was, of course, only a small proportion of all those seen. This maximum possible follow-up in time showed that of the 53 patients 45 were relieved on discharge, 40 remained relieved in 1931, and 39 still remained well in 1937. After making due allowance, from detailed scrutiny of other favourable factors which could have influenced the picture, the authors concluded that there remained 30 patients who improved directly as the result of psychotherapy and who had remained well for ten years or more; these had not only lost their symptoms and remained socially well, but also reported that their interests had widened and their efficiency had so much increased that in many cases since treatment or as a result of subsequent improvement they had progressed in socio-economic life out of all proportion to their own or parents' expectations before treatment. When these now adult patients were first seen they were not only severely handicapped, but were generally maladjusted, unhappy children with a poor record at school or work. It must be explained that in those days the Children's Department saw young people up to the age of seventeen, whereas the school-leaving age was fourteen. The overall follow-up of the 500 patients also disclosed the interesting fact that the majority of homes visited were comfortable, without obvious signs of financial stress. This made the authors express the view that the incidence and importance of neurotic factors in illness is, if anything, less in the poor than the rich. They also said that some children recovered in the face of apparently insuperable difficulties under therapy, and some retained their symptoms for reasons which often remained obscure even under quite good external conditions.

Looking at these reports thirty-three years later, we are, of course, struck with their relatively simple design, and particularly with the absence of untreated control series or series treated by other methods elsewhere, and so on. This would make much of this work unacceptable in our present more sophisticated, statistically minded era. None the less, it shows that the Tavistock in those days was not unmindful of the need both to verify what it was doing and follow as far as it could the cases that could be reached. At this time only one comparable survey had been done, by T. A. Ross of the Cassel Hospital. Many years later D. H. Malan was to take up with more scientific rigour follow-up and validation studies on his Tavistock patients.

(ii) *The Chronic Attender Problem*

In the pursuit of more effective, as well as of cutting wasteful, patient attendances and medical deployment we instituted supervision, not only as a training method for our clinical assistants, but also as a procedure which in the Soviet Union might have been called 'self-criticism'. This obliged every doctor, however senior, who had spent fifty interviews with a given patient to report and discuss the progress of the case with another senior colleague, himself under the same obligation. With the democratic atmosphere prevailing, this was perhaps less threatening than it might have been in other institutions of the period. It proved of the greatest help in the relief of guilt and anxiety in the counter-transference of some of the staff members which had snarled progress. With more uneven personal training, especially among the oldest doctors, than could be expected of a present-day psychotherapist, such situations were best tackled as routine rather than as being 'on the mat'. It helped to prevent the collusive development of chronic attenders the therapist dared not discharge.

In general, the trend of expectations was one of scepticism and warning against facile optimism; the more senior and more experienced, the less optimistic or omnipotent did our members become. One of our wisest men of that period, Dr Maurice Wright, was also the most pessimistic, but achieved individually much the best results of any of us. We had follow-ups on all patients for each staff member.

Educational Activities

A good deal has already been written about the internal training of clinical assistants in earlier sections of the book. The method, which is, I suppose, a pretty universal method of training psychotherapists, was continued and consolidated and made more systematic as the directors under the Medical Committee were able to use a certain amount of organizational ingenuity to secure that every clinical assistant had his weekly hour of supervision with the selected supervisor, that they all attended seminars and case discussions and went to the courses generally prescribed for them, and that they also learnt not only to keep good notes, but also to write reports to the referring agencies, which for a time were always vetted and corrected by their supervisors. We were anxious that our standing was kept high by first-class reports and constant liaison with the patients' general practitioners or other referring agencies. This liaison work was particularly well done and conscientiously accomplished in the Children's Department, where by this time we had five P.S.Ws under the direction of Mrs Phyllis Haml n and where, in addition to the senior physicians, there were some notable 'students'. In the mid-1930s Dr Mary Burbury, who never reached staff level in our clinic, became Director of Child Guidance for the city of Manchester, a post which she held with distinction until she went as a University senior lecturer in child psychiatry to Leeds after the war. Another of our 'students', Dr Margaret Methven, was appointed in the late 1930s to her present position as Director of Child Guidance for Edinburgh and a member of the University teaching staff. Dr H. Mary Capes similarly went to Southampton as Director of Child Guidance and became a distinguished member of the Child Psychiatric Services of this country.

Of greater volume and scarcely secondary in importance to our turning-out of adequately-trained psychotherapists in this era were our *extra-mural* courses, to which our internal students, naturally, had free access. In extra-mural teaching we provided extensive lecture experiences, intensive week-ends and the like for general practitioners and later on also for magistrates, probation officers and for ministers of religion. During one summer vacation we laid on a special course at the request of the University Department of Cairo for a number of Egyptian psychiatrists and psychologists. Professor Askar was a trainee with us. Our external lecturers were not only our own staff, but we always had contributors from our medical advisory board and other sympathetic leaders of the profession. Thus, we ran a course for general physicians on special aspects of neurosis in organic disease, in which the gynaecologists were Professor F. J. Brown and Mr Alec Bourne, the neurologist was Russell Brain (later Lord Brain), the dermatologist W. J. O'Donovan – each covering the borderland between organic and functional disorders in their fields.

In the non-medical area there were welcome developments which even brought us limited University recognition. Thus, Miss Simmins's course in clinical psychology for intending child guidance clinic staffs was so recognized. We also had many students from the London School of Economics in our social casework department for their practical work, which included the observation of play-groups and all that is implied by child study, which they shared with the post-graduate psychologists. We also instituted under the leadership of Professor (Sir) Francis Fraser, by this time Chairman of our Medical Advisory Group, a study seminar for young physicians from the teaching hospitals at recent consultant or at senior registrar levels. This was an exceedingly lively and fruitful piece of work, from which developed joint psychosomatic projects with our research staff, as will appear below. We continued our policy of celebrity lectures: C. G. Jung gave a week's course, very well attended, published in 1968. We also had Kretschmer from Tübingen, while in the field of child development Dr Maria Montessori, Susan Isaacs and Charlotte Bühler were contributors to a large course by our own department. Our staff members remained in great demand for outside engagements to speak on topics in our area. From time to time we arranged public lecture courses for the general public, which were financially profitable to the Clinic's exchequer.

Research

For reasons indicated, research was a relative late-comer in the Tavistock. In 1936 this gap in our work began to be closed. In that year the Rockefeller Foundation awarded a research fellowship tenable at the Tavistock, and almost simultaneously, but independently, the Sir Halley Stewart Trust also made us a research grant. Dr A. T. Macbeth Wilson became the Rockefeller Fellow and Dr Eric Wittkower the Sir Halley Stewart Fellow. Their work, which has been widely published, was mostly concerned with the then new psychosomatic method. Wilson took up the study of peptic ulcer in its psychological and social aspects. Wittkower collaborated with Dr Geoffrey Bourne of St Bartholomew's Hospital on cardiac pain, with Dr E. R. Cullinan on ulcerative colitis, and with Dr John Freeman of St Mary's Hospital and others on the pathogenesis of asthma.

Wilson was in close touch with Professor Millais Culpin and Dr May Smith at the School of Hygiene, and used some of the methods which Culpin had developed for mapping personalities of probands and of a control series of 100 patients with hernia.

Wilson's first paper was written in collaboration with Dr D. T. Davies (later Sir Daniel) of the Royal Free Hospital. Significant differences were found between the worrying, tense personalities in 95 % of the ulcer patients, compared with only some 30 % of the hernia group. Similarly, precipitating events of defined types occurred in highly significant excess in the ulcer patients. Wittkower's work developed on similar lines with personality studies of hay-fever sufferers, and later with psychological stress as a factor in *all* cases of heart pain, functional and organic. He showed that cardiac failure in rheumatic heart disease and even in coronary disease was related to the supervention of stress. In his collaboration with E. R. Cullinan, Wittkower studied chronic diarrhoea going on to ulcerative colitis, in which he found a preponderance of grossly unusual individual life histories and a tendency to a definite psychological personality profile. This is not the place in which to detail the results of papers published and still available, but rather to show that the type of research chosen was very much linked to major medical problems of the day. It was in fact chosen to emphasize the intimacy of the body-mind linkage to a highly 'mechanistic' medical generation. The aim was to make a contribution to holistic medicine.

It should be mentioned that in 1939 a second Rockefeller Fellow, Dr J. P. Spillane, of Cardiff, was nominated, but could not take up his duties owing to the outbreak of war.

Our research fellows had come from medicine and physiology. A. T. M. Wilson's job at the Middlesex Hospital and his publications had been in the physiological sphere before he became a trainee with us. Wittkower was already well known for his work in Berlin before having to leave Germany when the Nazis came to power.

Wilson and Wittkower made closer research links with various teaching hospitals. With Drs Geoffrey Bourne and Ronald Bodley-Scott of St. Bartholomew's Hospital, twelve cases of peripheral vascular disorder were examined, with negative results on personality findings – itself important. Quite otherwise was the case with certain skin diseases, in which Wittkower was to develop a very fruitful collaboration with the Dermatological Department of St Bartholomew's Hospital under Dr R. M. B. McKenna, beginning with acne rosacea and going on to other functional skin troubles. Similarly, at the invitation of Professor Brown of the Obstetric Department at University College Hospital, Wilson and Wittkower made an investigation of primary dysmenorrhoea, amenorrhoea and sterility, with primiparae as control cases.

A not unimportant piece of research was also done by Dr Alan Maberly in the Children's Department in 1936 on the results of sexual assault in childhood. This showed that the most important factor in producing or avoiding later traumatic neurotic reactions was the method of handling of the child after the assault, rather than the fact of assault itself.

During the same period our follow-up department did a special study of 496 cases of delinquency or potential delinquency seen in adults since the Tavistock was opened in 1920. Of these, 168 were given treatment, the remainder having only one consultation. Of the 168 patients it was possible to follow 104 patients for three years or longer. The cases selected for treatment were usually those estimated to have a sufficient intelligence to profit by 'talking cures'. The results, which never saw publication, are of some interest. Thus, of 62 treated cases of stealing, 43 could be followed up for three years, and of these 24 remained free from symptoms. Of sexual offences, i.e. homosexuality, exhibitionism, sexual assault, habitual prostitution and 1 case of transvestism, and also including female homosexuals, 73 were treated, of whom only 2 were under institutional care during treatment (1 of which was my case of the man handcuffed to his warder). Of the 73 cases 39 could be followed up for three years, of whom 25 remained free of symptoms. The improvement rate was higher in this group than in any other, suggesting that sexual deviations seemed particularly suitable for treatment by psychotherapy, contrary to psychiatric views. In the case of addiction, of 65 cases there were only 4 drug addicts, the rest being alcoholics, usually of long duration: 16 cases were treated, of whom 9 could be followed up and of these 7 remained free from relapse for three years. Lastly, a group of 41 cases of various forms of anti-social behaviour, such as violence, wandering, etc., 18 could be treated, of whom 13 cases were followed up for three years or more, and of these

7 remained free from symptoms. These are not impressive results, and they were not matched by the necessary controls. The report by the follow-up department said that a survey of the unsuccessful cases showed that a number were responsive to psychotherapy, but the difficulties of their continuing environment were too great for them to remain well. 'Under existing conditions the best efforts of social workers were unavailing in providing for them a sufficiently stable environment to give the background of hope and confidence necessary.' The general opinion of the staff at the Tavistock at that time was that delinquent behaviour was not a disease, but a symptom that may arise from a number of different causes, the treatment indicated varying with the cause. This self-evident proposition still had the ring of novelty to the medical and legal services of the period.

In a modest way there was also some laboratory research going on in the years now under review. Our pathologist, Dr Joseph Fine, made thorough investigations on fairly large numbers of our patients into possible connections between endocrine dysfunction and psycho-neurotic conditions as revealed by studies, especially of carbohydrate metabolism. This meant that he was investigating glycosuria in non-diabetic patients as an index of anxiety. Sugar curves were thought in those days to have opened up lines of enquiry into the aetiology of various endocrine disturbances, such as hyperthyroidism and its opposite, an excess of adrenal secretion, and also excess anterior pituitary activity, each of them producing a fairly characteristic curve. He found that 2 % of our total patient load had such glycosuria. Dr Fine's papers were published, not in psychiatric, but in pathological journals and seem to have left little impression. He also made the observation that anxiety states tended to have excess of oxalic acid in the urine – another of those many clues to bodily states associated with psycho-neurosis that seems to have become obliterated with the years. Dr Fine left us for higher spheres in 1937 and was succeeded by the late Dr H. Fleischhacker, who subsequently became the pathologist at Shenley Hospital.

Quite apart from these more formalized researches, the atmosphere of the Tavistock was one of lively enquiry and creative experimenting in the approach to psychoneurotic illness and personality problems. I was reminded again not only of the discussion groups centred around Ian Suttie and later continued by A. T. M. Wilson, G. R. Hargreaves, W. R. Bion, Grizel Thompson and others, who managed not only to crash the barriers separating us from the psychoanalytic movement, but also produced much new thinking which could be fed into the Tavistock's work on independent, psychodynamic lines, and in the face of our great case loads much more patient-and-reality-centred. Publications, both as papers and as books, flowed from the Tavistock in numbers and quality of which no university department need have been ashamed. In Miss Simmins's department the post-graduate psychologists working under the auspices of London University were also contributing a good deal to research not here listed under Clinic publications. Their work became theses in the University of London and suchlike. The climate was certainly more that of an academic post-graduate school with a busy clinical life than of some routine clinic or out-patient department in which people merely came and went. As already mentioned, much of the mutual stimulation came through the provision of a canteen and of a library, which was perhaps not always as silent as it might have been, but hummed with lively discussion.

Our educational work was greatly broadened by the friendly link we made with Dr W. J. T. Kimber, then Medical Superintendent of Hill End Mental Hospital, St Albans. Many of our younger doctors served there in salaried general psychiatric appointments, under an early example of the rotating internship or registrar scheme. The trainees were, as already mentioned, encouraged to undergo training analyses, the choice of school being left to them. The gradual drift of some of the ablest towards the Psychoanalytic Institute began in this period, and was later to become much more marked. At this time, however, the rival systems or deviations still had their supporters. Until 1939 there were always two or three strong Adlerians on our staff, though never many fully-fledged Jungians. It was my role for a short time to act as the not too well-tolerated supervisor to Dr M. S. M. Fordham, who has since become the leading exponent of Jung's system in this country.

Position of the Tavistock in the Community

I have already referred to J.R.'s great talent for public relations and 'promotion'. In 1934 the public standing of the Tavistock was such that our Council could achieve success in their request for Royal patronage. His Royal Highness the Duke of Kent, K.G., the youngest son of King George V, agreed on 26 June 1934 at a dinner in support of the Institute of Medical Psychology, to become our President, a position in which he remained until his premature death on war service as the result of an air-crash. In his speech at that dinner His Royal Highness said:

> When therefore I was asked to come here this evening and to take the Presidency of this Institute I at once accepted. . . . I am sure, Ladies and Gentlemen, you must be as interested as I am in this movement. . . .

He went on:

> It is really only since the war [meaning the First World War – H.V.D.] that the importance of academic, industrial and medical psychology has been realized. If we are to relieve suffering we must get away from purely physical conditions in dealing with patients and understand what medical psychology means. I believe that in the past the mere mention of the word 'psychology' was quite sufficient to prejudice financial support, but I am glad to say that in these days, when we are faced by countless individual, national and international problems, many of which cannot be solved without psychiatrical understanding, this is no longer the case.

His Royal Highness then went on to speak about the statistics of nervous and mental disease in the community and called it a national problem. After hoping that the work would rapidly increase because of the great need for help, he concluded:

> Having visited this Institution a few days ago and been much impressed by its organization and the work it is doing, I am convinced it merits every support.

He then went on to appeal for funds, which was the primary function of all such events!

In the report of the Chairman of the Council, Sir Henry Brackenbury, the event was greeted naturally with very great pleasure, and Sir Henry went on to say that the Duke of Kent watched as much of the work as could be shown to anyone on his preliminary visit – for example, intelligence-testing, the children's playroom and something also of the records, and so on. In that year the Duke of Kent had married the Princess Marina, who remained until her death in 1968 her late husband's successor. In the same year a bust in marble of the Duke by Professor de Ströbl, donated by an anonymous friend, was placed in the entrance hall of the Institute in Malet Place and has remained one of the precious possessions of the Clinic.

It will be appreciated that Royalty cannot afford to extend its patronage and active interest to organizations unless they are well established and of good standing. The patronage by the Duke of Kent therefore represented in a sense our 'arrival' on the medical and social scene after some fourteen years of labour.

Our efforts and activities in publishing, in extra-mural teaching and in achieving good communication with those doctors and other agencies who referred patients had the effect of enhancing our prestige, not so much as an academic than as a clinical institution in which much suffering was relieved in novel, person-respecting ways – more understandable and closer to general medicine than the still dreaded work of the psychiatric hospitals of the period or the strict analytical groups, both still regarded as on the fringe of respectability. It can be claimed that the Tavistock thus helped in breaking down the old image of psychological medicine and in integrating it in the minds of the profession and the public with the main body of medicine. For this it got scant credit from psychiatrists. This position was not to be repaired even by J.R. prior to the Second World War. There was too much irrational prejudice both ways in those days, with the Tavistock facing hostility and scorn from both sides – the orthodox psychiatrists and the orthodox analysts, a dismal picture of entrenched opinions precluding reasonable discourse. The Freudians were, in a sense, better off than the Tavistock. They were an international and quasi-monolithic body linked to similar institutes in other countries. They made little attempt to seek recognition, and their rigorous training requirements and self-containment commanded scandalized respect at arm's length. The Tavistock got it 'both ways'. It was neither a united group marching in step nor a 'proper' psychiatric institution – as it were, 'soft' on both counts: tainted with Freudian doctrines, but also 'do-gooders', choosing the easy option of neurosis.

It is part of the history of psychiatry in Britain to place on record these early divisions between its three main branches. The psychotherapists increasingly made informal friends with psychoanalysts proper and with each other. We have mentioned the forum of the British Psychological Society, the joint enterprise in founding the Institute for the Scientific Treatment of Delinquency, and the private discussion groups. Individual psychoanalysts such as Susan Isaacs and Karen Stephen defied the official ban on professional dealings with us and lectured in the Tavistock courses. In the sphere of official recognition of what we did and taught, not even Mapother's hostility and apprehension could entirely obstruct us. His own need to be perceived as moving with the times doubtless demanded some acknowledgement that psychotherapy existed. It is worth repeating that the University of London recognized the Tavistock as a centre where candidates for its Diploma in Psychological Medicine (of which Mapother was the Chairman) could obtain experience in the treatment of psychoneuroses which was a requirement for that more rigorous Diploma of the University in contrast to the D.P.M. Syllabus of the Conjoint Board of the Royal Colleges. In this limited sense, therefore, we were a recognized institution, although we never had medical staff recognized as University teachers. We did also have recognition for some of our clinical psychology and social work courses, as already mentioned. We ourselves wanted to be part of the University scene. There was in the middle 1930s an attempt made to affiliate the Tavistock to University College Hospital, whose consultant psychiatrist at the time was Bernard Hart. The negotiations, however, were not successful: the Tavistock was perceived as too big and powerful to be the psychiatric department of a teaching hospital. One U.C.H. man said: 'It will be a case of the tail wagging the dog if we take you over.'

We were more successful in colonizing and export than in the home base. The growing number of child guidance clinics in the provinces as well as in Greater London were largely staffed by the graduates of the Tavistock's Children's Department, medical and psychological. We strongly influenced the development of psychiatric social work. Sweden's first P.S.W. was trained by us, and became the head of the social work school there. It was also not surprising that as our staff members reached seniority and recognition they were in very considerable demand for committee work and as officers of the Psychiatric Section of the Royal Society of Medicine, the Medical Section of the British Psychological Society and Psychiatric Sections of the annual scientific meetings of the British Medical Association, as well as, of course, in the newer mental health activities, such as the Child Guidance Council and the National Council for Mental Hygiene, directly inspired by some of us.

The Tavistock staff was always fully represented in the British branch of the largely German-speaking International General Society for Psychotherapy, of which H.C.M. was Chairman and I was Honorary Secretary up to 1939. We organized a large and very interesting congress of this Society at Oxford in 1938 under the presidency of C. G. Jung, for which the late E. B. Strauss, then associated with the Tavistock, was the Organizing Secretary. At this meeting the tensions between the democratic nations and the German-Italian Fascist Axis representatives were already very marked. None the less, the Tavistock, as a new kind of model institution *sui generis* of psychotherapeutic service, gained a good deal in prestige among European psychiatrists.

Scarcity Economics

But while our medical prestige stood quite high, this could not be said of our finances, especially of the growth of capital funds which would free us from constant worry for our very survival in a world which had suffered the economic depression of 1929, and which still did not have a clear image of the role of psychological factors in health and disease. Official psychiatry (ultimately the policies of the royal colleges, universities, etc.) was very much dominated by the first new advances made in physical treatments (E.C.T. and Cardiazol). The overall conservatism of the medical profession despite the support shown by some of its London-based leaders, and the recurring claims for funds by much more obvious causes, such as blind babies, orphans or cancer and tuberculosis, made appeals difficult. The Medical Research Council at this stage took no interest in any psychiatric or psychosomatic work. A small contribution was made by King Edward VII's Fund for Hospitals, but only in respect of our in-patient department. It was only by a piece of double-talk that for their regulations we managed to be a hospital and at the same time not a mental hospital.

It is all the more fitting in the light of these difficulties that tribute should here be paid to some of the individuals who contributed so very greatly to the fund-raising and good-housekeeping efforts of the Tavistock. In 1935 the famous athlete, Mr Harold Abrahams, barrister-at-Law, consented to become the Chairman of our Finance Committee with a place on the Council, and gave unstinting service. The so-called 'Friends of the Tavistock Clinic' formed themselves into a very active Appeal Committee. Among them should be specially mentioned the Lady Cynthia Colville, Lady (Basil) Blackett, our Chairman, Sir Henry Brackenbury, and his wife, and Lady Whyte. The latter has remained a faithful and esteemed friend right to the present day. It was this Committee, served by our Appeals Secretary, Mrs Stopford-Douglas, who, with J.R.'s urging, organized the many dinners, bazaars, midnight matinées, and who persuaded cinemas to give the charitable part of their Sunday earnings (as required by law) to us. That Committee succeeded in getting prominent personalities to appeal for us on the now-developing radio services on Sunday-night programmes, and so on. This was indeed as much as the medical and scientific effort a part of the battle for survival of the Tavistock, as it was of many other voluntary hospitals. Some of the latter at least owned land or had other resources due to their long histories, or managed by reason of their much more obvious appeal to attract big donors. Nobody like Lord Nuffield or Mr Meierstein, who rebuilt and endowed new departments of great hospitals in the inter-war years, emerged to help the Tavistock to be free of its hand-to-mouth existence. This, however, is not to underrate the faithful and constant flow of small donations and subscriptions and an increasing number of seven-year covenants which had just then been invented, helping to balance our current expenditure and income account, and also sometimes to earmark funds for future development, which was never far from our minds.

It only took a very few years to realize that the Malet Place premises, which in 1932 had seemed so commodious and splendid, had become too small for us. Even the expedient of subdividing consulting-rooms into narrow and rather unattractive halves did not solve the problem of treating all those who needed treatment and training all those who asked for it. Our trainees never had corners of their own in which they could write notes or interview patients out of turn, because all rooms were booked every hour of the day and had to be vacated by the previous occupants on a strict sessional basis. In this situation it was characteristic of J.R. and the whole staff that they fervently went on believing in the future of the institution, and that, despite the financial stringency, we went ahead with planning the extension of premises and services which will be described in the subsequent section. Here are just a few more personal references. It was in 1938 that our revered Chairman of Council, Sir Henry Brackenbury, was forced by increasing age and deafness to retire. He was replaced by Lord Alness. This distinguished Scottish Appeal Court Judge was not one to be easily impressed. None the less, in his first report he wrote warmly of the contribution which he felt the Tavistock was making to medicine and the mental health services of the country, and was clearly caught by the spirit of enthusiasm, which made him a splendid successor to Sir Henry Brackenbury, who had made the cause of the Tavistock his own. Lord Allness was to stay with us as Chairman throughout the war years, greatly admired and a true friend of our work. When he came to us he had already behind him a long experience of the Bar, the Scottish Bench and the Court of Appeal, both Houses of Parliament and the Cabinet, in addition to serving many good causes. He was also a member of the Child Guidance Council and the Feversham Committee, which, it will be recalled, began its sessions around this time, concerned with the task of co-ordinating the voluntary mental health services in Great Britain. Lord Alness brought to us a 'new kind of respectability' which not even Sir Henry Brackenbury had quite managed to provide! In fact, the 1938 report by the Medical Director had to answer certain criticisms (one suspects from some of our opponents within medicine) that we were always beating the big drum and that we indulged in too much publicity and promotion to be in good medical taste. J.R. had to write:

> Our Medical [Advisory] Board have given us their backing and approval of what we have attempted and, in spite of a number of almost inevitable slips, a great deal has been done through the lay Press to bring the work of the Clinic and the needs of mental health in general to the notice of the public, and lay journals have in large measure followed the admirable lead given by the medical Press in recent years. Sir Henry Brackenbury had been successful as Chairman of the Council of the B.M.A. in interesting the profession at large and especially general practitioners in our affairs. We felt justified in this publicity because we occupied a difficult position in 'the no-man's-land' between the general hospital with its obvious appeal on the one hand and the mental hospitals on the other hand with their budgets and their functions laid down partly by legislation, partly by the provisions of local authorities who ran these mental hospitals.

Another criticism that was levelled at us was that we were apart from medicine and from official psychiatry, and this, of course, was true at the beginning, when we were an institution of a new kind fitting no existing pattern – neither fish, flesh nor fowl. It could be argued that we increasingly remedied this position, not only by our clinical and research links with the general hospitals and with general practice, but also by increasingly supplying specialist staff to certain mental and general hospitals. We also influenced a growing proportion of our staff to take the Diploma of Psychological Medicine on the one hand, while on the other hand also recruiting increasingly those with previous general psychiatric experience acquired in posts at mental hospitals or elsewhere. It was, and has remained to the present day, always difficult to maintain our image and our identity as a new model of institution with a philosophy and task of its own, neither quite in classical psychiatry nor yet fully committed to the psychoanalytic doctrines and practice. It is this position of a marginal or unusual, unconventional place in either terms which contributed to making economic survival difficult.

By 1938, when the threat of the Second World War was already upon us, the Tavistock offered its services to the Ministry of Health to man a neurosis unit for the expected civilian war casualties of a psychoneurotic kind, and also undertook to help with training in air-raid-precaution duties and so forth, as our contribution to mobilization. As a pointer to the solidarity and enthusiasm of the staff, in 1937 all staff members voluntarily gave up honoraria (always very modest) for their attendances, and the hours of work done by the senior staff none the less did not decrease. This was our gesture in trying to help the finances of the Clinic. Originally these honoraria had been instituted because of the very considerable number of hours which such psychotherapeutic staff had to give when they as yet had few other sources of income. We may, however, surmise that by this time most senior staff members were earning quite well in private practice. The public had recognized the usefulness of psychotherapy and so had G.P.s. There certainly did not seem to be any haggard faces among the staff members as of 1938!

In 1936, after six years of calling ourselves the Institute of Medical Psychology with the sub-title in brackets (The Tavistock Clinic), we reverted to our old name. Already, despite our relative youth, our older name had acquired permanence and firm usage. There were several arguments, one of which was that other institutes, not always reputably or responsibly staffed or sponsored, were springing up elsewhere and used appellations scarcely distinguishable from our 'Institute of Medical Psychology'. Further, there was also the realization that the Institute of Medical Psychology was a dream of the future, and that the name by which we were popularly known was more appropriate. We had now become the Tavistock Clinic, having dropped the 'Square' long ago, and we carried in brackets the sub-title (Institute of Medical Psychology). It will be seen in a subsequent chapter that this change was not without some significance for future developments.

To sum up the achievements of the Tavistock Clinic up to 1939, it can be said that it had made a very considerable change in British medicine by the pioneering of middle-of-the-road psychodynamic psychotherapy that could be flexibly applied to quite large numbers of patients. We had also established the notion of the multi-professional team for more effective work and for saving of medical time – only now (1969) coming to be talked about as the great innovation for medical practice. We had established training for these groups and sent out a good number of relatively experienced and trained persons to other centres at home and abroad and had budded off at least one daughter clinic in Edinburgh. We had influenced many students, general practitioners, magistrates, clergy and social-work students and workers in other fields, from the general teaching hospital to the local public health, maternity and child-welfare clinics. We had thus produced a certain climate of opinion favourable to the study and consideration of personality as the central factor in health and illness, as well as trying to link these factors to the body of established medicine. More lately we had also succeeded in creating a respectable – indeed, quite advanced – research unit, through which we influenced the development of the new psychosomatic method both in its research and in its teaching and treatment aspects. We had made many friends among the medical as well as the social establishment in Great Britain, and we had also contributed by teaching, committee work and many personal contacts to the eventual unification of several discreet aspects of mental-health endeavour in this country which, through the Feversham Committee, was achieved in the National Association for Mental Health. What we scarcely realized was how much we had also contributed to the growth of similar interests abroad, notably in North America. Among the many young postgraduates from America who attended the early Tavistock lectures on psychotherapeutic method and psychopathology were William C. Menninger, Brock Chisholm and Lawrence Kubie. These good friends reminded us later that they were influenced in their later distinguished careers by the kind of concepts and practice they had encountered in the squalid little building in Tavistock Square.

Aspirations for the Future

With these achievements to our credit and with an extremely live, coherent and friendly staff group in wide contact with the medical scene, it was reasonable to expect that we would before long achieve something like teaching hospital status – if not as a post-graduate 'hospital' in the accepted sense, then at least on the lines of a special institution, perhaps analogous to the School of Tropical Medicine and Hygiene, with academically-recognized courses and teachers for the subjects in which we had become expert. It was for this reason that in 1930 we changed the official title of the Tavistock Clinic to that of 'The Institute of Medical Psychology'. Plans had in fact already been drawn for a 'proper' building in which such an Institute could develop and flourish. Unfortunately, the economic depression around 1930 and the resistances to the wider implications of our work, which we underestimated, somehow always made it 'inopportune' between 1930 and 1937 to launch any large public appeal. In our minds the removal from Tavistock Square to Malet Place, while very welcome, was never regarded as more than a halfway house. The activation of the Extension Committee from among the body we called the Friends of the Institute of Medical Psychology had the express purpose of creating the financial base for such an Institute. By 1936 we had got to the point of asking Mr Graham Dawbarn (the architect responsible for adapting Malet Place) to prepare a plan and a model for the site which the Extension Committee, backed by Council, had acquired. This was quite close to our existing location, at the corner of Store Street and Ridgmount Gardens, just off Gower Street. The plan was for a building which was to contain on a number of floors 101 beds, forty of them reasonably-priced pay-beds, many more consulting-rooms than at present, with far better facilities for laboratory work and physical treatment, and also the necessary lecture-rooms and other educational and research facilities. We felt that a hospital and out-patient centre of this kind in central London could be of great importance in the development of studies expressly aimed at the group of disorders we had always been interested in (and had successfully relieved for fifteen years or more), especially as they affected the interaction of generations, with a great emphasis on children and on development of the personality in nature and society. Britain needed a school of this kind, because we now felt that it would be many years before the medical profession as a whole and psychiatry in particular would come up to our fund of experience and interest in this very large group of disorders, either aetiologically, epidemiologically or in clinical skill. Until such time as this knowledge permeated the whole of medicine, we felt it to be essential to have a special post-graduate training centre providing and developing the collective knowledge we possessed. We had gone a long way to meeting the objections that our staff were one-sidedly trained by making a creative link with the Hill End Hospital at St. Albans (see p. 80), and we also had by this time a proportion of our senior staff serving in teaching or other general hospitals in addition to giving time to the Tavistock.

However, the situation in Britain was in some ways never favourable for large-scale support for an unestablished form of therapy – something which Dr Alan Gregg of the Rockefeller Foundation called the 'lunatic fringe' of medicine for which he specifically endowed our research fellowships. It was his aim to counter the crude 'mechanism' of medical thought. Many excellent ideas already in our minds, therefore, had to be postponed or shelved indefinitely. Among them should perhaps be mentioned J.R.'s public-health-training inspired epidemiological and comparative study of treatment results. In this ambitious project equal numbers of matched psychoneurotic patients from the Tavistock, from a general hospital and from the London Clinic of Psychoanalysis would be studied in detail, and each would be compared to an untreated group of psychoneurotic patients. Similarly, our whole system of record-keeping and classification was such that we hoped to undertake various demographic and epidemiological studies of the distribution of various types of psychoneurotic and allied disorders and their responsiveness to various kinds of therapy. This work, however, was never done, nor indeed was the site where we hoped to do it ever built upon. The model, however, is one which has still to be improved upon. It was to have the beds partly as we had contemplated a larger intake of provincial as well as more seriously disturbed psychoneurotic and early psychotic patients. In the original plan it was mentioned that the beds were to be 'for a type of case for which there is often no choice now but the observation wards of the public hospital or else an expensive nursing-home, as the present accommodation in existing hospitals for psychoneurotic illnesses is so very limited'. In other words, we contemplated doing quite a lot of 'acute breakdown' treatment for persons in various psychiatric crises and emergencies. The knowledge of the action of the newer sedatives was already beginning to be established, and it was in the late 1930s that E.C.T. as well as the intravenous barbiturates for abreaction and for general therapeutic purposes would have made such a proposal both feasible and very interesting for psychodynamic study and evaluation. In the meantime, we regarded the site as a kind of nest-egg bringing in revenue from shops and a pub.

The plan made in the 1930s provided for a more or less self-supporting institution, which would contain private consulting-rooms for the part-time staff, paying economic rents to the Institute. Moreover, the plan aimed at preserving the existing shops and the public house on its ground floor, (some staff liked this prospect!), and using the rents against the overheads for the Tavistock premises in the upper storeys. It is not hard to imagine that those few years of medical enthusiasm generated especially by J.R.'s infectious optimism must have been very difficult to sustain for the Honorary Treasurers, first and foremost 'sound' men of finance, who quite often used to tear their hair at the scale of loan, overdraft and projected future expenditure which was gaily embarked upon in pursuit of the extension scheme. J.R. reported, not without some humour, that in the summer of 1939, when the imminent war situation led to contraction of our work and a decline in major donations and subscriptions, the then Chairman of the Finance Committee had suggested to him that the only way the Tavistock could meet its obligations was to declare itself bankrupt! J.R. responded to this by transferring the Tavistock account to another bank, and the latter agreed to accept our overdraft. By this desperate manœuvre, the actual closing of the Tavistock was staved off, in spite of our conservative financial advisers.

Instead, then, of the projected expansion and extension into a 'great new future', the staff settled down seriously to adapting the Tavistock to the threatened war. J.R. had been appointed in 1938 as Consulting Psychiatrist to the Army for the emergency and began scouting for his staff officers and for the recruitment of psychiatrists. The Tavistock group compiled a book, under the editorship of Emmanuel Miller, which appeared just around the outbreak of war, entitled *The Neuroses in War*. This drew upon the experiences of the older members who had seen war neuroses in the First World War. W. R. Bion, D.S.O., who had commanded tanks at Cambrai, H.C.M. and Maurice Wright were among these. There were also contributors from elsewhere.

I conclude this chapter by some personalia. Around the turn of 1938 and 1939 our most excellent Secretary, Miss V. J. Howard, was lost to us by the usual hazard of marriage, to Dr Eardley Davidson; we were fortunate in acquiring a male successor for her, Mr Conrad Ormond. About the same time we also lost, through ill-health, our Educational Secretary, Mr H. A. Downes, mentioned earlier. In his stead we were joined by a man who was to have great influence on the fortunes of the wartime and post-war Clinic, Mr G. Dudley Herbert, a gentleman of independent means who wanted to serve the cause of mental health without remuneration, and stayed to see the Clinic through the wartime period. The smooth transition from peace to war was as much as anything due to the excellent efforts of Conrad Ormond and Dudley Herbert, who also became good personal friends. Plans for the emergency were painstakingly complete and effective.

VI

The Tavistock in War

Westfield College

It was accepted, since the world learnt about the destructiveness of modern bombing, that our premises in the heart of London would not remain tenable for very long. It was therefore decided to evacuate on the outbreak of war to a suburb not likely to be a bombing target. An arrangement was made in good time with Westfield Women's College of the University of London in Hampstead that in the event of war we would occupy, furnished, one of their halls of residence, the University as a whole being scheduled for evacuation to various provincial centres. This was carried into effect. Most of the Committee records and some of the spare furniture were stored in a small office on the Store Street site which housed our Appeals Department. This was the one regrettable decision. Whatsoever was stored there was unfortunately destroyed by a later bomb. This is the main reason why the records for this history are so scanty; no correspondence, minutes of Council or of Committee meetings of pre-1939 survive. But our clinical records and some of our furniture were transferred on the very first day of the war by the co-operative effort of staff members, who somehow or other contrived to remain anonymous. We all suspected that a major share was taken by Ronald Hargreaves, by Winifred Doherty and by several others of the younger staff members, as well as by our secretarial and domestic staffs. The plan was that those staff members not designated under the National medical man-power plan for the Emergency Medical Service or the armed forces could choose to live as a community in the hostel-like building at Westfield, where by day their bedrooms would be their consulting-rooms, a common refectory would feed them, and where there were one or two largish rooms available for conducting any teaching activities and also as the 'common rooms'. In their rooms staff would also see private patients if they wished.

Our caretaker and cook, Mr and Mrs Harland, our loyal good friends since Tavistock Square, and their daughter, Mrs Betty Davis, agreed to transfer with us. Those electing to move in as residents were male and female members of our staff, including one or two of our refugee colleagues from Germany, Austria and Czechoslovakia. In 1939, within a few days of the outbreak of war, we received Dr Erwin Popper from Prague and his wife, Yana, at this stage an archaeologist, who soon took over the functions of house-mother. Dr Popper contributed to clinical work and later became also the consulting psychiatrist to the Czech Army in exile. Westfield was their first 'home' in England.

How this devoted and very coherent 'rump' group of our staff carried on uninterruptedly the services of the Tavistock forms a remarkable record of the working of a democracy with high morale. Personally, I have little doubt that one of the major factors in this excellent readjustment to new conditions was the fact that J.R., now in his role of chief of the psychiatric service of the Army, decided to live in one of these bed-sitting rooms. This enabled him to give moral support and counsel to his team in such moments as he could spare from his very concentrated efforts for the Army, which progressively involved more and more of the Tavistock staff.

In his 1939 report our Chairman of Council noted that the Clinic was not included in the Emergency Medical Service of the Ministry of Health. This was not, strictly speaking, correct. In fact, Stanboroughs Hydro, a Seventh Day Adventist Nature Cure establishment on the outskirts of Watford, had been taken over by the E.M.S. as a war neurosis centre. H.C.M. became its medical director, with Mary Luff and myself as the other two psychiatric specialists. Here we were preparing to receive a large number of neurotic air-raid casualties, such as we had been led to expect from the literature. In point of fact, during the long period of so-called 'phoney war', when there was no hostile action worth mentioning against the British Isles, Stanboroughs as well as the other three centres, Mill Hill in north London, Belmont in Sutton, Surrey (staffed from the

Maudsley Hospital), and Maidstone, Kent, had very little to do in this way. We therefore began to receive at these centres ordinary neurotic patients. At one time in 1939 there were at Stanboroughs three such patients, with three doctors and some thirty-five nurses, as well as lots of other ancillary personnel. Even with this formidable medical cover, of our three patients one managed to escape from our hospital undetected! In fact, so little was there to show for the war that Mary Luff was soon released to become the acting Medical Director of the Tavistock Clinic in its Westfield premises on a part-time basis. Dr Grizel Thomson replaced her.

A remarkable fact must be recorded. Owing to the financial state of the Clinic, which suffered catastrophically as the result of the reduction in numbers of patients, and therefore of patient payments, as well as in donations and subscriptions, the majority of our lay technical staffs who had been salaried could no longer be paid. None the less, they volunteered to continue their work for the Clinic part-time without remuneration. It is true that one or two of them were married women not needing money, but others certainly suffered very considerable hardship as the result of this self-denying action. This was the Tavistock of 1939.

The medical staff decided on a very interesting co-operative experiment. Before the outbreak of war those who intended to move in, as well as some that did not but were not likely to be called up, agreed to pool the earnings of their private practices and, by saving in a common fund, safeguard as far as possible the interests of mobilized junior members of staff, including non-medicals, who might otherwise at the end of war be forced to desert psychological medicine for some quick money-earning alternative. The pool scheme had no direct connection with the Clinic; it was based on private patients being seen at Westfield, a wartime practice adopted also by other hospitals. This pool was another self-denying ordinance which limited the takings of those who joined it to about £30 a month, the surplus earned being pooled for the benefit of colleagues on service pay. One of our wits, G. R. Hargreaves, present at a meeting at which this scheme was voted on, and learning that several senior members with large incomes and family commitments had decided not to join this scheme, made one of his characteristic quips. He exclaimed: 'This is the first time I have ever heard of a ship being sunk by the rats leaving it.' The ship, however, did not sink. The pool was able not only to benefit some of the less well-off members, but also assume some considerable responsibility for the overhead expenses of the Clinic itself. I think this scheme worthy of record, since it speaks louder than words of what kind of morale we had in those critical days. I know of no similar medical effort, and it succeeded in large measure throughout the period of the war.

I must record some losses during this time. William McDougall, a good friend and a Vice-President of the Clinic, died in 1938. In 1939 we lost one of our original staff members, Dr W. A. Potts, the first Director of the Children's Department, and Mr Wilfred Trotter of the Medical Advisory Board. Dr Hamilton Pearson, for many years senior physician in the Children's Department, retired – but not into inactivity. As stated, he decided to join the Merchant Service as a medical officer, in which capacity he was soon to become one of the doctors on board the ships which took our evacuee children overseas, a characteristically gallant expression of his personality. He wasn't going to be caught in a backwater with a war on! Alan Maberly was appointed Director of the Children's Department in his stead. He stayed throughout the war, and later took up other work in child psychiatry, in which he made a considerable reputation until a chronic illness forced his premature retirement. Maberly died in 1969.

The geographical change to the uplands of Hampstead was perhaps more abrupt than the change in routine for many of the staff. There was time to adapt, as patients were few. Among those mobilized on the first day were J. R. Rees and both Assistant Directors, Mary Luff and myself; but quite a number of people continued with their normal stint of work. So smooth had been the transfer that, like the famous Windmill Theatre in Piccadilly, the Tavistock 'never closed' in the war. At the risk of being a little parochial, it is perhaps worth describing the scene and life at Westfield. For patients and visitors there was easy access by the bus routes of Finchley Road. There was a good bomb-proof basement, containing a communal dining-room, which, with another room, also served as common rooms, also kitchens and stores, plus rooms for our caretakers. Here presided Mrs Yana Popper as our chatelaine, who brought a welcome touch of Czech cuisine to the wartime rations and turned a camp into a cosy home from home. Her dry humour and Mr Harland's (ex First World War Guards!) old soldier's sang-froid were notable ingredients in the prescription for weathering Goering's Blitz on London. On the ground floor was a reception office, the Secretary's office, where Conrad Ormond and Dudley Herbert were installed, one or two typing rooms and some bed-sitting rooms which by day functioned as consulting-rooms, including the divan beds, which by night received the bodies of the doctors who sat behind them by day. J.R., though resident when in London with very good effect, did not officially function as the Medical Director. Some twenty senior staff members and a number of psychotherapists and clinical assistants had disappeared at once. They joined their war stations in the Emergency Medical Service or the armed forces all over the country for which they had been earmarked by the medical manpower authority.

H.C.M. did not come to Westfield to work or visit from Stanboroughs Hydro. Mary Luff and I, however, did some clinical work and attended committee meetings from that easily accessible location. During the phoney war I used my ample spare time to start a Child Guidance Clinic at Stanboroughs with the help of a young P.S.W., Miss E. M. Goldberg, for the mounting neurotic casualties among evacuated schoolchildren. This Clinic survives as part of the Hertfordshire Child Guidance services, of which the post-war Director until her recent retirement was one of our staff members, Dr R. Evelyn Lucas.

This is by way of showing how peaceful were the early phases of the war. The Stanboroughs Neurosis Centre up to the end of the big air raids had admitted only a total of forty-one 'war casualties'. It was closed soon after for lack of work. Many E.M.S. psychiatrists now joined the Army – for example, myself. Some of these also used the Westfield College Tavistock as a *pied à terre*. My first military assignment was that of Command Psychiatrist for the London District, and Westfield was a convenient place. Westfield was open for lodgings to any

Army psychiatrists, e.g. Ferguson Rodger, Stephen MacKeith and several more when posted to London, also lived there. There was thus a constant coming and going of the Army group, with a stable core population. One gave a hand with the odd consultation, the odd seminar or evening discussion.

During the first winter, the 'phoney war', we held our regular staff meetings as heretofore. It was remarkable how, without any design, our interest seemed to shift from reporting on individual morbid conditions or cases to considering the larger problems of war and of human relations, the nature of hostility, the state of civilization and similar things which were to be very much reflected in the philosophy, first, of the Army psychiatric service and later on in our post-war planning and policies. I remember giving an address for which I apologized, entitled the 'Anal Sadistic Basis of Our Culture'. However, it went down well, as it was this kind of thing which preoccupied the Tavistock staff in this era. The paper, I may add, became the theoretical basis for my later work on German prisoners-of-war which had not then been contemplated.

While the Tavistock was open daily in much the same way in its new premises as it always had been, there were not only fewer doctors working, but there was also at first a very sharp decline in the number of patients seen. Whereas in 1938 we saw 1,071 new patients, in 1939 up to 31 August we saw 750, and in the next four months, from September to December, we saw 243, making a total of 993. In the first week of the war, the number of treatment hours fell to its lowest level ever, registering just over 100, but mounted steadily to over 350 hours per week. A decision had therefore to be made that, with the diminishing number of doctors available, the standards for the selection of patients must be more rigid. The Tavistock as such had not been designated an emergency hospital. Hence its role was to serve the 'ordinary' non-war traumatic cases, although obviously the stresses of war both altered and intensified some clinical pictures. This was particularly true in the Children's Department, which was the only child guidance unit to remain open in London at the outbreak of war. At first it had to deal largely with difficult children returned as unmanageable from the reception areas almost before the war began, and with cases referred by the Courts. But in the absence of air raids during the first months of the war many parents brought their children back to London. The activities of the Department in consequence began to approximate to their pre-war character.

As in 1938 after the Munich Crisis, so at the beginning of the war the staff considered it their duty to give as much education in emergency psychiatry as possible. Three short courses of lectures on neuroses in wartime and the like were given for doctors and for other personnel manning first-aid posts. Nearly sixty doctors attended each of these courses. The regular post-graduate training was continued during 1939 and 1940, and of the twelve doctors enrolled seven completed the full two-year course. It had been necessary to abandon the course beginning in 1940 because of the dispersal of the would-be students on war assignments. There none the less remained a substantial medical audience for our systematic lectures in psychopathology. The staff contributed a good deal to lectures on neuroses at the Post-graduate Medical School and elsewhere until hostile action cut these short. As the University was evacuated, all our other University courses were cancelled. The research work by Wittkower and Wilson came to an abrupt end. Dr J. D. Spillane, our second Rockefeller Fellow, never started.

The difficulties of attendance in the blackout, etc., brought some losses among our older staff members; Dr Mary Ferguson and Dr Shirley Adams left us. The resignation of that indomitable sexagenarian, Dr Hamilton Pearson, has already been reported. How lucky for some of the dislocated children on those long voyages to have him as their medical officer! Dr W. J. T. Kimber, head of Hill End Hospital, St Albans, joined our Advisory Board, a good friend with whom we had long worked to mutual advantage. Valuable wartime accessions to the Council into some vacancies were Mr Christmas Humphreys, now a judge, and Mr (now Sir) Leslie Farrer, who was to give many years of distinguished service to the Tavistock Clinic and later to the Tavistock Institute of Human Relations.

It was on the Council and Finance Committee that from the beginning of the war, and deepening as it proceeded, there was pessimism. The site for our new Institute premises in Bloomsbury, instead of being an asset, had become a millstone round our necks. There was the large mortgage; the rents from it dwindled to zero as shops closed or were later destroyed by bombs. Subscriptions and donations, especially those earmarked for the Extension Fund, fell catastrophically, as can be imagined. All drives for fund-raising stopped. The public were in no mood to subscribe to an extravaganza like a psychotherapeutic clinic. Despite J.R.'s coup with the banks, the general situation was such that the honoraria which we had, as mentioned, at least paid to clinical psychologists and social workers had to be stopped. Notwithstanding their loyalty, economics told, and as the war proceeded we saw an attrition of our devoted staff, particularly among social workers and clinical psychologists, who had to find paid work elsewhere. Losses of staff were therefore not only due to the call-up, but also to the necessity for some to find paid work outside, and to the difficulties for others in getting about, with severe petrol-rationing, etc. The year 1940, for example, shows fewer than ever staff members in residence and active clinical work.

Paradoxically, we had some belated good fortune at a time when we could not use it effectively. Somewhat ironically, the recognition from London University for approved teachers in the Tavistock came through after a prolonged gestation. To relieve the financial gloom hanging over us, there arrived an unexpected legacy of £14,000 which abolished the overdraft and made our bank smile again. The changes in management and direction of the Clinic owing to repeated call-ups were also characteristic of this year and 1941. Conrad Ormond was drafted for National Service and Dudley Herbert, for so long a voluntary worker and Lecture Secretary, gallantly took on the Secretaryship of the Clinic. About him more further on. Mary Luff, released from the E.M.S. to be Acting Director, had to give up to take her children for safety to the United States. She was succeeded by A. T. M. Wilson, who in turn was soon called up to the R.A.M.C. He was followed by Jane Suttie, the widow of Ian, but she soon had to retire to Ireland for family reasons. Now Margherita Lilley was appointed 'Executive Medical Officer' without being accorded the rank of Acting Medical Director. The Council could meet but rarely, and delegated responsibilities to a small Emergency Committee for the period of the war, which managed to meet monthly. Our Chairman, Lord Allness, became Emergency Regional Commissioner for Scotland and had to depute the Chairmanship of the Council to Mr J. A. Thompson, a member of Council who during this period gave generously of his time and his business acumen to the Tavistock. This was the period of the first Blitz, very intensive and as yet unadapted-to air raids, and naturally patient attendances in the last quarter of 1940 fell to about one-third of what they had been in the first three; attendances fell from about 4,000–4,500 per quarter to just over 2,000. This, however, was also the period when some people revealed their quality. Our new Secretary, Dudley Herbert, seemingly the most diffident and retiring of men, not only magnificently organized the maintenance of the Clinic and its medical as well as social amenities for patients and staff, but was also the air-raid warden for the building, with wider Civil Defence responsibilities in the area. Fortunately, we had chosen a pretty safe location, and no bombs fell anywhere near Westfield College, but its roof, overlooking London, provided for those of us who lived there and spent the nights fire-watching a magnificent and macabre spectacle of the great fire raids on inner London. The staff pool of income-sharing continued. It included even several of those who for family or other reasons had to withdraw from participating in the work of the building itself. 'Daughter colonies' of a temporary kind developed. Thus Dr C. Boenheim ran a psychotherapeutic service in Reading General Hospital, laying the foundations of a future psychiatric out-patient department, and Dr Winifred Doherty established a similar service in the Maidenhead area. Allusion has already been made to the foundation of a Child Guidance Unit in Watford which became a permanent feature of that town's services.

1940 and 1941 were for those staff members now in the Army Psychiatric Service still years of incubation and shaping the ideas which were to emerge from it. None the less, we already see Eric Wittkower deserting psychosomatic research to explore the possibilities of personality studies for military personnel-selection at Edinburgh in conjunction with Scottish psychiatrists, who were to assume a more prominent part later on. We see Hargreaves and A. T. M. Wilson, already called up in the Army as command psychiatrists, while mastering the sociological and disciplinary structure and set-up of the armed forces (which served us in good stead), also digesting much social psychology, from Moreno to Kurt Lewin. J. R. Rees has described most of what went on in the Army Department of Psychiatry in his book,[1] so I here merely record some of the roles played by individual Tavistock staff members in the build-up of the Department of Army Psychiatry, in so far as this can be reconstructed largely from memory. Our earliest effort was the creation of a neurosis hospital, which was activated at Bishop's Lydeard, near Taunton, as the 41st General Hospital, commanded by a regular R.A.M.C. officer, but staffed by such men as J. A. Hadfield, Emmanuel Miller, Alan Maberly (soon to be released for duty at the Clinic), Geoffrey Thompson and several others, including Barrie-Murray, who stayed with that hospital as medical specialist over a long period. The history of that hospital, being part of the Army, will not be related, except to state that it was largely Tavistock-staffed and remained a psychodynamically oriented unit throughout, until its closure in Palestine after V.E. Day. I have already alluded to the preparatory work, notably of G. R. Hargreaves, who, in the Army setting, found his real *métier* and genius. Hargreaves, while waiting for his call-up, made himself a tremendous expert in all Army matters, from the history of regiments to King's Regulations, from staff structure to weapons training, and so on. With Wilson, he was to be one of the 'psychopathological snob' resources men behind J. R. Rees, which they did brilliantly. He first served as Command Psychiatrist under that distinguished man who later became the Adjutant-General of the British Army, General Sir Ronald Adam, a soldier-scholar, then G.O.C. at York. Hargreaves' personal liaison with Sir Ronald was a fortunate beginning for the collaboration between combatant officers and medical psychology in the experiments which the Army Psychiatric Department was destined to undertake under the Adjutant-Generals' Branch, which looks after all personnel matters, including recruitment, welfare and medical services. When Rees created the Directorate of Army

[1] *The Shaping of Psychiatry by War* (see Appendix III).

Psychiatry, known to all of us as A.M.D. 11, under Brigadier H. A. Sandiford (referred to in J.R.'s book), Hargreaves became Assistant Director of Army Psychiatry and launched the scheme for officer selection, and also selection and job analyses of other ranks' roles. He wisely foresaw that, for this, a separate department 'outside' psychiatry would be more useful. J.R. and Hargreaves persuaded Sir Ronald Adam to create the Directorate of Personnel Selection. Here there was concentrated a wealth of psychological talent from all over Britain. It also contained psychiatrists of psychodynamic outlook who could make something of personality studies and inject this viewpoint into the psychometric techniques of that Department. Their presence helped to give an aspect of therapeutic community to the residential Officer Selection Boards.

Many other creative schemes in the Army could be traced to Hargreaves's inspiration and backroom work, by which he was able to give J.R. the necessary intellectual ammunition and literature with which to implement the socio-psychiatric work which was destined to permeate British psychiatry after the war in a number of ways.

Hargreaves decided, after his experience of the fruitfulness and the broad interest of the new developments described by Rees in his book, that he would forsake 'straight' clinical psychiatry. He became an epidemiologist and social psychiatrist in his dreams and talk. After the war was over he was invited to become Chief Medical Officer of the Unilever Corporation, whence his friend and warm admirer, Dr Brock Chisholm (at one time Assistant Adjutant-General and later Director of Medical Services of the Canadian Army, and a psychiatrist) recruited Hargreaves as the first Chief of the Mental Health Section of the World Health Organization in Geneva. This was, as Hargreaves in his humorous and humble way said, one of the best post-graduate educations that could be had. At the end of Brock Chisholm's tenure of the Director-Generalship of W.H.O., Hargreaves decided he wanted to bring his family home and accepted the Nuffield Chair in psychiatry at Leeds, once again vacant when my first successor, Douglas MacCalman, had been taken seriously ill. In this post Hargreaves died prematurely soon after his wife, a much-loved colleague and human being, one of the brightest spirits that the Tavistock helped to shape, and one of the great contributors to the creative ideas in post-Second World War psychiatry in the world. Many of us will never cease mourning him.

In all the scheming, planning and contact-making for which I have just praised Hargreaves, he was ably seconded by his good friend, A. T. M. Wilson, our erstwhile Rockefeller Research Fellow. Wilson also was responsible for many creative schemes. Later in the war he joined Brigadier Frank Crewe, the eminent Edinburgh geneticist, in a special Army research department called the Directorate of Biological Research, whence issued such things as operational research groups and many slightly 'undercover' operations, contributing to military statistical and epidemiological research. The military effort for which Wilson should chiefly be credited was the development of the Civil Resettlement Scheme, the prototype of one aspect of the therapeutic community. Beginning in 1943 with the first return of prisoners-of-war under the 'men of confidence' and wounded provisions of the Geneva Convention, after a disastrous beginning at an R.A.M.C. depot and based on the experience of a pilot unit at Derby, he supervised this important rehabilitation work until his demobilization and return to the Tavistock. Eric Trist joined Wilson in the later stages of War Office planning and stayed in civil resettlement units until he too came to the Tavistock. Wilson, Trist and Adam Curle (a young anthropologist) later designed a follow-up study which was published under the latter two authors' names, and later republished in Theodore Newcomb's second volume of *Readings in Social Psychology*.

Wilson became one of the key figures in post-war developments at the Tavistock, until he too went to Unilever as Adviser to the Corporation in the Use of the Social Sciences. After ten years in his post, he is now Professor of Organizational Behaviour at the London Graduate School of Business Studies.

Leonard F. Browne, a staff member from the earliest years of the Tavistock, at well above military age, became the Command Psychiatrist for the Eastern Command. This Command contained a lot of 'young soldiers' battalions', special new intake units for difficult adolescents, to whose better handling and morale he made considerable contributions. After the war Leonard Browne became an Alderman in the London County Council and Chairman of its Special Education Committee, in which capacity he was responsible for the overall administration of London's child guidance and similar services, and subsequently became one of the Vice-Chairmen of the L.C.C. He had been associated with Crichton-Miller at Bowden House. Edward A. Bennet, M.C., after being Command Psychiatrist at Aldershot, was promoted to Brigadier and became the psychiatric consultant for India Command, in which capacity he established the many procedures which had been worked out for the home Army, with suitable adaptations for the Indian sub-continent. After the war Bennet became a teacher on the staff of the Maudsley Hospital, like our other colleague, Dr Emanuel Miller, who, after being at 41st General Hospital, worked in War Office selection boards. The latter provided one of the more fruitful outlets for a number of Tavistock-trained psychiatrists. Wittkower, who had helped to clarify the psychiatric role and techniques for officer selection, later switched to morale surveys, showing the connections between the incidence of V.D. and malaria, and their connection with depression and apathy in soldiers long abroad. W. R. Bion, D.S.O., a tank-commander of the First World War, was also seconded to the first experimental War Office Selection Board (or the Research and Development Centre), which, because it was quartered in a country house near Watford called Wall Hall, was referred to as 'Valhalla'. Bion not only contributed his first-hand knowledge of tank warfare, but also brought real authority to any discussions with reluctant combatant officers, to whom he could speak from experience. It was the impressiveness of this first group of Tavistock men which, I am sure, 'sold' the idea of the respectability of dynamic psychiatry to a number of unbelievers. This, however, would have been difficult without having some quite exceptional senior Regular officers on our side. Apart from Sir Ronald Adam, among such notable friends was Lieut.-General Sir Alexander Hood, Director of Army Medical Services. At somewhat less exalted level we encountered Colonel R. S. Rait-Kerr, Secretary of the M.C.C. in peacetime, another 'intellectual' soldier who became the

Colonel commanding the Research and Training Centre of the War Office Selection Boards; likewise Colonel Richard (Dick) Rendel, who under his deceptively military bearing, including a monocle, hid a close connection with 'the Bloomsbury Group', a delightful intellectual left-wing character who became a great promoter and friend of Army psychiatry and later on of other schemes, of which more anon.

It is impossible to name all the Tavistock staff members individually for their contributions. Some began as area psychiatrists, became command psychiatrists, moved to a military hospital and then into War Office selection and vice versa. There was a certain amount of rotation: some, as already mentioned, went to India, some to North Africa and later on with the Eighth Army to Italy, and so on. Among these was a relative newcomer and not yet full staff member, J. D. W. Pearce, later to become head of the Department of Psychological Medicine at St. Mary's Hospital. Jack Pearce for a time also commanded another experimental hospital set up when 41st General went overseas. This was Northfield, housed in one of the Birmingham mental hospitals, where Bion, amogh others, was to develop some of his work on groups which was to form the basis not only for the Tavistock's clinical policy in the post-war era, but also for the work with therapeutic communities and the handling of institutional group relations problems.

But it would be grossly unfair to attribute all that was interesting, new and creative in psychiatry to the unaided efforts of the Tavistock group. From the days of 'Valhalla' onwards there came into being what we have often privately called the 'invisible college'. This was the collection of men from many hitherto scattered walks in psychiatry and psychology who met and became firm friends under the unifying and cementing influence of J.R. and the common work. Among the senior research and development officers now recruited to what became known as the R.T.C. (Research and Training Centre) under Colonel Rait-Kerr's command was J. D. Sutherland, a man with a Ph.D. in psychology and a D.P.M., the product of the Edinburgh Psychology Department and Gartnavel Hospital, Glasgow, who functioned as senior research psychologist.

His subsequent contribution to the growth of the Tavistock will be taken up later. Another such was a young and energetic child psychiatrist and psychoanalyst by the name of John Bowlby, who showed by statistically validated methods that officer selection done our way reduced the failure rate from 45% to 15%. These follow-ups of psychiatric prediction experiments made not only a deep impression on the War Office, but also a contribution to methodology of psychodynamic research. Also recruited into R.T.C. from Mill Hill Neurosis Centre and ex St. Andrews University was a clinical and social psychologist, Eric L. Trist, another personality destined to become one of the pillars and innovators of the post-war Tavistock organization. Also among 'selectors' among military psychologists were Major Ben S. Morris, who was to become a post-war Tavistock builder, and a still younger man, Major (at first Sergeant) Herbert Phillipson, now the Chief Psychologist to the Tavistock Clinic. Another notable accretion to the strength of the Army Department and forming at that time very much part of the 'invisible college' was T. Ferguson Rodger, also a Gartnavel product, who became the second Assistant Director of Army Psychiatry for a time, having been Command Psychiatrist in Scotland, until he was promoted Brigadier and Consultant Adviser to the Allied Land Forces in South-East Asia (A.L.F.S.E.A.), in all of which posts his contribution was outstanding. Another such 'bright young man', the Deputy Superintendent of one of the Northumbrian mental hospitals, Major Thomas F. Main, was one of our number to gain his parachutists' wings. His field for a time was that of a roving expert in studies of morale, battle training, and especially in the selection and management of parachute troops, which were then being developed. One of his later contributions was to follow A. T. M. Wilson as senior medical officer to civil resettlement centres, where another future Tavistock consultant, John Kelnar, was one of the earliest men to practise group therapy. These were Army models of rehabilitation in a transitional therapeutic community, all based on the developing work by Bion and others on group dynamics.

Among many other such friendly and highly esteemed persons who one thought of as forming part of the 'invisible college' were Stephen MacKeith, afterwards head of Napsbury Hospital, then a consultant at Norwich, later head of Warlingham Park Hospital and now the moving spirit of the new school for psychiatry of Wessex Region, based on Knowle Hospital; also Neville Copeland of Warley Hospital and Bernard Gilsenan of Shenley Hospital, and many others who made great contributions and changes in the shape and content of psychiatric institutions and their curative work. Also shortly to belong to this group was Major John Rickman, the eminent psychoanalyst and at that time Editor of the *British Journal of Medical Psychology;* and Dr S. H. Foulkes, pioneer in group therapy and subsequently a teacher of psychotherapy at the Maudsley Hospital, who took part in the Northfield experiment.

Many women colleagues also donned uniform and played a considerable part in the medical and psychiatric services of the Forces. Mary Luff, on her return from the United States, became a Major and took part in Army selection work with the Women's Service. Dr Caroline Nicholson joined the Air Force medical service and Drs Kathleen Horton-Williams, Amy Thoms and Margherita Lilley were also Majors in the psychiatric service. We had our 'deviants': B. W. Crowhurst-Archer rejoined the Navy, in which he had already served in the First World War, as a Surgeon-Commander psychiatrist; and Dr R. F. T. Grace became a Wing-Commander and Clifford Allen a Squadron Leader in the Royal Air Force psychiatric services. Some of our other members remained in the Emergency Medical Service; others were in large armament factories (also at the time nationalized) as medical officers, and contributed to morale studies and maintenance in that important sector of the war effort. Among these were Grizel Thomson and Letitia Millard. Alfred Torrie, who joined the Army relatively late, being by no means young, was destined subsequently to follow Brigadier Sandiford as Director of Army Psychiatry in the immediate post-war era, after which he took on a number of consultant psychotherapy posts in which he still works.

In 1941 I was seconded for the extraordinary and highly secret duty of looking after that notable visitor to wartime Britain, Rudolf Hess, whence issued a book written under the editorship of J. R. Rees. As the result of this experience, a good contact was made with Military Intelligence, which took me off the developments which I have just sketched into a hush-hush realm in which it became my duty to study the social structure, morale and cohesion of the German *Wehrmacht* as reflected in interviews and statistical studies of prisoners-of-war and other methods available to Intelligence. From this beginning there developed some further studies in German psychology with Wing-Commander O. A. Oeser (now at Melbourne), which led us to create a selection centre in the British element of the Control Commission in Germany to pick 'non-Nazi' future leaders and administrators among Germans. Colonel Dick Rendel became the Commandant of this Centre at Bad Oeyenhausen. My small contribution to officer selection was the procurement of a captured German document on selection methods for the Nazi armoured forces, which was subsequently studied as a deterrent example by R.T.C.!

The Army psychiatric group became in fact an alembic in which, through the core of the Tavistock group and especially through the personality of J. R. Rees, a number of hitherto somewhat disparate types of specialists were at least temporarily welded into a harmonious team. The prospect seemed bright for a holistic broad approach in which the concepts and scientific tools and methodologies of social science and of depth psychology could be integrated in a future science of psychiatry and mental health.

So much, then, for a brief sketch of the contribution of the Tavistock to the wartime Army psychiatric service, with apologies for many omissions. We must now return to take up again the story of the vicissitudes of the much less glamorous but in some ways more heroic group of those who kept the Tavistock Clinic's identity in being and in good repute. I have already mentioned the effective and self-effacing leadership provided by our Secretary, Dudley Herbert. The community at Westfield continued throughout the war years to do its duty by the civilian population, and to do such teaching as was possible. We had some sad losses to record, most poignant of all the tragic death on R.A.F. service on 29 August 1942 of our Patron, His Royal Highness the Duke of Kent, who had given so much moral as well as actual support to our Institution. We were honoured and touched by the fact that his relict, the then Duchess of Kent (Princess Marina), in her bereavement very quickly assumed the Presidency of the Clinic in his stead, and that in the midst of war she paid us an informal visit and familiarized herself with the work that we were doing and with the theoretical positions underlying it, the first of many visits which she from time to time continued until her own death in 1968. More reference will be made to this gracious lady and to the part she played in more cheerful times. Another staunch friend, Sir Henry Brackenbury, died in 1942, having been until 1938 Chairman of our Council.

By 1942 we were already beginning, in such spare time as we had, to plan our post-war shape and policies, and most of all to worry where we should be. This was before the National Health Service had even been mooted and when we expected to return to the scarcity budgets and shoe-string finances of our pre-war and current existence. I have already alluded to the shift in interest within the Tavistock staff early in the war, when our seminars were apt to deal with social themes. In 1942 J.R., who usually wrote the annual reports, put on paper some reflections on future planning, the result of many informal staff discussions, which he headed 'Social Psychiatry'. In this report he refers to an article which he probably wrote himself and which appeared in the *British Medical Journal* around the turn of 1942–3, entitled 'Three Years of Military Psychiatry in the United Kingdom'. In the Tavistock report on future planning which largely duplicates this article, he lists personnel selection, surveys of the extent of psychiatric disorders, the role of area psychiatrists as some sort of 'medical officers for mental health', covering the country from a military point of view, and other similar matters. The trend of Tavistock thinking in terms of a broad mental health programme is clear: selection and aptitude for a job as a stress-reducing measure could beneficially be transferred from the Army to industry and civilian life in general. Concerning these proposals, J.R. said that there were many districts in which mental health services were lacking, that indeed for many years a policy of the Clinic had been to encourage a movement of post-graduate students to such areas on completion of training. An increase and co-ordination of provincial work would lead towards a more satisfactory psychiatric service for the country as a whole.

As regards survey he says:

> All surveys of the extent of psychiatric disorders in the general population have shown how widespread they are, their frequency being so great that any schemes for treatment appear inadequate. Prevention of future trouble is therefore the only rational method of dealing with the wide problem. The avoidance of occupational and environmental stresses cannot be looked upon as a perfect panacea, but it can undoubtedly do a great deal.

Speaking of our aspirations for post-war life, he concludes:

> Members of the Tavistock Clinic staff are active, and in some cases leaders, in these developments of psychiatry. There is no doubt that in the post-war future the Clinic will play its part in the further advances which will grow from the experience of these years of stress. The exact form which this work will take cannot yet be foreseen, but the possibilities are unlimited.

By 1943, when major air raids on Great Britain had virtually ceased, the number of applications for treatment from new patients was as high as it had ever been in peacetime, and it was a real anguish for the now minimal staff that survived being drafted to have to refuse so many. The new patient applications for 1943 totalled 1,164 (of which 570 were children), but the total of treatment hours was only 10,000, so that a very large number obviously had to be simply seen and counselled or given very sketchy psychotherapy, while many had to be refused altogether.

This may also be the place in which to pay tribute to our secretaries, some resident, some non-resident, at Westfield College, who carried on with astonishing cheerfulness and efficiency the administration and the case-reporting and contact work with the medical services throughout the war. First a few words about Miss Margaret Ingle, who had worked with us for many years, but who now resigned to take up an important administrative post in the Red Cross in that year. Miss Ingle was the Departmental Secretary of the Children's Department and for some years a popular and important member of the staff. As in the sisters of a teaching hospital, so it is in the secretaries of a place like the Tavistock that much of the mystique of a department resides. They are the 'continuity girls', who stay while professional staff come and go. It was Miss Ingle who stood in this way for the self-esteem and functional autonomy of the Children's Department of the Tavistock. Next I want to recall Miss Beulah Varney, who joined us after leaving school, and became later the first Administrative Secretary under Mr Gray in the new Institute of Human Relations, and finally, to our great pleasure, Mrs Eric Trist. Another great acquisition of the wartime period was our senior receptionist, who retired only a few years ago, Mrs Stanger, whose reassuring and serene personality, presiding over the reception desk, radiated an atmosphere of welcoming warmth and calm at the very first contact of patients with our somewhat frightening institution.

Here I also record the devoted long services of another member of the secretarial staff, Miss Violet Watts ('Wattie'), who had been with us since 1927 and was to stay with us for many years after the War. Wattie was the Secretary to the Adult Department and was indeed its super-ego. She kept the waiting list. No doctor dared neglect or forget any patient or any appointment or report, or any promise about any of these, or Wattie would ask the reason why. She was the patients' secret weapon, especially of those not yet seen, with a computer-like memory and a never-failing sympathy for the suffering. Wattie will be remembered with affection as a most typical representative of the Tavistock spirit since its earliest home. She began a tradition which her successors, Winifred Hunt, Bertl Roe and many others, have well kept.

The quality of secretaries and receptionists at all times has been an essential feature of the Tavistock. We have been most fortunate in the committed, mature and intelligent ladies (not all of whom I can name here) who have filled these posts, which, at any rate to the writer, seem as important as the roles of the technical staffs, whose work can easily be undone by wrong handling at the reception desk or in correspondence. In this volume I want to praise the vital part played by our reception staff and our secretarial colleagues in nourishing the particular climate and informal humanity of the Tavistock, which H.C.M. was so concerned to create and which his successors jeopardize at their peril.

By 1943 and 1944, when it was becoming apparent that Britain and her Allies would win the war, the annual reports reflect our forward-looking and somewhat anxiety-laden uncertainties about our future. 1944 saw a very considerable aggravation of air attacks on London with flying bombs. Many children were again evacuated and life in the capital, despite the apparent winning of the war, was at a low ebb. Whereas we had seen unprecedented numbers of new patients in 1943, now the figures fell greatly. Epidemiologically, this patient population contained a large proportion of demoralized housewives discouraged by the renewed bombing that seemed to belie the news from France; also some extremely disturbed and rudderless children; and, thirdly, the earliest referrals of neurotic ex-Servicemen by the Ministry of Pensions.

The staff resident at Westfield College was also at its lowest strength, although by no means disheartened. It may be interesting to summarize the relation between this group and those called up for military service. The two groups mingled to a very considerable extent throughout the war because of the 'caravanserai' nature of Westfield as a transit depot in which various members of the military group were always welcome, spent a night or three months, took part in the odd vacation case-taking and talked. We should remember that quite a few of the 'called-up' continued to draw bonuses through the private practice pool, which was only wound up after the end of hostilities in Europe. Dr Rosalind Vacher, subsequently Child Guidance Consultant for Hertfordshire, was by now the Acting Medical Director. In 1944 we again had eight students working for the academic Diploma in Psychology Course of London University; there were also between one and three medical Child Guidance Fellows in residence and working.

Our extension hopes suffered a final blow when the Council

of the Clinic decided to sell the Store Street site in order to remain in business at all. The sale fetched something like £71,000, which just about extinguished our indebtedness and in fact lost us a few hundred pounds on the deal. However, the finance officers could breathe again, while we had to think seriously where and what we were going to be when peace came and the staff now on war service returned to claim back their appointments and place of work.

Peace Plans and Anxieties

It was during this latter part of 1944 that the change, started through military service, in the relationships between official psychoanalysis and the Tavistock group was carried a long step further, with considerable repercussions on all our subsequent history. I had a private meeting with John Rickman and John Bowlby, both influential psychoanalysts, and all of us in the Army at the time, to discuss possible collaboration and the shape of things to come. Rickman and Bowlby felt that, with the likely prominence or policy-making roles of certain of our staff members, all of whom they now knew personally, there could be no difficulty in joining forces and possibly having psychoanalysts serve on the future staff of the Tavistock Clinic, in marked contrast to the hitherto prevailing official interdict against the Tavistock as a place where true psychoanalysts might not work. Rickman and Bowlby shared the common viewpoint of the 'invisible college' and saw in the Tavistock a ready-made centre for implementing the new dynamic social psychiatry.

While the day-to-day affairs of the wartime Tavistock at Westfield College were run by a small medical executive, from time to time the pre-war Medical Committee would also meet in order to deal with longer-term prospects. Unfortunately, the records of these meetings hardly exist, but around the end of 1944 it became clear that we would need to sit down and plan seriously for the future. It was already obvious that a very considerable change had occurred in orientation and basic value systems in relation to the work the Clinic had hitherto been doing. For example, the 1944 report states that 'in the post-war period the Clinic will need to expand very greatly in order to meet the increased demands on its services.' Apart from this 'nod' to our traditional role – training and treatment – there is the following:

> Lastly and perhaps of greatest importance, the developments in preventive work that have grown as a result of wartime experience must be carried on by the establishment of a department of social psychiatry in which the fundamental causes of psychoneurosis would be explored. These plans can only come to fruition if adequate finance is available. . . .

This kind of thinking originated not only from the Army work, but also from the epidemiological observation of the phenomena of what would nowadays be called 'alienation', the disruption of behaviour resulting from frequent changes of school and from broken homes on children, the difficulties making themselves apparent 'as evacuees return to homes into which many come almost as strangers. With the end of the war this aspect is likely to play a larger and larger role.' Another interesting observation was that the analysis of routine intelligence-test results confirmed that there was a very high proportion of children above the average among our patients. This contrasted markedly with figures given by other clinics, where the majority of cases referred directly from schools were often dull, if not defective. The case was made that among disturbed children the highly gifted ran in some ways greater risks of mental breakdown than those who were average or just below average. This was especially true of our cases referred by the juvenile courts, often with the label of backwardness and truancy. We ascertained that these children were suffering not from faulty intelligence, but from frequent changes of school, social disruption and lack of reference groups or 'belonging'. The backwardness, then, was a social effect on personal integration and not due to constitutional intellectual defects. This is quoted here not only as a sidelight on the trouble with I.Q.s, but also as an index of the kind of thinking which emerged as a new dimension in the consideration of individual cases, for our future as therapists and diagnosticians. It is this stress on the social-psychiatric dimension that becomes overt in the preamble to the 1945 report, which includes part of the post-war era. Here it says (and doubtless this was written by J. R. Rees himself): 'Until the end of the war the work of the Clinic continued on much the same lines as during the past few years. The end of hostilities, however, brought forward many problems to be faced, involving change and reorganization'.

A scheme was therefore devised for the election by the whole staff, whether in the services or working at the Clinic itself, of a new *Interim Medical Committee* of seven members which would eventually supersede the old Medical Committee, but was primarily to advise the Council of Management on future policy and staffing of the Clinic. This was a democratic decision taken quite early in 1945, before the end of the war. It will be part of the next chapter's purpose to describe the work and the ensuing policies of this Committee.

With the impending end to the war, however, the most urgent fact was that we had notice to quit, as Westfield College were coming back into their building in the autumn of 1945. An anxious search began for new premises. For a brief time conflict revolved round a final choice between two buildings, both large, cumbersome and old-fashioned, one in the Finchley Road near Westfield College, and the other, a derelict private nursing-home, at No 2 Beaumont Street, in the Harley Street area, which had been used as a wartime hostel for temporary civil servants and now stood empty. In the autumn of 1945 the Council decided in favour of the purchase of No 2 Beaumont Street, which thereby became the third home of the Tavistock Clinic.

A summary of the wartime activities of the Clinic staff divides itself conveniently into two sections. The first –

Staff at Westfield. Probably the core of the Tavistock staff who remained on the 'Home Front' and who enabled the Clinic to live through the war years had both the hardest and the most honourable time. At various times the various members were temporarily demobilized or released and went off again, but the following were those who worked at Westfield throughout nearly all of the war and until the date of the move to the new building:

Doctors

C. Boenheim
Grace Calver
Stella Churchill
H. de L. Crawford
Hilda de Peyer
Mary Ferguson
Karl Friedman
Alice Hutchinson
Desmond Irwin
Evelyn Lucas
Alan Maberly
Lois Munro
W. Nunan
Erwin Popper
Mary Hemingway-Rees (Mrs J. R. Rees)
H. C. Scott
Leopold Stein
Rosalind Vacher
Hilda Weber

Among the non-medical technical staff Miss Gwen Chesters, Mrs Phyllis Hamlyn, Miss Rowlands and Miss Constance Simmins all stayed devotedly with this group, despite salary cuts. Among the non-professional staff, Mr and Mrs Harland had followed the Clinic through its various moves and borne the brunt of the domestic and catering work under all the wartime difficulties. No tribute to this couple who had endeared themselves to generations of Tavistock staff can be too high. It was my sad duty to represent the staff at Mrs Harland's funeral shortly after the war.

The Services. The Royal Navy had two, the Army had thirty-one, the Royal Air Force three of our staff members. The ranks held in the Services by members of the Tavistock staff included two Brigadiers (J. R. Rees and E. A. Bennet), twelve Surgeon Commanders, Lieut.-Colonels or Wing-Commanders, and nineteen Majors or Squadron Leaders. In addition, the non-fighting services had from us four or five staff members, the Ministry of Supply (which means industrial health in the great arsenals) had two, and the Ministry of Pensions, dealing with veterans' and discharged soldiers' affairs, also had two. This, however, was not all, as several of our staff members at Westfield gave part-time service to the armed forces. Thus, as already mentioned, Dr Popper acted as part-time consultant to the Czechoslovak Armed Forces, being himself a Czech. Dr Leopold Stein worked as part-time consultant for speech disorders for the British Army. Miss Theodora Alcock became the Child Guidance Officer for Huntingdonshire at the beginning of the war and rendered great service to countless evacuee children.

The end of the war also saw a number of resignations, some already mentioned. Dr Mary Ferguson, Dr Shirley Adams, Dr Clifford Allen, Dr Eleanor Montgomery and Dr Joyce Stephen retired at this point. Some of our younger staff went to exciting rehabilitation jobs. Gwen Chesters and Grizel Thomson to U.N.R.R.A. J. C. Mackwood was appointed to the Prison Service as a psychotherapist at Wormwood Scrubs – a pioneering role at that time. J. A. Hadfield also left us – one of the 'early fathers' of Tavistock doctrine and training, Director of Studies since 1934, but associated with its teaching programmes since 1920. Dr Hadfield only died at the end of 1967, ripe in years, with several volumes of contributions to the theory and practice of psychotherapy to his credit.

Two of our most illustrious medical supporters, Lord Dawson of Penn and Sir Humphrey Rolleston, Bart., died in 1944. Both were past Presidents of the Royal College of Physicians and Personal Physicians to the Sovereign.

Mr J. A. Thompson, who had stepped into the breach for Lord Allness (who retired in 1945), had to cease from his acting Chairmanship of the Council. In his place we welcomed a new Chairman-designate who was to play a crucial role in the affairs of the Tavistock up to the present day. This was Mr Leslie Farrer, to whom we owe a special debt of gratitude for coming in to serve during difficult years and to preside over the changes which were about to be implemented.

While we could take pride in the contribution which the Tavistock made both at home and in the various services to the war effort, one reflected that, like many organizations and families, we had lost more than we had gained in pride and prestige. We had lost our building and our hope of extension, most of our records, most of our library; we had had to stop most of our training activities and research, which was beginning to pay off so handsomely both to the Fellows themselves and to our reputation as a serious scientific institution. We had a paltry sum with which to restart. We were once more a beggarly small outfit by no means in the main stream of British psychiatry and anxious to find a role in the post-war world. University status, nearly within our grasp, was again far away. What we did have, retained from the early days of Crichton-Miller, was a remarkable spirit of group cohesion and a broad consensus on the kind of aims which the Tavistock should pursue. We were still resolved to work in that part of the field which now could be subsumed under the name of 'interpersonal relations', on family and children, on neuroses and personality disorders. We would not attempt to 'catch up' with large psychiatric hospitals in the management of the total spectrum of psychosis and organic neuro-psychiatric disorders in which we were not expert. We had also gained the co-operation and respect of many general psychiatrists and social scientists, and the confidence of the younger, more scientifically-minded and progressive wing of the psychoanalytic movement, whom, together with the Jungians, we could now reckon as friends anxious to work with us in a more unified movement towards psychodynamic psychiatry and preventive mental health work in the community, including the family, industrial relations and even the political sphere.

VII

'Operation Phoenix'

The move to No 2 Beaumont Street, was carried out in August 1945. This building, though shabby, had a great deal more space than Malet Place, with increased scope for our activities. It was soon after this move and some well-deserved vacations that the Interim Medical Committee[1] began to meet. As the result of staff elections the Committee consisted of Wilfred Bion, Leonard Browne, myself, G. R. Hargreaves, Mary Luff, J. R. Rees and A. T. M. Wilson. Mr G. Dudley Herbert, Secretary to the Council, became the Secretary to this Committee. Its first meeting was held on 5 October 1945, when Bion was unanimously elected Chairman to hold office until December – a reflection of his very high standing among us at this time. We held weekly meetings. At this meeting we agreed to co-opt two hitherto non-Tavistock personalities: Lieut.-Colonel Eric Trist, clinical and social psychologist, and Lieut.-Colonel J. D. Sutherland, psychiatrist, graduate psychologist and soon to qualify as a psychoanalyst, who had both been members of the War Office Selection Board research staff. It was agreed to invite suggestions about the future of the Clinic from all members of the staff who had elected us, and that we should endeavour to communicate with our colleagues by frequent reports. Our proposals could then be offered for staff discussion before implementation. Contact with the Council was also made in this way when their authority was necessary on any point. We assumed powers to appoint *ad hoc* sub-committees for special purposes, but these were not to become permanent.

A typical Tavistock resolution read that the Committee should not work by majority decisions, but through the common

[1] This Committee will be referred to by the initials I.M.C. in the following pages.

consensus of the group. Before this meeting a quite elaborate memorandum had been drawn up by several of us which set out all the matters on which the I.M.C. was to reach recommendations for the future. Typical of the new focus formed during our war service was the considerable attention given to our internal structure. For example, there was the Committee's own procedure 'whilst engaged in planning', which was to be decided first. Secondly, there were the short-term and long-term perspectives. We were to consider how far the Committee was bound by what the Council (recruited, of course, mostly pre-war, and not a party to the conceptual revolution which many of us had undergone during the war) had themselves set down as objectives for the post-war Clinic. I have not been able to unearth this Council memorandum itself. From the extracts of annual reports and the like, it seems clear that the Council had planned to continue the Tavistock on pre-war lines, only more so. There were to be more staff members, beds were to be reopened, training intensified, the Research fellowships taken up again. The Council saw the Tavistock continuing to expand along the lines which had seemed to be so successful and had led to limited University recognition, to a constant flow of post-graduate students and other signs of a useful role.

By comparison with such old minutes as one recalls, the memoranda and minutes of the I.M.C. read like documents from a different world. Not only is there a very considerable awareness of an all-round socio-politico-psychological point of view in relation to our growth, but resources, public need and political tactics are all taken into consideration. We had become a more sophisticated group. Short-term routine activities were left to the normal Medical Committee, which was still in being and had several of us on it. The latter's decisions, we said, need merely be watched for consistency with the long-term plans of the I.M.C.

I reproduce below the skeleton outline of the memorandum drawn up to illustrate succinctly the scope and trend of thinking in the I.M.C. in 1945. From it can be seen that it was based on extensive consideration of the community's needs, and provided a sort of agenda for discussing the priorities therein which we were capable of responding to, and the ways of achieving these goals. I make no apology for including this document, especially the irrelevant parts of it, because it was our 'complete blueprint'. It embodies a trend which has since permeated a good deal of British psychiatry and the mental-health movement. This was to become obvious in the contents and transactions of the 1948 International Congress for Mental Health and other bodies concerned with these great issues of public weal in a non-political spirit.

From this memorandum can be seen also the very considerable pains to which we went to mould the internal structure of the new Tavistock to meet public needs and to achieve a balanced staffing, interpersonal relations of the staff, and especially the relationship between the medical and the non-medical technical scientific and administrative personnel to achieve a spirit of co-operation. Mental health and human relations, we hoped, would begin 'at home'. I now think that the preoccupation with the need for achieving this 'new model' of an institution differing very considerably from medical models of the past became too absorbing of our limited manpower.

INTERIM MEDICAL COMMITTEE OF THE TAVISTOCK CLINIC

Draft of Planning; Programme

I. *Committee's own Procedure whilst engaged in Planning*

1. Chairmanship
2. Co-option of other members, medical and lay.
3. Minutes and secretarial.
4. Times and places of meetings.
5. Sub-committees and delegation of functions.
6. Procedure and method of decision.
7. Reporting and contact with staff and Council.

Note: Committee will have to sit frequently to get through all that follows by 1 January.

II. *Short-term and Long-term Planning*

1. Consideration of how far the Committee is bound by the Council's Memo., 'The Postwar Tavistock Clinic'.[1]

[1] This document has not been traced. H.V.D.

2. Decision as to priorities for implementation –
   (*a*) on a politico-tactical basis,
   (*b*) in the light of public need,
   (*c*) in the light of the Clinic's resources,
   (*d*) in the light of the characteristics and achievements of the Clinic group.

Notes on 2, above

It appears to the writer that the considerations run somewhat as follows: The main priority in decisions must be on a long-term policy, i.e. the kind of activities and subjects which the Clinic will undertake and study.

On this will depend the sort of personnel they would wish to attract and appoint for various branches of work, and on this, in turn, the policy of selection to be adopted, of training and of administrative set-up.

Financial policy will also depend on all the above considerations.

Thus, despite the apparent paradox, it would seem that consideration and decisions as to major, long-term policy – i.e. what kind of place the Clinic should grow into in the years to come – must precede *ad hoc* short-term plans, which can be left to the Medical Committee still in being. The latter's decisions should be watched for consistency with the long-term plans of the Interim (Planning) Committee.

The sense in which short-term points of view must, nevertheless, also guide the I.M.C. is that of urgency – e.g. the launching of a piece of research, the appointment of certain key personnel before others, etc., where delay might involve the missing of opportunities. That is to say, though in the long-term view we shall visualize an 'ideal' scheme as if it were rounded-off, in practice we shall have to decide on and implement successive steps in policy in a certain order, according to the political omens, the needs of the social situation and the practicability of the steps in the light of finance.

Note on scheme below

The outline that follows is not necessarily in order of priority, but is a general outline of matters for consideration by the I.M.C. on which its agenda would be based.

III. *The Place of the Tavistock Clinic in British Medicine and Social Science*

A. *Below are some of the chief needs*

1. *The Integration of Social Science with 'Dynamic Psychology* –
   (*a*) at the level of interpersonal relations between workers,
   (*b*) at the conceptual level,
   (*c*) in methodology,
   (*d*) relations to other schools,

2. *Theoretical Psycho-pathology*
   (*a*) Bridging the gap between structural and functional concepts of disease processes.
   (*b*) Relationships between individual and social psychopathy.
   (*c*) Integration of psychopathological concepts and terminology.
   (*d*) The relations between guilt and shame in social psychology.
   (*e*) The nature and role of identification, introjection, etc., in the transmission of parental attitudes.

3. *Individual and Societal Health Studies*
   (*a*) The nature and control of aggressiveness.
   (*b*) The role of the taboo on tenderness and irrational processes.
   (*c*) The nature and control of acquisitiveness.
   (*d*) The study of projection mechanisms in interpersonal and intercultural relations.
   (*e*) The study of authoritarian and democratic groups and leadership.
   (*f*) The study of reality evasions.
   (*g*) The role and nature of social ideals.

4. *Training of Suitable Personnel for Sociatric Work*
   (*a*) Medical Psychologists.

(*b*) Sociologists (psychologists, anthropologists, economists, historians).
(*c*) Social workers (psychiatric, industrial, health visitors).
(*d*) Educationalists (general and special, e.g. play-therapists, testers).

5. *Education*
(*a*) General public enlightenment in mental hygiene and cognate subjects.
(*b*) Medical profession, jurists, criminologists, clergy, industrialists.
(*c*) Influence on legislative and governmental agencies.

6. *Psychotherapy of Individuals and Groups*
(*a*) Definition and involvement in methods in relation to indications.
(*b*) Relationship to social processes.
(*c*) Actual radical therapy of patients – selected or unselected.
(*d*) Desiderata for selections: Who needs treatment and why?

B. *Aims and Objectives*

The Clinic must decide the proportion of effort, personnel and outlay it should devote to the above needs of social science and psychological medicine, i.e. its definition of aims and field.

1. *The Provision of a Centre of Thought and Work*
(*a*) Degree of priority of this idea.
(*b*) Degree of 'selecticism' and toleration.
(*c*) Degree of admission of non-medical disciplines.
(*d*) Clinic, college or institute?
(*e*) Public relations, affiliations and orientations.
(*f*) Type of internal relations: homogeneity, hierarchy, anarchy.
(*g*) 'Pure science' or ethically inspired pioneering?

Note: This must of necessity be a very general decision, more of an aspiration, but is perhaps the most basic of all, since from a definition of aim, the open forum, the closely-knit fellowship, the focus of free and intimate discussion unafraid of unorthodoxy and speculation, etc., new lines of development and progress will follow.

2. *Research (i.e. Theory and Fundamental Concepts)*
   (*a*) Priority over other aspects and activities.
   (*b*) Sociatry versus 'medicine'.
   (*c*) Priorities within sociatry, in the light of the possible.
   (*d*) Priorities within medical psychology, within the limits of the possible.
   (*e*) Invasion of the field of structural disease?

3. *Training*
   (*a*) Priority over other activities.
   (*b*) Priorities as between types of personnel in medico-psychological and sociatric work.
   (*c*) Spirit and syllabus of training for various types of workers.
   (*d*) Competition, overlap and affiliations with other post-graduate training centres.

4. *Psychotherapy (in the Hitherto Usual Sense)*
   (*a*) Priority over other activities.
   (*b*) Numbers or quality?
   (*c*) Relation to teaching and research aims.
   (*d*) Consideration of selection.
   (*e*) Place of new group concepts.
   (*f*) Competition, overlap and connections, especially in relation to physical methods.
   (*g*) Children or adults: priorities?
   (*h*) The problem of pre-psychotic, psychotic and 'psychopath'.

5. *Social Investigation (i.e. Social Diagnostic Techniques, as distinct from Theory)*
   (*a*) Priority over other activities.
   (*b*) Priorities between various aspects (selection, field surveys, man-management problems).

(*c*) Practical jobs versus improvement in method. (Not very real conflict in this!)

(*d*) Competition, overlap and delimitation of Clinic's field.

6. *Education of the Public*

(*a*) Priority of this over other activities.

(*b*) Definitions of sections of public most usefully educated.

(*c*) Type of education: direct or indirect, technical or non-technical.

(*d*) Relationship to political bodies or movements.

(*e*) 'Objectivity' versus partisanship and alignment with ethical values?

Note on B, 1–6

The above are complementary or possibly conflicting *aims* which the I.M.C. might have in their minds. The next sections will be concerned with the *means* for their accomplishment. Those include the decisions on the type of staff to be selected and appointed, the internal professional and administrative structure, the provision of an in-patient service, the desirability and degree of priority for paid whole-time or part-time staff, with the consequent adjustment of financial policy, type of assistance and co-operation of the Council, etc.

Prior definitions and decisions under B will enable consistent and clear planning of the organization, to which the rest of the programme is devoted.

IV. *Means of achieving the Agreed Aims, thus meeting Public Needs*

A. *Internal Structure*

1. *Varieties of Function on the Clinic Staff*

(*a*) Outline of structure in terms of departments.

(*b*) Definition of 'job analysis' of types of person and experience required for above.

(*c*) Consideration of terms of employment for each (e.g. salaried, voluntary, etc.)

(*d*) Likely sources of personnel for each.

2. *The Status of the Clinic in View of Desirable Aims and Functions*
   (*a*) Voluntary hospital versus non-profit corporation ('Menninger'). Private wing. Pool.
   (*b*) Rate of transition from one to another, if any.
   (*c*) Financial and legal review of powers and resources.
   (*d*) Changes in Council arising therefrom: policy and personnel (for discussion only).

3. *Leadership in the Clinic*
   (*a*) Directorate or Committee 'rule'.
   (*b*) Methods of choosing both and their relations.
   (*c*) Powers and functions in outline.
   (*d*) Handling of personal problems of staff and disciplinary powers.
   (*e*) Relations with Council.

4. *Appointments for Key Posts*
   (*a*) Definition and role of heads of functional divisions.
   (*b*) Methods of selection and appointment.
   (*c*) Priority of appointments (e.g. Director of Studies).

5. *Composition of the Staff*
   (*a*) Medical.
   (*b*) Non-medical scientific.
   (*c*) Technical auxiliaries.
   (*d*) Administrative and clerical, in so far as it affects technical efficiency of the Clinic.
   (*e*) Methods of selection applicable to each.
   (*f*) Optimum size and balance.

Note on 5

While all the above raise difficult issues, the problem of choosing staffs in terms of the outline of structure and future role will raise the thorniest personal issues. It will mean the possible non-appointment of some existing members, and the thorough consideration of status anxieties, old loyalties and in-group versus out-group conflicts.

It also involves, together with 1 and 2, the possible abrogation of the Clinic's status as a 'purely medical' institution.

6. *Terms of Appointment of Staff at Various Levels* (Detail of 1(*c*), above).
   (*a*) Period of tenure, i.e. reappointment, revision, etc. Age limits.
   (*b*) Time given (whole-time, part-time).
   (*c*) Remuneration.
   (*d*) Consideration of various categories and the status, dignity and security needs of each.
   (*e*) Discipline, dismissal, etc.

7. *Integration of Staff*
   (*a*) Morale-building factors.
   (*b*) Common-room and interchange facilities: staff meetings.
   (*c*) Group versus individual kudos.
   (*d*) Team, 'firm' and individual in relation to functions.

8. *The Role and Fate of Present Goodwill Appointments*
   (*a*) Medical Advisory Board.
   (*b*) Vice-Presidents.

B. *Practical Implementations of Policy*

1. *Research Policy*
   (*a*) Accommodation and assistance.
   (*b*) Facilities of access.
   (*c*) Tactics and practical aspects of choosing research projects.
   (*d*) Direction, supervision and integration with other activities.
   (*e*) Funds.

2. *Specialist Training*
   (*a*) Outline of syllabus.
   (*b*) Consideration of panels of supervisors and training analysts.
   (*c*) Methods of selection of students.

(*d*) Methods of selection of teachers and analysts for them.
(*e*) Balance between tutorials, lectures and personal tuition.
(*f*) Integration of students in the Clinic group.
(*g*) Time and money factors.
(*h*) Co-ordination with other clinical activities.

3. *Non-specialist Medical Teaching*
(*a*) Types of courses (G.P.'s refreshers, M.O.H.'s, consultants, industrial J.O.'s, etc.).
(*b*) Criteria for selecting teachers.
(*c*) Precautions against improper representation of specialist training, etc.

4. *Non-medical Teaching*
Selection, syllabus and practical considerations in arrangements for –
(*a*) persons falling under III, A.4(b) to (d),
(*b*) persons under III, A.5 (b) (other than doctors).

5. *Clinical Policy*
(*a*) Selection of patients in practice.
(*b*) Consultation service.
(*c*) Waiting lists.
(*d*) Considerations of allotment of cases to doctors.
(*e*) Supervision, interference in treatment, transfers.
(*f*) Almoning and social work.
(*g*) Failures and chronics.
(*h*) The pros and cons of an in-patient service.

6. *Sociatric Service Policy*
(*a*) Social surveys.
(*b*) Vocational selection.
(*c*) Consultative services.
(*d*) Prolonged loans of Clinic staff.
(*e*) Extra-mural activities.

7. *Publications*
(*a*) Desirability.
(*b*) Nature and frequency.
(*c*) Production.

Note on IV, B

It is not intended to convey that the I.M.C. will work out all the above to the last detail, but begin to implement those steps which are essential and to formulate fairly definite directives for its own later stage of becoming the new Medical Committee.

C. *External Relations*

1. *Research Affiliations and Links*
   (*a*) at Home.
   (*b*) Abroad.
   (*c*) Methods of contact.
   (*d*) Finance-seeking.

2. *Training and Education: Relations with* –
   (*a*) other psychiatric post-graduate schools and courses (notably D.P.M. schools),
   (*b*) the problem of recognition,
   (*c*) diplomas and certificates,
   (*d*) post-graduate medical centres (non-psychiatric),
   (*e*) undergraduate medical schools,
   (*f*) academic bodies (non-medical),
   (*g*) voluntary organizations,
   (*h*) the Press.

3. *Clinical*
   (*a*) Hospital affiliations.
   (*b*) Government schemes.
   (*c*) Other clinics in London and provinces.

4. *Sociatry*
   (*a*) Industrial bodies.
   (*b*) Psychological services and institutions.
   (*c*) Voluntary organizations at home.
   (*d*) Governmental agencies at home.
   (*e*) International organizations.

5. *Interchange of Staffs and Students, Home and Abroad*
   (*a*) Own arrangements.
   (*b*) Sponsorship by other agencies.
   (*c*) Precautions.

6. *Publicity*
   (*a*) Vigilance measures in relation to Press.
   (*b*) Standards and sponsorship of publications by staff.
   (*c*) Appeals.
7. *Medical Ethics*

After perusal of this document, some of the recommendations and decisions which emerged from the intensive labours of the I.M.C. will become more meaningful. They were all made between the end of the summer and the New Year.

The staff had instructed the I.M.C. to lay its recommendations before them at the turn of the year 1945–6, when they were to be criticized and discussed. At this date the old, largely wartime, Medical Committee was to be superseded by the I.M.C., which would now become the 'substantive' Medical – or, as we were to call it – Professional Committee.

In November 1945 a modest official ceremony took place inaugurating the new building, with many guests and well-wishers from other medical and academic or learned institutions. The retiring Chairman of our Council, Lord Alness, Sir Ronald Adam, Adjutant-General to the Forces, and J. R. Rees spoke. At this ceremony we were able to announce that the Rockefeller Foundation had granted the Clinic the sum of £22,000, to be expended over three years, with effect from 1 February 1946. This money was given to develop 'work in social and preventive psychiatry'. A memorandum for the Rockefeller Foundation had been prepared by the I.M.C. (in fact, largely by A. T. M. Wilson) as a top priority, covering some of the points made above. The detail will appear as I report the decisions of the I.M.C. Already at this time the announcement was made that the Council had agreed that the new social and preventive psychiatric work would be carried out by a new division under the title of 'The Tavistock Institute of Human Relations', which would function within the matrix of the psychotherapeutic Clinic. Thus by the end of 1945 we had already gained an encouraging acceptance for our new ideas, promising well for the future. As always, the Americans saw more in our work and ideas than our own people.

The National Health Service Bill had only just been published at the end of that year. We were uncertain how we would be affected by its provisions. Whatever our place in such a projected National Health Service, confidence was expressed that the Clinic would continue to play an important part along its own lines in the wider spheres of mental-health work.

Meantime, however, the early meetings of the I.M.C. dealt with many requests from industrial firms for help with various mental health and industrial relations projects in which we were asked to supply technical advice or to suggest suitable staff psychiatrists for such enterprises. Such requests came mostly from industrialists demobilized from Army service, where they had met our work, such as officer-selection or morale studies, and had been impressed with the potentials for civilian applications. It was in part on the existence of such a demand and clientele that our good friend, Dr Alan Gregg, that great man who was Medical Director of the Rockefeller Foundation, recommended to his governing body to make us this most generous further grant, by which we were enabled to start our new activities. Dr Alan Gregg visited us in November 1945 and, after receiving the memorandum, was able to meet and discuss our plans and ideas with us personally. In parallel with the developments in the I.M.C.'s thinking, the Council underwent a decided change in composition, reflecting the aspirations or needs of the professional staff for a new supporting group. I think it important to record that the Council which sanctioned these far-reaching changes and welcomed them at the end of 1945 was composed as follows: The Right Hon. the Lord Alness, P.C., K.C. (Chairman), Mr W. Leslie Farrer, Mr Owen Hugh-Smith (Vice-Chairman), Lord Hollenden, J.P., Mr Walter F. Roch (Hon. Treasurers), General Sir Ronald Adam, Bart, G.C.B., D.S.O., O.B.E. (a new appointment), Dr Leonard F. Browne, J.P., Mrs Margaret Cole (wife and collaborator of the distinguished economist, G. D. H. Cole), Professor H. R. Hamley, M.A. (then Director of the Institute of Education, London University), Mr Douglas Hamlyn (Chartered Accountant), Mr W. J. Hinton (Banker), Mr J. L. Hodson (an eminent journalist), Mr R. A. Howden, Mr Christmas Humphreys (Senior Treasury Counsel, now a

Judge at the Old Bailey), Colonel R. S. Rait-Kerr, C.B.E., D.S.O., M.C., Mr Conrad Ormond (our former Secretary), Miss Leila Rendel (Director of the famous Caldecott Community for handicapped children), Mr R. Lloyd Roberts, C.B.E., Mr C. H. Scott (Chairman of the Finance and Executive Committee, a banker), Mr John F. Watson, J.P. (a Metropolitan Magistrate) and Lady Whyte. Earlier in the year Sir Dougal Malcolm, K.C.M.G., and Mr J. Albert Thompson, J.P., already mentioned in these pages, had retired.

I want to stress that it was within our Council's power, had it so decided, to veto some of the quite revolutionary and fairly ruthless-sounding recommendations of the I.M.C. We certainly made proposals unprecedented in any medical institution devoted in the narrower sense to the relief of immediate suffering and the treatment of the 'sick poor'. There is little doubt that J.R.'s infective enthusiasm and capacity for presenting these new ideas played a very large part in convincing the Council that these were both reasonable and creative changes. Doubtless they were also impressed, not only by the backing given to these policies during these early months by Dr Alan Gregg of the Rockefeller Foundation, but also that two anonymous British donors, one of them closely connected with the Council, demonstrated their support of the new developments with handsome donations of £1,500 and £2,000 respectively.

It was not to be expected that all members of the staff would be able to accept the proposals which were promulgated from time to time during 1945. Already during 1945 we began to see resignations from the senior staff, not only by weight of years. It is probably true, although this is my conjecture, that the kind of talk about social psychiatry which animated and perhaps dominated the scene seemed like a reversal and denial of the priority of the sick person and the rights of the individual as the prime consideration at the Tavistock. Our activities must have looked suspiciously like some kind of 'Politburo' riding roughshod over individual clinical points of view and methods of work. Nor can it be denied that there was a certain reality in such an image: the impatience on the part of the I.M.C. with the older sort of psychotherapists, who in some instances had come out of general practice, with their highly individual methods based on rather inadequate training and concepts. But this cannot be said of all the staff members who at this point became apprehensive about what would happen to 'the old Tavi' as they knew it. There was also the shadow of the coming State Medical Service, against which they wished to preserve their individual identities. We saw this in many doctors, unaccustomed to teamwork and highly individualistic as a profession. There was probably also some element of suspicion about our negotiations and much closer relation with the psychoanalysts. In the light of the former enmities between the Tavistock, with its 'eclectic' non-doctrinaire attitudes towards psychotherapeutic work, and official psychoanalysis, this might have seemed like a capitulation or a 'take-over'. Some substance was given to such apprehensions, however ill-founded, by my meeting with John Rickman and John Bowlby (as already reported in Chapter VI), and discussing possible closer peacetime links already forged in the Army between psychoanalysts and the Tavistock staff, as with many others from the mental-hospital services and University departments. John Rickman's role in mediating our rapprochement with official psychoanalysis was crucial. The closer link with psychoanalysis as the most serious and most rigorous method of study, training and treatment within the psychotherapeutic sphere could have appeared as a considerable threat to the older Crichton-Miller and Hadfield traditions among us. But it also functioned the other way. The more orthodox, old-fashioned Freudian group were also alarmed at the hobnobbing with the Army group, and regarded it as not far removed from a betrayal of their principles. As a gloss to this statement I record a meeting in 1968 at dinner with one of these now very senior psychoanalytic figures, when the following conversation took place. We were discussing the work of W. R. Bion. The analyst in question, when told that he had written a most important book on experiences in groups, exclaimed, 'Oh, but I always thought Bion was a nice man'. Bion, who started as a Hadfieldian many years ago, subsequently became a fully-qualified member and high office-holder in the Psychoanalytic Society and Institute. It obviously did not take much straying from the straight and narrow path of orthodoxy to become a bad object in some psychoanalytic minds. Playing with innovations like group therapy and other 'perversions' of Freud's technique was very dangerous 'deviationism'.

It should be stressed that in the I.M.C. the developments of the Tavistock organization were conceived very much as a whole. The applications of psychodynamic ideas to social techniques and industrial relations and surveys, etc., which were to be the role of the Institute of Human Relations, were seen as part of a unified conceptual scheme. This unified approach was clearly expressed in the memorandum we had written to the Rockefeller Foundation. The memorandum began by stating that certain workers from the fields of psychology and psychiatry in the British Army were proposing to employ their experience to meet certain urgent needs of their civil community. The group hoped to grow into a permanent organization, we said, from a base in a reorganized Tavistock Clinic, and realized that to achieve its aims it must eventually become self-supporting. I now quote:

> (*a*) The pressing military needs of 1939 to 1943, combined with the slowness of developments in ordinary medical work, produced for military psychiatrists and psychologists opportunities to tackle large-scale problems not previously regarded as falling within the scope of orthodox medicine or psychology. Experience of a variety of problems has led to the formulation of a confluent body of knowledge and experience which appears to be relevant to certain expressed civil needs.
>
> (*b*) Concurrently the senior staff of the Tavistock Clinic, who have played a part in these developments, have been faced with the need to recast their social role as the result of a number of factors. Among these are the development of a State Medical Service which will of necessity undertake psychotherapy, and the acceptance by the Ministry of Health of the Goodenough Report on medical education, which recommends that State-subsidized post-graduate training in psychiatry in England shall be confined to the Maudsley Hospital. In these circumstances the staff of the

Clinic recognized the necessity to reorganize its functions in order to cater for expressed needs unlikely to be adequately met by the State service. It is thought that these will centre round family affairs, problems of group relations and the provision of opportunities for advanced study and training in dynamic and social psychiatry.

The large positive part which military experience has played in the reorganization of the Tavistock Clinic has been commemorated by naming this process 'Operation Phoenix'.

(*c*) The Army psychiatrists and psychologists concerned with social problems form a functional group based on chosen working relationships and basic agreement on psychodynamic concepts. After full exploration, they have decided to identify themselves with those of their number who form the Interim Medical Committee of the Tavistock Clinic and further to associate themselves with the future work of the reorganized Clinic. To restate this position, after two co-options, the Interim Medical Committee of the Tavistock Clinic has now become the parent body of a larger group of former military psychologists and psychiatrists which it is now convenient to refer to as 'The Tavistock Group'.

In this preamble, therefore, the I.M.C. clearly pointed to a new source and affiliation of personnel by no means identical with the old Tavistock staff of pre-war days, the resignations among whom were the first symptom of this very considerable revolution affecting not only ideology or conceptual thinking, but also ideas on where the relevant personnel for these new operations was to be drawn from. Let us now look, in slightly greater detail, at what this memorandum had to say on the Tavistock Clinic in particular. I quote again:

The 'Operation Phoenix' at the Tavistock Clinic

The reorganization of the Tavistock Clinic which is now under way is so much the result of military experience that there is more than a mere joke in the military name, 'Operation Phoenix', given to it by the participants. By 1939 it had become obvious that in the post-war world the Tavistock Clinic could not hope directly to continue the role which it had endeavoured to fill since 1920 when it emerged from the

> experience of World War One. It must, if it were to survive, open up new fields of work and raise the professional standards of its work to a very high level.
>
> Between 1939 and 1944 this problem was discovered at intervals . . . the need for change and for action was strongly underlined by a realization that the forthcoming State Medical Service would at least claim to undertake psychotherapy; and such a State Service, necessarily conservative, would preclude a field for activities of a progressive nature not yet recognized within the scope of orthodox medicine.
>
> The present staff of the Clinic have joined in discussions with the Interim Medical Committee, whose intention it is to encourage members of staff to co-operate to the full not only in planning, but in working in the transitional phases of the new fields of group work with the much greater demands which they make. Army experience supports the view that by exposing the staff to group problems, those who are unsuited to work in these new fields will inevitably realize this for themselves and make plans accordingly, and thus reduce to a minimum formal exclusion from the new staff.

The memorandum now proceeds to tell us who were the 'Tavistock Group'. In addition to the now nine members of the I.M.C. resulting from the co-option of Dr J. D. Sutherland and Mr E. L. Trist as people whom we felt must at all costs not be allowed to be lost to us, there was a second group consisting of the following: Major Harold Bridger (psychologist), Major Martin Doyle (psychiatrist), Lieut.-Colonel T. F. Main (psychiatrist), Lieut.-Colonel B. S. Morris (psychologist), Lieut.-Colonel A. Torrie (psychiatrist), and Major E. Wittkower (psychiatrist). The two last-named were, of course, already staff members of the old Clinic. In various other places in this report there are mentioned other names in accordance with the kind of military experience in which these men had stood out. Among command psychiatrists we see the name of R. F. Barbour (of Bristol), J. D. W. Pearce, already at the Tavistock since before the war, and Brigadier T. F. Rodger. These names are brought together because the memorandum tried to outline the areas of work in which this common concept had been built up. First, there was the experience in area psychiatry, with its analysis of morale-building and its study of human relations. Secondly, there was the work of the Directorate of Army Psychiatry, which taught us how to promote general psychiatric and mental-health policy in relation to changing military needs, and how to deal with the inevitable resistances of the 'Establishment' in a situation of lack of psychiatrists experienced in these social roles. Thirdly, there was the group who developed officer-selection and personnel-selection in general. In this field there occur the additional names of John Bowlby and John Rickman. The latter had also been one of the first to test our group techniques in a wartime psychiatric hospital setting. Fourthly, there was mentioned an inter-Allied study group formed by myself in co-operation with Edward Shils, the Chicago sociologist attached to the O.S.S. of the U.S. Army in Britain, Drs J. M. Meerloo of the Royal Netherlands armed forces, and Erwin Popper, adviser to the Czech Army, Drs Kemball Young, Otto Klineberg and Theodore Newcomb of America, and Eugene Schreider from France. This group was particularly concerned with post-war international problems, such as displaced persons and the work of U.N.R.R.A. Fifthly, there was a group which had been concerned in the so-called 'Northfield Experiment' at the military psychiatric hospital near Birmingham, where, in addition to Bion, Rickman, Doyle, Bridger, Main and Torrie, we meet the name of S. H. Foulkes. The report says that this experiment was concerned with intra-group tensions and group therapy, and later with the developments, internal and external, of social relations, responsibilities and activities in a community devoted to the treatment of neuroses. (This is perhaps almost the first mention of community psychiatry, very much a baby of the Army group who now called themselves the 'Tavistock Group'.) Finally, there is mention of the most recent military group of psychiatrists and allied professions concerned in the development of civil resettlement units. Here are mentioned four new names: Miss Barbara Boyle (social worker), Colonel Ian Dawson (who was to play no further part in the post-war Tavistock developments), Miss Isobel Menzies (basically an economics graduate, but about to be trained as a psychoanalyst) and Mr Hugh Murray (psychologist, and now a senior staff member of the T.I.H.R.). I have previously mentioned the roles of Tommy Wilson, Tom Main and John Kelnar in this connection. The Tavistock as such was not in a position to develop these ideas.

Even while Main, Kelnar and Trist, with others, were still working to perfect these communities, the scheme for their continuation collapsed. The Ministry of Labour was to have taken over six of these civil resettlement units as industrial rehabilitation centres. In the event, institutions with beds – the Cassel Hospital and Belmont Neurosis Hospital under our friend Maxwell Jones – were the more natural locations for the development of these innovations, for which they rightly take much credit. Here the 'common origin' of this work is recorded for history – ultimately from Bion's theoretical contribution.

In this chapter I propose to concentrate on that part of the new Institute which carried on the clinical aspects of the Tavistock organization. It should be stressed that between 1946 and 1948 the whole of the new 'Phoenix' which arose from the old Tavistock Clinic was conceived as the Tavistock Institute of Human Relations, which had as its base, as well as its parent, the Tavistock Clinic. In a subsequent chapter Mr Sidney Gray will deal with the main steps in the developments of the Tavistock Institute of Human Relations as a separate organization designed to safeguard its persistence after the Health Service came into being. It is the older medical side of the Tavistock which is celebrating its golden jubilee! Its new brain-child was not born until about 1946. Its full history deserves a volume to itself in 1996.

I will now continue with some of the essential points made in that historic Rockefeller memorandum. It stressed that we regarded our kind of social science development as closely linked with our analytic and psychodynamic insights. Thus it argued that there was a present situation in civil life with regard to social psychiatry which corresponded to that which existed in the Army. Combatant and administrative officers were on the whole more ready to value psychiatric and psychological help than the medical authorities. This analogy was also likely to hold in the civilian sphere. The memorandum goes on:

> One further lesson learnt in the Army should be mentioned here. Military experience has led to a recognition of the principles which should govern the relationship between a technical group with diagnostic and therapeutic interests and, so to speak, a 'patient' group with internal tensions and internal problems. Experience suggests that an effective relationship between a group of social therapists and a social organization whose problems they are asked to tackle bears a stronger resemblance to those between patient and doctor than may at first be obvious. It is particularly necessary for the social therapists to help the 'sick' organization to formulate and evaluate the real nature of its 'symptoms' (i.e. the problems) and to be careful to assume and implement a therapeutic role from the start of their relationship. It is by now only too obvious that attempts to fulfil a purely diagnostic function (i.e. 'research') leads inevitably to bad relations between 'patient' and 'doctor' unless it is complemented by therapeutic measures.

This was a declaration of the well-known Tavistock doctrine, 'No research without therapy; and no therapy without research'. The first element in the proposition is of course partly ethical and partly technical, of the widest relevance in medicine. The latter was the aspiration that a research component should be 'built in' to all current work done, in order to refine knowledge and to feed the conceptual refinements back into the subsequent activities of the institution. In this way we hoped to avoid becoming at any level, clinical or socio-therapeutic, a routine body adding little to scientific development. The memorandum further records the Tavistock Group as agreeing that it should 'train for everything that it does'. This would involve post-graduate teaching in psychodynamic theory and psychotherapeutic practice, in group dynamics and group therapy, in clinical psychology, such as methods of assessing personality, and in social psychology, which was clearly meant to imply also the techniques of social casework.

Among the recommendations which had been made both to the Council and to the Rockefeller Foundation, the following seem particularly relevant to the developments in the 'new' Tavistock Clinic:

> (*a*) The Tavistock Clinic should in 1946 expand its activities so as to deal with patients over the whole income range. In this expansion the role of the 'family clinic' will be to undertake various individual and group projects . . . these projects and activities will arise naturally from the present work of the Clinic and will cover a wide field of advice on family problems. They will also include the supply of whole or part-time participant technical members of the staffs to a pattern of selected medical institutions, such as Infant Welfare Clinics, Obstetric Units, as well as to such organizations as a Nursery School and a Juvenile Employment Agency. This represents an evolution from the present work of the Clinic, with an altered emphasis in relation to individual casework and increased collaboration with paediatricians, obstetricians, local authorities and education authorities.

This development was stated to be urgent on the British social scene by reason of the widespread family-resettlement problems of the post-war phase, the changed and still changing status of women and mothers in Britain, anxieties over the birth-rate and population problems of the future, and the growing awareness of the significance of childhood in individual and social development and consequently an increased sense of parental responsibility.[1] Here follows the argument adopted in 1945:

> One of the ways in which psychiatrists, psychologists and sociologists can make a contribution in this field would be by an approach to 'sick' families and 'sick' communities, so as to throw light on present deficiencies and build up knowledge which would help to plan prevention of such sickness. Among the phases and sources of family anxiety for which there is at the moment no adequate provision either by way of prevention or treatment are the following: (i) problems of engagement and marriage; (ii) anxieties of the newly married in relation to home-making and the development of

[1] Spock had not yet published.

family mores; (iii) the difficulties in social integration of new families, particularly in suburbs or where there are moves from town to country, etc.; (iv) anxieties of the ante-natal period; (v) deficiencies in obstetric services from a psychological and social point of view; (vi) the inadequacies of present infant welfare methods and services; (vii) misconceptions about the nursery school, the need for group experience for the child; (viii) problems of 'school leavers'.

These problems, we argued, formed an integrate within the fields of work of medical and social psychologists. This part o the memorandum, which was longer than the excerpts here quoted, ends as follows:

> The suggestion of growing a family clinic of this kind in a specific community of suitable size and structure must inevitably be considered on sociological grounds, but for the immediate future its development outlined can be accomplished within the present set-up of the Tavistock Clinic [i.e. as part of the existing clinical services and available skills – H.V.D.].

The next clinical development which has its sociological and research repercussions is that of group dynamics and group therapy. Here the memorandum makes some of the following points (now summarized):

> Psychiatrists have long been concerned at the expense of psychotherapy; it is costly to both patient and doctor. They have also been aware that money matters often provided a centre of anxiety and conflict in the human mind. Recently it has occurred to them to question the psychiatric basis of a situation that was, on the surface at least, equally unwelcome to both parties. This, however, has not been the only foundation of recent developments of a group approach to therapy, though undoubtedly such an approach, if successful, would at one stroke simplify the economics of psychotherapy.
>
> A few psychiatrists, remembering that man is a political animal – that is to say, an animal whose fulfilment can only approach completeness in a group – and aware also that neurosis manifests itself as a phenomenon of personal

> relationships, have sought to treat neurosis as a group phenomenon rather than as a purely individual one.
>
> This has developed into a form of group therapy which is also an occupational therapy; but the occupation deemed to be therapeutic is the study by the group itself of the tensions within it.[1] So far it seems clear that in this procedure real problems of both individual and group are made manifest and the group shows signs, according to the capacity of the individuals composing it, of mastering an approach to the problems of human relationships which stands them in good stead in everyday life and sets them on the road to a progressive liquidation of their neurotic disabilities after they have left doctors' care.
>
> Such a development indicates that a creative, evolutionary process may soon be offered to the community as an alternative to apathy on the one hand or revolutionary discontent on the other. The individual for his part is offered the possibility of development rather than 'neurasthenia or psychoneurosis'.

The Tavistock Group was also impressed by the possibilities of the methodology I had used in my wartime 'ideology and personality' study of Nazis, differentiating them by a cluster of significant variables from non-Nazis. The Rockefeller memorandum made the following comments:

> The method opens up many new fields of enquiry into the relation of domestic and nursery culture to later political and economic behaviour on a large scale. It provides a possible link between intimate personality study and political attitudes and group dynamics. It ties up childhood patterns with later political and social projections, applicable to any group or institutionalized behaviour.

This aspect, however, did not in fact become a major concern of the Tavistock, because for obvious reasons of demand they

[1] This is a clear reference to the paper which was published by Bion and Rickman under the title, 'Intragroup Tensions in Therapy', *Lancet* ii, 27 November 1943, pp. 678–81.

became more interested in new insights into industrial developments and relations, more likely to attract money than my work on political psychology.[1] But the principle of the link between primary and infantile learning and socialization processes and later culture patterns and social attitudes formed part of our conceptual framework.

Lastly, in this memorandum the I.M.C. made very strong recommendations that funds should be allotted for the immediate appointment of certain full-time or part-time paid senior staff together with several junior workers, who would at once launch work on the major problems of the family and its therapy, vocational selection and guidance, both in industry and for school-leavers, and research and training for which the necessary time would not be found if these people had to earn their living in private practice as in the past. It is a reflection of the change in monetary values that the paragraph said 'it will be necessary to offer at least £1,500 a year, since these are all senior men with considerable family responsibilities'. The sum, even in 1945, represented less than the pay and allowances of a Lieut.-Colonel specialist in psychiatry, and much less than the salary attached to positions outside the Tavistock already offered to certain individuals among us or to their pre-war earnings in private practice. The proposals for junior staff on training fellowships were at the same level as the so-called post-war 'Class III' registrarships offered by the Ministry of Health to some categories of demobilized young doctors to complete their training, for which the Tavistock (not being recognized as a teaching hospital) was not eligible. We also stressed the need for considerable secretarial services, which at that time were not considered among the necessities of a psychiatric service – a lack from which we had suffered and had managed to remedy in the Army. It must again be emphasized that these recommendations were not made to supplant what had gone on hitherto in the Tavistock Clinic, but to supplement it. The normal clinical services to both children and adults suffering from neuroses, personality disorders, etc., were of

[1] I have only since 1965 had the opportunity to return to this field under the aegis of the Centre for Research in Collective Psychopathology, based on the University of Sussex.

course to continue on the old basis until we knew what the mental-health provisions of the National Health Service Bill would bring.

Around this period, I was deputed by the I.M.C. to call upon Sir Francis Fraser, still head of the Emergency Medical Service in the Ministry of Health, who was then planning the new post-graduate developments for the National Health Service. We wanted to confirm or disprove on Sir Francis's authority the rumours of there being only one projected post-graduate institute of psychiatry for Great Britain – namely, at the Maudsley Hospital. In a long interview with the man to whom I had been houseman and whom I knew well, who had been Chairman of our Medical Advisory Committee before the war, it was made abundantly clear that the Tavistock was much too small an outfit, had no beds and could not hope to be designated as a post-graduate institute with teaching status. 'We will let you do some G.P. refresher courses – that kind of thing' stands out in my memory. This at least cleared our own thinking in terms of the choices before us when the National Health Service came into being. We must so plan as to be able to be a completely independent institution, still offering clinical services as in the past, but at the same time also developing the new social psychological and related projects we saw as the next advance. The one thing we knew with little discussion was that we could not become an independent University teaching school, and that if we opted for teaching status, it would be refused. We could not have predicted that in post-war Britain each medical speciality would only be granted *one* post-graduate teaching institute.

Considerations and Changes of Structure and Staffing

While the Clinic had got going with its primary service to patients, and with organizing group therapy including Dr Stein's speech-therapy groups, and while a number of industrial projects were handled by our staff as then constituted, we felt it essential to clarify what our optimal long-term staff requirements in the new phase would be. We needed suitable people to carry out these 'non-clinical' projects. As mentioned, this went hand in hand with a review of the composition and functions of the Council. The emphasis for the latter was on a new image, on personalities drawn from industry and science, especially social science, from public health; in general, from among people who were known to support the new developments on the basis of their experience of them in the Army. Among those approached, not all accepted our invitations to serve.

An 'anti-Establishment' tendency was in the air. Thus, at one of the I.M.C. meetings, when it was reported that the old Council had hoped that the Finance Committee would soon be reconstituted, doubt was expressed whether our pre-war financiers and bankers were still the best people for our post-war Council. If they were of high enough level, they would most likely not have time to attend regularly or work on its sub-committees; and the conservatism of lesser 'safe men' might be too inhibiting to our new development. These were the 'sound thinkers' who had proposed to bankrupt us. There was also a feeling that the kind of Society figures that had been the Vice-Presidents and members of Council might no longer suitably represent the new image of the Tavistock. We wanted no Lady Bountifuls for the 'sick poor'.

By October we were debating the size and nature of future permanent senior staff. To facilitate these discussions, Mary Luff and I resigned from our posts as Assistant Directors. The large and very part-time unpaid staff which had carried the burden of the Tavistock's professional work before the war was not thought to be sufficiently committed or coherent to give continuity to the development of the new programme. Persistent suggestions came up for a nucleus of some eight highly qualified senior staff to work at the very least half-time, but preferably full-time. We were constantly labouring under the fear that the most essential members of the 'Tavistock Group' would drift away unless concrete proposals could be made to them very soon. We felt it to be of prime importance that the salaries paid should be sufficiently high to attract 'the right people'. We needed university level psychologists and social scientists. On the other hand, to pay for them we had to canvass the idea of taking fee-paying patients, and this would jeopardize the future of the Tavistock as a registered charity. In these circumstances, J.R. suggested that within the organization the Institute of Human Relations be created as a separate department, to remain in the closest association with the Clinic, but distinct in that it was able to earn income from private fees and from industrial and Government departments. These moneys would be ploughed back into a central fund to pay full-time salaries to professional core staff, and they in return would help with the training and research side of the Clinic's work. This, however, raised the difficulty about the relation of this full-time nucleus to voluntary staff – that is, to the people who worked on an unpaid part-time basis on the pre-war model. If they were treating the 'sick poor' on an honorary basis while making their living in private practice, they would obviously be in competition with the full-time paid staff, who, it was visualized, would also be doing some psychotherapy, group treatment or analysis as well as giving part of their time to the industrial and other projects in social psychology, etc. We were worried about a split between these two kinds of staff.

On the problem of a unified point of view, one of the questions in our 'skeleton memorandum' quoted earlier, we resolved that an arrangement should be made with the Institute of Psychoanalysis under which Clinic post-graduate students and junior staff would obtain their training analysis at that Institute while having some of their wider clinical experience at the Tavistock. It was reaffirmed that all post-graduate students in training at the Clinic should have training analysis as a base of insight from which to launch into group projects, either of an industrial or a therapeutic kind. The precise routine of the order of training or of procuring training analysts for our students was not settled so quickly. These arrangements were made in the face of the knowledge that the Tavistock would get no support from the University of London or from the Post-Graduate Federation now springing into life under Sir Francis Fraser. The salaried 'Class III' psychiatric registrarships were to be tenable on Government grants only at the Maudsley Hospital and at Guy's Hospital. Despite this prohibitive situation, we already had a list of twenty-four young ex-Army psychiatrists who had opted to have further training at the Tavistock Clinic. We thus had to consider exactly how they should be financed and taught, both sides knowing that their training would not be officially recognized. This training programme will be described later.

Among the problems of replacing old methods and men by new ones was that of our Children's Department. This, under Alan Maberly no less than through all our history, had always been a strongly 'separatist' or autonomous body, despite J.R.'s efforts to integrate the whole Clinic. By November 1945 the I.M.C. recorded its feeling that 'there was a total difference of outlook between the existing Children's Department and this Committee'. We had concluded that the orthodox type of child 'guidance' clinic, closer to 'education' than to medicine and psychiatry, was out of date. At this time there was no specialist in child psychiatry on the I.M.C.[1] As already mentioned, the notion of a much more inclusive family clinic with a multi-faceted approach to parents, children, adolescents, young mothers, etc., something of an integrated neighbourhood health centre, was our favourite image at this time. It was felt that even if the State were not to take over such a service the municipal authorities, closer to the grass roots, might accept and help pay for it. It was in this connection that the name of John Bowlby emerged as the right person to head such a 'new' family service. Besides being a qualified psychoanalyst, Bowlby had a degree in natural science and psychology, had trained at the Maudsley and the Child Guidance Training Centre, and had been on the staff of the latter before joining the Army. Those also considered included Dr Donald Winnicott and Dr Evelyn Lucas, herself one of the earliest Child Guidance Fellows training in the U.S.A., but working with us in the Adult Department. The situation was pointed up for us very much by the knowledge that the Rockefeller Foundation, before making us a grant, would need to be satisfied, not only by our policies (as described above), but also with the persons to carry them out. This meant a firm decision as to who should be the responsible leaders of the Tavistock's thinking and actions.

Among the other people we rated highly, and not yet on our

[1] John Bowlby advises me this was a misconception by people not expert in the field.

staff or on our Committee, were T. F. Main, T. Ferguson Rodger and Harold Bridger, the latter a non-medical colleague drawn from the War Office Selection Board (and now a senior member of the Tavistock Institute). Bowlby agreed and was recruited to start work in January 1946. But Colonel Main was soon to become the new Director of the Cassel Hospital. In that role he remains a good friend, close to our own concerns, developing excellent therapeutic community services, psycho-social nursing training and much else. Similarly, Brigadier Ferguson Rodger preferred to return to his native Scotland as Commissioner for Mental Health in the Scottish Health Office, which he left to become Professor of Psychiatry in the University of Glasgow, where he created one of the most progressive schools.

We were looking not only for medically qualified experts. Besides Bridger, we therefore invited Ben S. Morris (now Professor and Director of the Institute of Education at Bristol) and Herbert Phillipson, educational psychologists who had shown their qualities in Army selection. We also formalized the adherence of J. D. Sutherland and of Eric Trist, from clinical and social psychology, who had been co-opted to our Committee and were from the beginning in all but name integral members of the planning group, and 'musts' for our new staff.

These changes were from time to time reported to meetings of the whole professional staff, usually assembled at two levels of seniority, consultants at one meeting and people junior to consultants at another meeting. In the main the plans were pretty cordially endorsed, even though they carried an only too real threat to the status and even appointments of a number of people. The staff appreciated the need for a much more compact staff structure and for a nucleus of persons mainly and predominantly identified with the Clinic in research, teaching and clinical or social practice, as against the old pattern of 'visiting consultants' 'dropping in' for a few hours a week in order to see a few patients and attending the occasional staff meeting, but not identified with the Tavistock as their economic and working base, even though loyal to its ideals. The experience of working in the Army or Emergency Medical Service had made the majority of us no longer favour this loose, part-time system. We wanted a fresh start. We therefore obtained sanction from the staff to advise the Council to terminate literally *all* professional staff appointments of the old Tavistock Clinic in July 1946, when the Council would be asked to appoint a new staff. Among them we would expect to see a number of former staff, but no one person could take the appointment to the staff of the new Clinic and Institute for granted. Lest this should appear even more of a 'purge' than it indeed was, I should add that the principle of annual re-appointment of all medical staff had always existed in the Tavistock. Recommendations for the new staff were now drawn up by the Committee. The question of full-time salaries was also considered, putting the more experienced psychologists on the same level as psychiatrists at not less than £1,500 a year, but the final decision was left to Council. It was felt that Colonel Sutherland, Colonel Wilson, Dr Bion, Dr Mary Luff and myself were among the psychiatrists essential to retain, together with the newly nominated Dr Bowlby. Hargreaves, we knew, had his own plans – to our great regret.

The whole staff group showed excellent objectivity, more concerned with the substance of our proposals than with their personal fate. Critical concern was expressed over the viability of the new integrate. A typical rejoinder by J.R. stands out: 'If the Clinic got a sufficiently live group working they would eventually infect these other bodies'. Others canvassed the advantages and disadvantages of our not having beds, a very important consideration for the status of the Clinic as a 'proper' hospital. Hargreaves, among the iconoclasts of the Committee, considered the lack of beds no handicap, but suggested that a settlement on 'psychiatric Papworth' lines would be more valuable. There was no lack of Utopian proposals. The bed-promoters, however, were not easily discouraged. In the event, we know that the possession of a large number of beds is still the surest passport to high psychiatric status, even in 1970! Several members regretted the scrapping of facilities for short-term in-patient therapy of serious crises as envisaged in our pre-war development plans.

What emerges from the minutes of the I.M.C. is the close and mutually trustful working relationship of this group and its electorate. The wartime spirit of *camaraderie* persisted. For example, we undertook to put any casual earnings, such as lectures or broadcasts, into a common fund. We also established the custom for publications issuing from the Tavistock to be first submitted to the staff group. Again, a minute for 17 December records that I asked the Committee's views on the propriety of pursuing appointment to the newly advertised Chair of Psychiatry at Leeds, and that the Committee approved! Similar entries occur in later minutes about other people taking part-time jobs or doing other things outside, as to whether this or that would advance our group's new purposes. A sidelight on our feelings at this time is also thrown by our discussion whether future applicants for posts on the senior staff should or should not possess higher medical qualifications, such as the M.D. or M.R.C.P., as recommended by the Council. Our conclusion was that these qualifications were not in themselves a test of adequacy to carry the new kind of socio-psychological expertise and had little relevance to proficiency in our sense.

In January 1946 the I.M.C. became the new Medical Committee of the Tavistock Clinic. Among its first decisions was to call itself the Professional Committee and to rule that senior non-medical technical staff should be represented there on a basis of equality with the medicals. This demonstrated a real desire to abolish the to us unpleasant distinction in status between medical and so-called 'ancillary' disciplines. The Professional Committee did not appoint a permanent Chairman, but decided that its members take the chair in rotation. Among its first acts was to establish an Education Sub-committee and also a small technical executive to co-ordinate all the work done, composed of representatives of both the sociological and the psychotherapeutic wings. Discussion arose about whether we needed another medical executive officer to the Clinic whilst we still retained a Medical Director. The decision was that the Medical Director should in fact be the Chairman of the Professional Committee and its executive officer. J. R. Rees was elected by the Committee to this role. When this problem had been settled, and with J.R. installed as representing the continuity of the old and the new, we felt we had the authority to tackle the final selection of those whom we should retain and those whom we felt to be not readily assimilable to the new, more intensive and primary service to the new institution. Those whose reappointment we did not recommend after July 1946 were to be informed before we submitted the names to Council, so as to give them the opportunity of resigning first. This must have seemed a very harsh measure, and in some instances, indeed, it was. There was good personal contact with staff members, and the Professional Committee knew pretty well what the views of most colleagues on the old staff were. There was, for example, disapproval of group therapy; there was difficulty in understanding that a community view of psychiatric disorders did not imply disrespect for the sanctity of the individual therapeutic relationship; or that the skills of analysts might be used, for example, in industrial or other group settings. It seemed that these lines of demarcation between the 'ins' and 'outs' for the staff were fairly clear. About the same time there appeared another line of cleavage between those who wished and those who did not wish to enter the National Health Service. This made the task of selection easier, since the first set of 'conservative' attitudes was often associated with the second attitude – namely, not to become 'civil servants'.

It was the same spirit that moved the new Professional Committee to recommend to the Council the latter's own revision of its membership, so that we might be able to count on support for our new psychosocial policies from these representatives of the community. We ruled that members of the Clinic staff as such should be ineligible for Council membership, in view of a possible clash of roles; also that the Council should form a small sub-committee to dovetail with the new four-man technical executive of the staff.

Rumours of the revolutionary goings-on in the Tavistock were now reaching other interested bodies. We exchanged views with the then Sub-Dean of the Maudsley Hospital, Dr Aldwyn Stokes, on the subject of joint part-time training for interested registrars at the Maudsley Hospital. These friendly talks led nowhere. We also had to reassure the National Institute of Industrial Psychology that our work was not to be primarily in the field of vocational competence, but in the field of social hygiene and human relations. Our image as a powerful new force seemed considerable. We may be criticized for not using our high standing for external leadership, because in the main this period developed into one of rather intensive internal 'parochial' restructuring. We visualized the Tavistock's new structure as itself a social experiment, which, if successful, would soon be copied (shades of H.C.M.!). Lip-service was paid to our need to co-operate in the activities of wider professional groups, such as the British Psychological Society and the Royal Medico-Psychological Association, but in fact we were intensively preoccupied over a number of years with developing our own skills and our own institutional structure and did not play our full parts in these bodies. Well-wishing critics often expressed the view that by this 'withdrawal' (not, of course, complete) the Tavistock lost some of the opportunities for widely influencing psychiatric development just after the war. It is probably right to attribute this introversion to the fact that many of the leading personalities were completing analytic training, particularly the new professional ex-Army group. An exception to this was not unexpectedly our relationship with the Institute of Psycho-Analysis, which was becoming very close. This was not only due to the just-mentioned post-war psychoanalytic training of many staff members, but also to the wartime co-operation with senior psychoanalysts of the calibre of John Rickman and S. H. Foulkes. It resulted in a very considerable revision of the original reserve, if not hostility, of the psychoanalysts towards the Tavistock.

We continued, as a Professional Committee, to keep in close touch with the ongoing activities of our not yet demobilized staff – for example, in the civil resettlement units and other aspects of the Army's rehabilitative and therapeutic work, which continued in the post-war period. These were, after all, *our* creations of socio-psychological service to disturbed and displaced men and women. There was considerable public interest in these experiments, now known to be associated with the Tavistock. We hoped this might lead to considerable donations and at the least to valuable liaisons. Whilst the interest was great, the donations on any large scale were not forthcoming. It was once again a bad period in which to tap private British resources for endowing so unorthodox and unusual an institution as the Tavistock had always been and had now become to an even greater extent.

The position was different with local authorities, who were favourably inclined to pay for specialists' work of the Tavistock Clinic's Children's Department. This seemed to promise that at least the children's work was going to be in a fairly good position to meet its outgoings. The Middlesex County was our best supporter at this time.

Getting Ready for the National Health Service

In April 1946 J.R., in company with Mary Luff and our Secretary, Dudley Herbert, had an interview with the two senior Commissioners of the Board of Control (now incorporated in the Mental Health Division of the Ministry of Health) on the likely role of the Tavistock in the National Health Service plans. One of the Commissioners was the late Hon. Dr W. S. Maclay – an ex 'Tavistock man'. The impression then gained was that the Clinic would definitely be taken over and allowed to go on doing what it had always done. It had also been suggested that it might be wise for the Institute of Human Relations wing of our post-war activities to become a separately incorporated body, as already envisaged by J.R. Equally, the Rockefeller Foundation intimated that they could not give money to a Government agency of a foreign country. This hint was acted upon seriously and quickly, and the Council was informed that the Professional Committee considered it necessary to take the required legal action for a formal separation between the two aspects of the Clinic. The older part – clearly related to medicine – would enter the N.H.S., whereas the other, unlikely to be perceived as obviously so related, should stay outside and develop with the help of Rockefeller funds. The result of these changes in the autonomous growth of the Tavistock Institute of Human Relations will be described by Mr Sidney Gray in ch. ix. Thereafter I shall continue mainly with the history of that part of the total institution which was taken into the Health Service under the old name, although some of its major activities were closely linked to the new Institute, as will appear.

The Professional Committee now gave serious consideration to the National Health Service Bill, and how best to shape its provisions for the optimal mental-health benefit to the nation. Our group was requested by the then Labour Government, and by some private Members of Parliament, to prepare a memorandum examining the mental-health provisions of the Bill from a scientific and sociological point of view. Eric Trist was entrusted with the report.

We now had the reassuring feeling that we could see where we were going, and the roles we might be playing. The task of sharing our varied experiences for our mutual education was initiated by weekly staff meetings. We also laid the foundations for the publication of a quarterly 'house' journal, which came into being in the following year under the title of *Human Relations*. From the outset it was a joint enterprise of 'both sides', as well as with the new U.S. Centre for Group Dynamics. Clinic and Institute were, it was hoped, to remain intertwined, partly by overlapping staff appointments, partly by the typically British solution of association between a private organization and a statutory body. (The same symbiosis was developed at the inception of the N.H.S. by the Institute for the Study and Treatment of Delinquency and its clinical aspect – the Portman Clinic – with continuing co-operation between the mother and daughter institutions.) The link was implemented, as will be seen in subsequent chapters, by the formal establishment of an 'Association' with its own structure and with certain executive organs by which the Health Service moiety and the non-Health Service part of our group continued to share a common allegiance as well as a body of concepts and methods, and differentiate out between themselves clinical services, training and research functions.

What remained still in some doubt was whether and in what capacity the Clinic should enter the National Health Service. We knew we had the option to enter. It was our determination to secure conditions under which we could pursue our sort of psychiatry. We knew that official post-graduate teaching was to be concentrated at the Maudsley Hospital under its new Professor, Dr Aubrey Lewis, Mapother's former right-hand man, who was not expected to share many of our views and priorities on the future of psychiatry. Decisions for our future were entrusted to an extensive meeting of all those now working at the Clinic.

These discussions continued within the Professional Committee and the staff as a whole over some months. In 1947 there were some who even questioned whether the Tavistock should go on being a therapeutic institution at all, so great was the deflection of our interest in the direction of the new social psychiatry and social research, and so promising were the many demands and contacts coming to us from industrial and other reconnaissances of all kinds. Our advise and expertise were sought on various personnel-selection schemes and various mental health institutions; there were contacts with the international wing of the New Education Fellowship, which contained some of the germs of the future U.N.E.S.C.O.; there was the International Committee of the Society for the Psychological Study of Social Issues, with its journal; there were many demands for writing, for broadcasting, for advice on making mental-health and similar films, and all the rest of it. Despite all this, there was never any doubt about our decision that we should continue to be a psychotherapeutic institution and should enter the N.H.S.

The next problem was in what form we should enter the National Health Service. Despite the discouraging news from the Post-graduate Medical Federation, we did not surrender our intentions of becoming an independent post-graduate training school in those elements of psychological medicine and medical sociology which we practised and in which we were experts. Indeed, we received a good deal of encouragement from the impact of Eric Trist's document prepared for the Ministry of Health, for which J. R. Rees took responsibility. This paper made Sir Ralph Glynn, M.P., Chairman of the Committee on Estimates of the House of Commons, ask for more detailed advice on mental-health needs and provisions under the coming National Health Service. Several Members of Parliament, as already mentioned, expressed interest and promised to promote our cause as a 'teaching hospital', but they had to be warned that the Minister's advisers were certain to be against any such course of development for us. In view of our

1946 policy memorandum on aims, we ourselves did not feel unhappy about the second path of development, that of an 'ordinary' regional clinic in the Health Service, serving, as we hoped, our own sector of the community in all aspects of mental health, co-operating closely with the local health authority in such fields as maternal and infant welfare, schoolchildren, young families resettling, war veterans and the like. In the event, as will appear, this was to be one of our roles, except that the really integrated community mental health service for the given area has yet to be carried into effect. We devised a model for 'community mental health' in 1946! It was not the fault of the Tavistock that so little came of it at the time, but of the separation between the hospital, the local authority and general practitioner services which had been written into the new National Health Service Act. The effect of this trichotomy was most severe in the Metropolis.

The topic was left open for the best part of another year, and perhaps wisely so, because we had time to enter into various regional negotiations and establish operational links with some of our sister institutions. It will be remembered that before the war Dr Kimber of Hill End Hospital had had a fruitful two-way training arrangement with the Tavistock. We now invited him to convene a meeting of the major psychiatric units located within our likely future area (which, in fact, turned out to be the North-west Metropolitan Regional Hospital Board area), to explore whether we could not devise a common training school and generally pool our resources for the improvement of psychiatric education and services. This collaborative effort resulted in the future North-west Metropolitan Region having virtually a psychiatric advisory committee before the National Health Service came into being, and at all events a very fraternally functioning group consisting of consultants at the great mental hospitals around St Albans, with such good friends as Drs O. W. Fitzgerald, Stephen McKeith, J. H. Patterson, Alexander Shapiro, and D. H. Thomas as well as Dr Kimber. We had debated whether to include the Psychoanalytic Clinic, and decided to leave them out, as they would certainly not come under the National Health Service. All this is stated here to show that at this time we did exercise very considerable initiative and influence upon the shaping of the mental health services, partly through J.R.'s influence at top level, partly through our work for the regional organization, and also in conceptual model-building through our prestige and achievements as a wartime Army group. Thus the first meeting after the war of the regional South-eastern division of the Royal Medico-Psychological Association was held in the Tavistock, and was addressed by Tavistock members on their new formulations of social psychiatric problems. Our staff were greatly in demand for lectures and seminars of this kind, both in the learned societies and at local professional levels. Psychiatrists and others were extremely interested in what we had been doing, and we did something to satisfy the many demands, both in London and the provinces, carrying on the pre-war Tavistock tradition in this respect.

By the second half of 1946 the staff changes, the comings and goings, new appointments and resignations were still going on as those we wanted and were demobilized joined us, and those who were either unwilling to join in the new development of the Institute of Human Relations within the Tavistock Clinic or were reaching superannuation were leaving. In addition, there were some resignations to take up new posts. In a sense, the most important of these was my own departure to become the first Nuffield Professor of Psychiatry at the University of Leeds in October 1946. Several of our most senior colleagues were made honorary consulting physicians: E. A. Bennet, J. A. Hadfield, E. A. Hamilton Pearson, Alice Hutchison, Emmanuel Miller and Maurice Wright. J. R. Rees remained Director and Chairman of the Professional Committee. The latter now reflected the new integrated disciplines and contained at the end of 1946, in addition to its Chairman, J.R., John Bowlby, Leonard Browne, myself (co-opted), G. R. Hargreaves (himself shortly to leave the active staff of the Tavistock and join the Unilever organization as its Chief Medical Officer), Ben S. Morris, J. D. Sutherland, E. L. Trist and A. T. M. Wilson. These were the new core staff of nearly full-time men who carried most of the policy decisions. Mary Luff did not seek re-election. On the adult side the part-time honorary medical staff at senior level were Leonard Browne, Evelyn Lucas, Mary

Luff (who had to resign from her near full-time post because of domestic responsibilities), J. D. W. Pearce, Geoffrey Thompson, Amy S. Thoms, Alfred Torrie and Eric Wittkower. Assistant physicians with permanent-staff status were Hilda de Peyer, J. R. P. Edkins, Erwin Popper and Joe Purser, and Kenneth Soddy in the Children's Department. An acquisition with considerable influence on the Tavistock organization at this time was the recently demobilized young Canadian-born psychiatrist, Elliott Jaques, with an honours degree in psychology from Harvard, who became the Secretary to the small staff executive already mentioned earlier. Among senior 'trainees' at this time were Henry Ezriel, originally a Child Guidance Fellow with us, and Gerald Caplan had some advanced training under John Bowlby in our Children's Department. Leopold Stein was given charge of the Speech Therapy Unit with consultant status; and several men shortly to be appointed to senior staff positions were already with us since the Army, but 'new' as compared with the pre-war Tavistock. These were J. J. M. Jacobs and F. T. Shadforth. Dr J. Barrie-Murray rejoined us as our diagnostic physician and Dr Ronald McKeith, a rising paediatrician with considerable psychosomatic interests, joined the Children's Department in a similar capacity. On the clinical psychology staff there remained Miss Constance Simmins as our chief psychologist, with Miss D. C. Chaplin and Mrs Yana Popper, who had by this time qualified in psychology, to help her on the children's side. On the adult side, in addition to the part-time services of Eric Trist, we had appointed Herbert Phillipson as a clinical psychologist. Our psychiatric social work staff was completely new. We were fortunate in securing Miss Noel Hunnybun, formerly of the Child Guidance Training Centre, as our chief P.S.W. tutor. We also appointed Miss Elizabeth Brown in the role of second children's P.S.W. On the adult side we acquired Mrs Mary Williams and Mrs Marjorie Sprince as psychiatric social workers, to be followed shortly by Miss Doris Tamplin, who had up to then been working at Shenley Hospital. At this time the professional staff concerned almost exclusively with the Tavistock Institute of Human Relations aspect consisted of Harold Bridger, Elliott Jaques, Isobel Menzies, who had learnt much social psychology with the civil resettlement units, Ben Morris, Eric Trist and A. T. M. Wilson, in addition to the part-time services of Herbert Phillipson and J. D. Sutherland. It is of interest that during this period we employed three staff members concerned with writing, the mass media and publications – namely, Mr T. S. Fairly, Mr Frank Frost as our General Editor, and Mr J. Harvard Watts, with the special task of promoting the newly formed publications company ('Tavistock Publications'), which was also to run our journal, *Human Relations*.[1] This necessity arose from the overwhelming demand for writing of articles, pamphlets and in some instances requests for books which these men were to help us with on the publishing and editorial side. In fact, there was at one time a project that the Tavistock staff should publish such documents of public interest anonymously under the pseudonym of 'Frank Beaumont', the Frank relating to Mr Frost and the Beaumont to our new address.

A picture of how the Tavistock Clinic and Institute looked in 1946 may be of interest, because in some respects this structure has remained the basis for subsequent development. Firstly, it is noteworthy that the staff lists were printed without any distinction of seniority; the professional staff, the secretarial staff, the administrative staff and the refectory staff are all in the same type and with the same degree of emphasis. This was part of the new egalitarianism and determination to make our institution as proud and self-respecting in all its aspects as possible. The same went for the identical salaries for medical and non-medical full-time staff. The honorary sessional staff, those who continued in the tradition of the old Clinic, were receiving no remuneration during this transitional phase, though several of them were to become part-time salaried consultants, etc., when the National Health Service came into being.

Emergent Institutional Structure

By the end of 1946 the report for that year describes in some detail the way in which the I.M.C. (later Professional Com-

[1] The original Directors of this company were J. D. Sutherland, A. T. M. Wilson and John Harvard Watts.

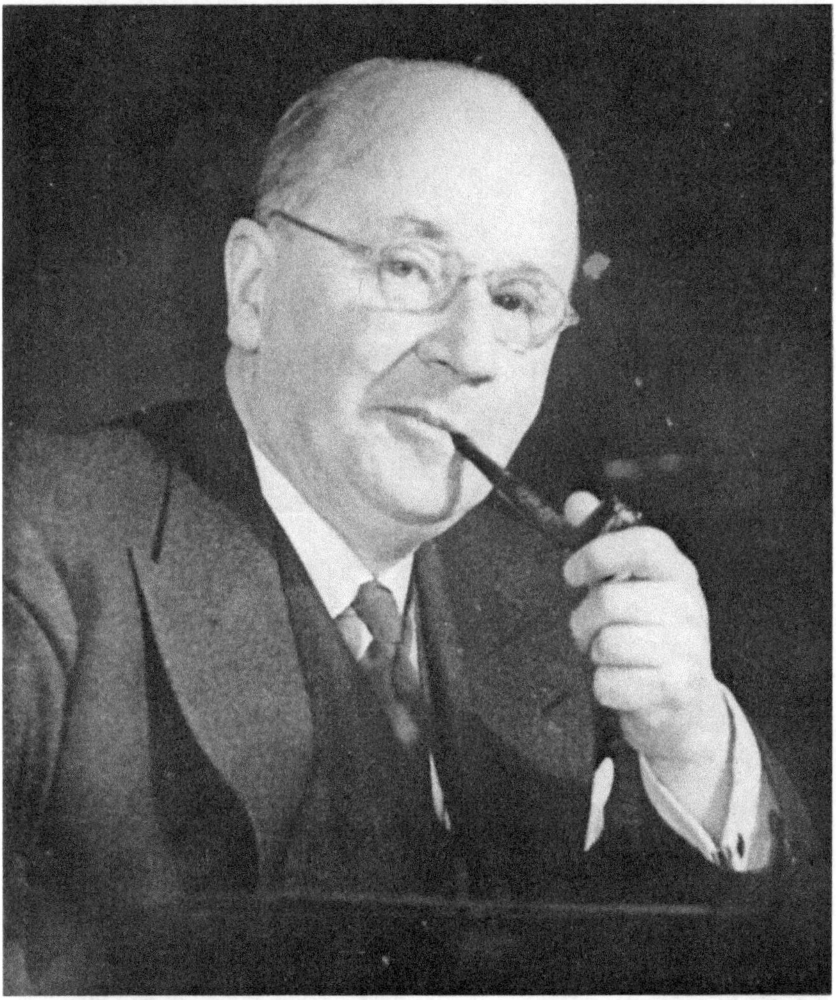

J. R. Rees, C.B.E., M.D., F.R.C.P.
Medical Director 1933-1947

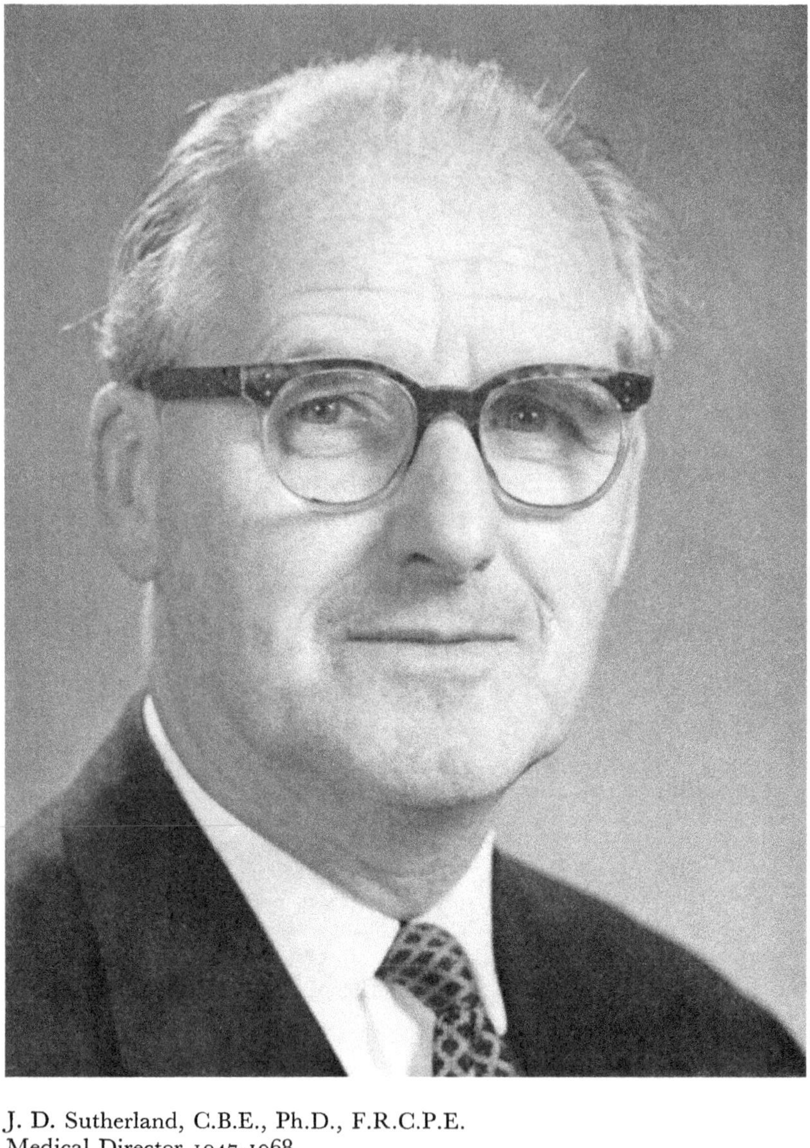

J. D. Sutherland, C.B.E., Ph.D., F.R.C.P.E.
Medical Director 1947-1968

mittee) had done its work and structured the new Tavistock. In essence, what follows will be taken from that report, although much of what happened is, of course, vividly within my memory as a participant in the decison-making right through that year. The structure was consciously designed to facilitate and streamline the institution for its now confidently expected entry into the National Health Service in a year to two's time. We wanted to hand over an organization in good working order rather than conserving our resources or dispersing them in expensive ventures. As already mentioned, the form of organization was approached by the Professional Committee as a research problem, because we had learnt that the social structure of a technical institution in the field of human relations is a decisive factor in any work that it is able to do.

Here are some of the principles: Every member of staff whether voluntary or paid, full-time or part-time, domestic, secretarial or professional, was to be a member of one or more work groups known as 'units'. A senior full-time member of the staff who was also a member of the Professional Committee would be responsible for one or more of these units. These members constituted a management committee of the activities of both the Clinic and Institute. Below this, all units were on the same level, but a co-ordination unit stood in the relation of a secretariat to the others, and was to carry out the day-to-day work of the management committee. This was the group presided over by Mr Herbert, later on with the assistance of Mr Sidney Gray, who in due course became the Secretary of the T.I.H.R. It contained such people as the receptionists and the assistants to the Clinic Secretary, Librarian when appointed, and so on.

Though the various units differed in size and role, the underlying design was common. Each was scheduled to carry out actual projects or operations in its own field, and at the same time to contribute to training and research, and each had its own internal micro-administration. The integration of these four functions in each unit was regarded as a fundamental principle, the question of 'how' being a problem for the group concerned. As regards staff, executive responsibility was in the hands of the member of the management committee in charge of that unit, supported by a policy panel which might include advisers on a sessional basis, not necessarily members of the paid or voluntary staff, but possibly drawn from outside as well as from within the Clinic or Institute. The work of a unit was to be carried out by a varying number of staff, who might spend either the whole or part of their time in its activities, allocations being made by the management committee in relation to an overall view of the priorities. Administratively, each unit had a secretary, who might be supported according to requirements by other clerical personnel. Research and training needs were discussed by unit meetings known as 'workshops', in which students as well as members of the unit participated. Students also participated in work assignments. So much for the principles.

In 1946 we only had our administrative and refectory units, in addition to the three major operational units, the Adult Unit, the Child Guidance Unit and the Institute Unit. We emphasized, however, that the variety of operational units in 1946 was no more than a start in organization. The development of operational units was limited by what could be budgeted for, though we were aware of the immense demand on us. This came from the public, not only for counselling and treatment, but equally for industrial consultations, management and selection problems and social surveys, etc. We therefore hoped to move towards tackling more of these problems when we knew our role and our resources in money and manpower more clearly after the coming of the National Health Service. Before describing the work of the two major clinical units, a word in passing on the relationship of our refectory and administrative units to the rest, which may seem faintly ludicrous to some readers. The professional staff took their relationship to our secretaries and our refectory and domestic staff very seriously, and, moreover, had senior staff members in charge of the improvements and facilitation of good catering, good morale, work distribution and staff relations in these very important supporting services. We remembered the importance of smooth 'A. & Q.' services for the welfare and efficiency of operational troops.

I will first describe the Children's Department, where John Bowlby, with characteristic energy, had got to work, in a slightly more well-defined field, more quickly than the adult services. By the end of 1946 this unit, with a relatively small staff, had seen 313 new patients, referred mostly from local health authorities, although quite a number, however, also came privately or through general practitioners, since we now, by a decision of the Professional Committee, accepted patients in all income groups and were competing with private practice as part of our determination to stay solvent. The Education Act of 1944 had put an obligation on the local authorities to provide child guidance services. This was taken by the Children's Department as indicating that training for the great increase in need for qualified workers was going to be the top priority for a skilled team of teaching status. Hence the Child Unit took the decision to limit its intake of patients to the north-western quadrant of the Metropolis and concentrate its resources more on training child psychiatrists, educational psychologists and P.S.W.s. The newly constituted National Association for Mental Health had made itself nationally responsible for the selection and allocation of Fellows in child psychiatry and in educational psychology to the few teaching centres. At the same time, the training of social-work students taking the Mental Health Course at the London School of Economics, which we had done before the war, resumed under our tutor, Miss Noel Hunnybun. The training was so designed as to give all the three professional groups plenty of opportunity for clinical experience with thorough discussion and supervision, including two weekly case conferences, two seminars on theory and one conference on general child-guidance problems; in addition, each student had one hour's private supervision or tuition per week. Despite her intended resignation, as she wanted to do more private work and writing, Miss Simmins stayed on and continued to take responsibility for the educational psychology training, of which she was a pioneer. Money was coming in to some extent from private fees, to some extent from local authority reimbursements for our services. A trenchant line in the annual report castigates the authorities: 'no Ministry or public authority assumes responsibility for training the workers for the new obligation and a few centres at present undertaking it, of which the Tavistock is the second largest, are still entirely dependent on private funds.' Thus Bowlby's Child Guidance

Unit, not yet re-christened the Department for Parents and Children, was a very lively and going concern doing an immense amount of extra-mural teaching in addition to training the above-named grades.

The Adult Department also had got going in the last quarter of 1946. There were 252 new patients and in all 456 patients under treatment, with attendances for that quarter totalling around 2,400. The report here also emphasizes that we were now seeing patients from all income levels, and that they were charged fees according to their means. The 1,000 new patients per annum were mostly referred by general practitioners. The Adult Department had not yet felt able to restrict its intake geographically because of the remaining scarcity of other facilities for psychotherapy. Our old friend the waiting list was already re-established and was the anxious concern of all, but especially of Miss Watts, whose heart always bled for every patient not yet cared for. The new feature in therapy was our concentration on groups. This was largely due to Bion's presence and influence. While we resumed the customary consultation and counselling services, which also included a good deal of vocational and social resettlement work, and while also offering individual therapy, long and short, in the traditional manner, the enthusiasm and desire to learn lay in 'group discussions', not yet dignified by the name of therapy. The 1946 report says that in an effort to give help to patients 'who seemed unlikely to benefit from counselling alone and for whom individual treatment is not possible or not indicated', interest had been devoted to group methods dealing with psychological difficulties. As the result of experience in the armed forces, where these problems became for the first time manifest on a large scale, there had been a considerable amount of clinical work in this sphere. The report continues:

> During the past year a number of group discussions with patients of various types have been conducted in the Adult Unit. In these groups the psychiatrist meets 8 to 10 patients for 1½ to 2 hours once or several times per week. In such group discussions experience has shown that patients can gain considerable understanding of their own problems and

> sometimes acquire increased ability in handling the difficulties they experience in their interpersonal relations – relations which have often been seriously affected by their psychological illness. In this connection it should be remarked that to look upon group methods as merely affording an opportunity of dealing with a larger number of patients or as a substitute for individual forms of treatment in no way does justice to the intrinsic psychological and social value of group methods. They demand to be appreciated as an essentially new orientation in therapy implicit in the newer and more social orientations in the psychopathology of interpersonal relationships.

The report then cautions:

> The *tentative* nature of the opinions on the value of group methods must be stressed. It is too early as yet to make any adequate evaluation of work of this kind, and whilst psychiatrists engaged on group methods believe that they are of value in certain cases, all are agreed that a means must be found of testing the validity of this belief. For this reason a programme of both extensive and intensive objective scientific research into the manifold problems associated with group methods, particularly their validation as a form of treatment, has been planned in the Adult Unit.

Unfortunately, this validation work was to hang fire for years, except for the very obvious summarizing of results under the old scheme of 'much improved', 'improved', etc., and we had to wait until the late 1950s for Sutherland and Phillipson and others to undertake some part of the spade-work required for such validation. To continue with the quotation from the report:

> A further development of the group discussion method in therapy has recently been initiated – for experimental purposes – of combining group discussion with psychodrama, an experiment which will be watched with interest.

Teaching and Training in the Adult Department

During the early months of 1946, between my demobilization

and my departure for Leeds, the Professional Committee appointed me Training Secretary, the equivalent of the job which Hadfield had been doing before the war. Here is an outline of the programme of educational work which was started at this time in the Adult Unit for psychiatrists and clinical psychologists – a term which had now come into usage. It is essentially that which had already existed pre-war and which, with additions and refinements, must be a basic plan for psychotherapeutic training anywhere. Teaching and training was conducted by means of (*a*) participation in diagnosis, counselling and short-term treatment; (*b*) supervised handling of short and long cases; (*c*) experience in therapeutic groups; (*d*) attendance at case discussions of diagnosis and counselling and at 'Unit Workshops'; (*e*) individual tutorials; (*f*) guided reading; (*g*) seminars in theory and methods of (i) technique in consultation and counselling, (ii) principles of out-patient psychiatry, (iii) psychopathology, (iv) techniques of psycho-diagnosis, including the use of projection methods. The adult clinical work was at this time divided into a Consultation and Counselling Unit in charge of one member of the Professional Committee, and Treatment Units, both group and individual, which were different projects, although, of course, closely linked by overlapping personnel. The rationale of this division was largely the need to differentiate between techniques of intensive treatment and those in which patients were not to be involved in deeper transference relationships, with all that this entailed. In the diagnostic and counselling service the handling was different, and the clinical psychologists played a much larger part, not only in psychodiagnostics, but also in vocational and educational counselling and so forth. Here the continuity of seeing the same doctor, etc., was regarded as less important. Trainees were familiarized with these two contrasted methods. In the same way the group methods unit was largely a separate project, at first mainly concerned with development and validation. Each of these three projects had their own 'workshops' for improvement of method and their own case conferences, but all of them joined together in general teaching case conferences and staff seminars.

As yet research was scarcely resumed, except in aspiration.

The Adult Department, as we saw, stated its intention of doing controlled validation studies on the effectiveness of psychotherapy, comparing group and individual methods and methods and criteria for selection of patients for these different treatments on a rational basis. We also hoped to formulate hypotheses about the more important variables affecting the outcome of group therapy and so on, but these proposals remained very largely in the 'pending file' for some time, until we would be able to afford the luxury of paying for research.

We resolved that very few patients were to be offered long analytic therapy, not only because of staff limitations, but because of the impropriety, as we saw it, of investing scarce resources on very few. There was a social-value judgement behind this decision, somewhat at variance with Crichton-Miller's and the classical psychoanalysts', although not with J. R. Rees's, nor with his former associates' wartime decisions about the Benthamite doctrine of 'the greatest happiness of the greatest number' rather than *de luxe* therapy for the few. Psychoanalysis in a 'mass clinic' was justified mainly as necessary training, which could only be gained on the basis of long and deep contact with some patients. At the same time, we were quite clear that such treatment was to be offered to certain selected patients where diagnosis along thorough social and psychodynamic lines indicated to a case conference that nothing less would do. On the whole, the Adult Department had greater difficulty in 'getting going', partly owing to the later demobilization of some staff members, and also because the group techniques with which we were experimenting were as yet tentative and met with some resistance and doubt from a number of honorary staff.

One clinical trial which began around this time was in selection of patients for groups. This led to our experimental use over some years of the so-called *group reception* technique. It consisted in having new patients sit together for both intelligence and some elementary projection tests with the psychologist (who was expected to observe their reactions to the group) before being seen by the psychiatrist. At one stage the joint reception technique also involved a subsequent group session with the diagnosing consultant on the model of the War Office

Selection Boards. This was meant to offer the setting for an initial appraisal of patients' capacity for making interpersonal relations in a social setting. It illustrated our conceptual shift to include interpersonal as well as purely intra-psychic processes in the evaluation of degrees of neurotic disability. From these techniques Phillipson, who was largely concerned with this development, began to devise new tests, culminating in his now well-known Object Relations technique.

I read in a minute with some satisfaction that in 1946 I had already advocated psychodynamic training for general practitioners in seminar groups of ten, and a similar teaching event for junior hospital officers in psychosomatics; and that I had also proposed one for medical officers of health for their work in future community mental health. These proposals were to see implementation several years later, when in the early 1950s we inaugurated with Balint our first general practitioner seminar on these lines.

Looking at the training arrangements for 1946, the annual report stated:

> The Professional Committee was aware of the difficulties which would be met, owing to the fact that the training arrangements would have to be tentative while the organization as a whole was developing rapidly, having to work out its own structure in the process of doing so. Training was therefore regarded as in itself a research project of top priority. Difficulties of an immediate beginning were matched by the urgency of the need to train people capable of independent work in the fields in which the Institution is interested. The pioneer nature of the courses was made very clear in initial talks with all intending students. For the same reason it was decided to take only a limited number of students that year and to select only those who it was felt would be sympathetic to existing difficulties and able to withstand the stresses caused by growing pains. The difficulties of the situation were thus turned to some advantage in providing a means of selection of students.

We saw ourselves at that time both in a teaching and in a learning role. We instituted regular group discussion or, one might say, experimental group therapy for ourselves under Bion's leadership. Most of the staff took part in these 'teaching and learning' roles. These regular staff groups were important in reducing internal tensions and in welding the staff together. A number of colleagues from certain other institutions interested in this field were invited to participate in these training groups. Thus, some members of the staff of the L.S.E., the National Institute of Industrial Psychology, the Industrial Welfare Society and certain research students from the Department of Psychology at Birkbeck and Bedford Colleges joined in these experiments.

We classified our courses into (1) individual methods, mostly offered to applicants in medicine or psychology, usually as an introduction or a supplement to specialist study in psychological medicine or clinical psychology; (2) social methods, designed for graduates in medicine, psychology, education, anthropology, sociology or economics, as an introduction to the study of principles of social psychiatry and social psychology applied to the community, and to educational or industrial problems. This was the more novel venture we often termed 'sociatry', following Moreno. It was in these experimental group discussions that Wilfred Bion presided in allegedly 'leaderless groups' of students, meeting to record their own experiences and to experience the tensions generated in such social situations. The main purpose of this series was to provide an opportunity to study the emotional phenomena of interpersonal relations as experienced by the students themselves. Here was the core of the new social dynamics training which has had very considerable impact on British psychiatry and many other fields concerned with interpersonal and human relations. Theory, however, was not neglected, and each week the whole group of students had a seminar on new developments in psychopathological theory in which, in addition to the staff, the late Dr John Rickman, then Editor of the *International Journal of Psycho-Analysis*, and myself, then Professor at Leeds, participated in a teaching role.

An explanation of how these enterprises were financed is not out of place. The Treasurers and Council decided that the development merited a fairly liberal use of the Clinic's reserves, preferring, as mentioned, to hand over the Tavistock Clinic as an efficient organization practising as many of the 'new' skills as its funds would permit. In consequence, it was decided to spend £10,000 or so of the remaining assets, as well as some of the Rockefeller grant, augmented by some £4,000 of British donations. The question how the staff lived during this transition period may be briefly explained. Some were still in the Army on the work of civil resettlement (centred on Richmond) or finishing various other projects in the Army, and were not in fact released until 1946. This was the case, for example, with J. R. Rees and myself, A. T. M. Wilson, Ben Morris, and some others. Those who were released were partly in receipt of our salaries out of the funds mentioned, and, if senior enough, had resumed part-time private consulting or psychotherapeutic practices. It has already been remarked how modest by modern standards were these salaries of the new core staff. This was, of course, in expectation that by 1948 the State would make itself responsible for the day-to-day running expenses and salaries of those appointed to the staff, on the basis of the Spens Report.

'*The old order passeth*'

It will have become apparent from the description of the preceding pages that the balance of power within the new Tavistock organization had undergone a considerable shift from a fairly equal distribution among a staff uniformly honorary, part-time and giving only such services as they could spare from other pursuits to a new full-time or maximum part-time staff, who had become both the policy-makers of the Professional Committee and the nucleus of the Institute of Human Relations. This latter group was a technically competent and also a conceptually coherent body committed to the new developments in the emerging social and dynamic psychiatry, many of them in their late thirties or early forties. This resulted in quite a strong line of demarcation between the old-style honoraries and this new group who, through the regular meetings of the Professional Committee, through the creation of the technical executive, and so on, were translating the new ideas and methods into daily action in the Clinic.

At this time J. R. Rees was Chairman and Medical Director, but he was not really in this group, and he had many other commitments. One also knew that he was not fully in sympathy with the influx of these younger psychoanalysts. He had experienced in his own evolution the very considerable hostility and rigidity of the inter-war psychoanalytic powers-that-be. The same new generation who had between them carried under him much of the creative development within the Army and whom he had loyally and most generously supported now appeared as the 'young Turks', the 'psychopathological snobs' who seemed to be making decisions and acting without his always having the time or the information to question or approve. Even before I went to Leeds this was at times becoming apparent. J.R. not infrequently suffered from the feeling that 'nobody told him anything'. Whether there was an element of the erstwhile more humorously expressed sense of technical inadequacy, or whether it was a generation gap (for he was by some fifteen to twenty years older than the average of the new nuclear staff) is a matter of surmise. Probably both elements as well as fatigue after his Herculean labours during the war may have had an influence. By the end of 1946 and in 1947 it became clear that he was no longer the effective head of the new institution, and it was perhaps to those in the know no surprise that he offered his resignation as Medical Director to the Council, who accepted it with great regret. J.R. motivated this by his increasing commitments, particularly of his appointment as a member of the North-west Metropolitan Regional Hospital Board. He also expanded on this in a letter received by the Professional Committee around November 1946. I was asked to meet Dr Rees as one not now immediately involved, by reason of my appointment in Leeds, and I reported back after the conversation that J.R. felt he was anxious in no way to embarrass the work of the Clinic and Institute and that he found difficulties in the changed status and function of the Professional Committee. This essentially confirmed the point made above about his feeling that the younger group were not really looking to him as the effective leader. He just had not been in the building enough and taken part in the intensive work of planning and discussion which men committed full-time to the institution were able to give, and he therefore felt 'out of it'. One felt that his mission had become wider, and he needed a different setting.

Here, then, was a second 'palace revolution', with the Medical Director feeling compelled by the pressure of the younger generation to give up his post, whilst still at the height of his own powers at the age of fifty-six or fifty-seven. Comparing it to the events of H.C.M.'s resignation in the early 1930s, there was, however, a great difference. J.R. not only presided over the meeting at which his own resignation was discussed, but also volunteered to remain until the reorganization had taken place, and that he would then review his position. He would in any case be prepared to work for the new institution at Council level. His bearing was generous and co-operative, and his given reasons for resignation nicely formal. During the following six months I was very busy organizing the new Leeds Department and was rarely in London. My contact with the inner life of the group was not close, but 'ideologically' I was with them. I had failed to persuade J.R. to stay. I cannot help feeling that J.R. was deeply hurt by the way in which the new group were taking power unto themselves, by-passing him and probably not communicating in the correct 'sociatric' sense with the democratically appointed leader of the group. Since this event his animus against 'psychoanalysts' in general certainly became more marked. It was probably inevitable that the young men whom he had recruited and brought together and given the opportunity of developing their ideas in the Army and in the first months after the war must in the end supplant him. This seems to be one of those relentless historical processes by which the succeeding generations displace each other. Many people, particularly those who loved J.R. best, felt that he was not given a really fair deal in this turnover, especially as he was not then doing any active clinical work on the honorary staff and, by resigning a year before, missed his opportunity of appointment as a consultant at the Tavistock under the Health Service. He was not slow to find fresh fields.

This is no place to write a full biography of J.R.'s great achievements or career, but it may have been for the good of the world that by this internal revolution of the Tavistock the international mental health movement gained what the Tavistock lost. It is a moot point whether his continued directorship would have made more or less of the Tavistock in the post-war era. What is certain is that a man of that vigour and with those broad international connections would not long be idle and that he now carried the notions of social psychiatry, a term he had used as far back as 1942, into the broader scene, first of British, and later of international psychiatry. It is well known that he was the inspirer and creator of the 1948 Mental Health Congress in London, out of which came the World Federation for Mental Health, which he nurtured and master-minded for many years, and in the upshot of which many less developed countries and many countries stuck with one-sided, antiquated mental-hospital services were moved a long way forward in their awareness and policies about mental health. The 1948 Congress, with so many of its topics suggested directly or indirectly by J. R. Rees to the planners and the programme committees, owed a good deal to the work which he had directed during his years at the Tavistock, which he carried forward with the help of this now dominant younger group during the war and had incorporated into his own broad vision of 'mental health'. This blue-print can be read in the reports he wrote during and just after the war for the Tavistock, and which have also, of course, remained the programme of development for the Tavistock itself.

It now seemed almost as if J.R. represented the 'old' orientation begun by H.C.M. and carried on by himself, which was now replaced by a more intellectual and scientific as well as psychoanalytic conceptual climate. I sometimes wonder with varying degrees of guilt and self-reproach whether, had I been able to be present throughout these events, J.R.'s resignation would have taken place at all, and at any rate if it would have happened in quite the hurtful way to him and to those for whom J.R. *was* the Tavistock. Through these his many friends, his withdrawal had a quite damaging effect on the image of the institution.

By July 1947 John D. ('Jock') Sutherland had been democratically elected by the staff as the new Medical Director of the Tavistock Clinic, giving up his hitherto more Institute and sociologically oriented work. At the same time he also took charge of the overall supervision of the Adult Department. John Bowlby, another psychoanalytic newcomer, was chosen as the Deputy Medical Director, with continuing charge of the Children's Department. We once again had a Medical Director with an Edinburgh tradition, carefully trained both in educational and academic psychology and in psychiatry, psychoanalytically grounded, but deeply affected by his experience in social psychiatry in the Army, an 'introvert', and the reverse of either a paternalistic or a promotional character. Both he and John Bowlby represented, as leading members of the Army's psychiatric team, the 'new era'. They were grounded in the neo-psychoanalytic object-relations theory, with which were fused, in a remarkable way, the concepts of family psychiatry in both its adult and children's forms, and a broad spectrum of their place in psychology and sociology. Neither, I feel, intended the separation of adult from children's work, but, as happened earlier, the pull of techniques, the greater use of non-medical therapists in the children's service and the divergent social involvements determined a good deal of functional separation.

In Sutherland's first report, which is also the last written under the voluntary system before the National Health Service came into being, the need for devising effective short therapy, whether in groups or in individual session, and the need to train psychiatrists, psychologists and social workers in these techniques were foremost in the new Director's thinking. He at once, with the Professional Committee's backing, proceeded to decentralize the work of the Adult Department into more or less self-contained clinical units, each with a consultant in charge, an assistant who might be a senior registrar in later days, one psychologist and one psychiatric social worker, together with a pool of sessional staff attached to each unit. Dr Mary Luff and Dr John Kelnar were appointed physicians-in-charge of these clinical units, which were completely autonomous, with the Medical Director in the Adult Department providing only the necessary co-ordination. Hope was expressed for a follow-up unit for the whole of the clinic's work, with the Medical Director, in addition, undertaking the functions of establishing the necessary external relations with regional and local medical authorities and other outside bodies. Bowlby had made his changes in the Children's Department earlier. He emphasized valuable links with potential client agencies. Both men, with the Professional Committee, spent most of 1947-8 in building up the services for the now impending Health Service. It was hoped that staff members, now sessional and unpaid, would be taken into salaried posts, leading to more work. We expected the Health Service to expand establishments so that our primary task in the Service – namely, psychotherapy – could be carried out under better conditions with more personnel and without the reproach of long waiting lists. In the 1947 report the aspiration was expressed that, whilst there were unlikely to be great changes in the scope of the Clinic's work, the Health Service would encourage people to work full-time, giving them the leisure to do more research and training. Only in this way, it was felt, would healthy growth and the pioneering tradition be continued.

At this point we can say that 'Phoenix' had risen from the ashes, and the National Health era began.

VIII

The Tavistock and the State

It is well known that the National Health Service took over on 5 July 1948. What is not realized is that there had been an earlier mooted inception date – namely, 31 March. The Tavistock Clinic and Institute had budgeted their money for salaries and overheads for the earlier date, and our coffers duly ran out by 31st March. However, like ourselves, many 'broke' hospitals about to become part of the National Health Service had to be kept in operation. The North-west Metropolitan Regional Hospital Board (hereinafter referred to as No. 5 Board for brevity) was already in being. On our showing of need, the Ministry and No. 5 Board made their grants retrospective to 31 March and in some cases back-dated salaries to October 1947. In fact, we may say that the National Health Service began for us as a kind of 'honeymoon'. It seemed that the authorities, especially the Central Middlesex Hospital Management Committee, under whom the Tavistock was grouped, were most anxious to impress with their helpfulness and their goodwill. We gaped when a supply of excellent reproductions of fine paintings arrived to decorate our bare and dingy rooms, and when in other ways it was made clear that the Management Committee were there to be good parents. There was great tolerance towards our strange amalgam of non-Health Service Institute and statutory Clinic, which reverted to its old name of the 'Tavistock Clinic'. The Ministry of Health had accepted the potential value of this hybrid, which, through awareness of our Army activities, they had learned to see as highly relevant to preventive and social medicine. Thus an arrangement was made for the Institute to retain space in No 2 Beaumont Street, the 'fourth floor', by which its work was frequently called, with its

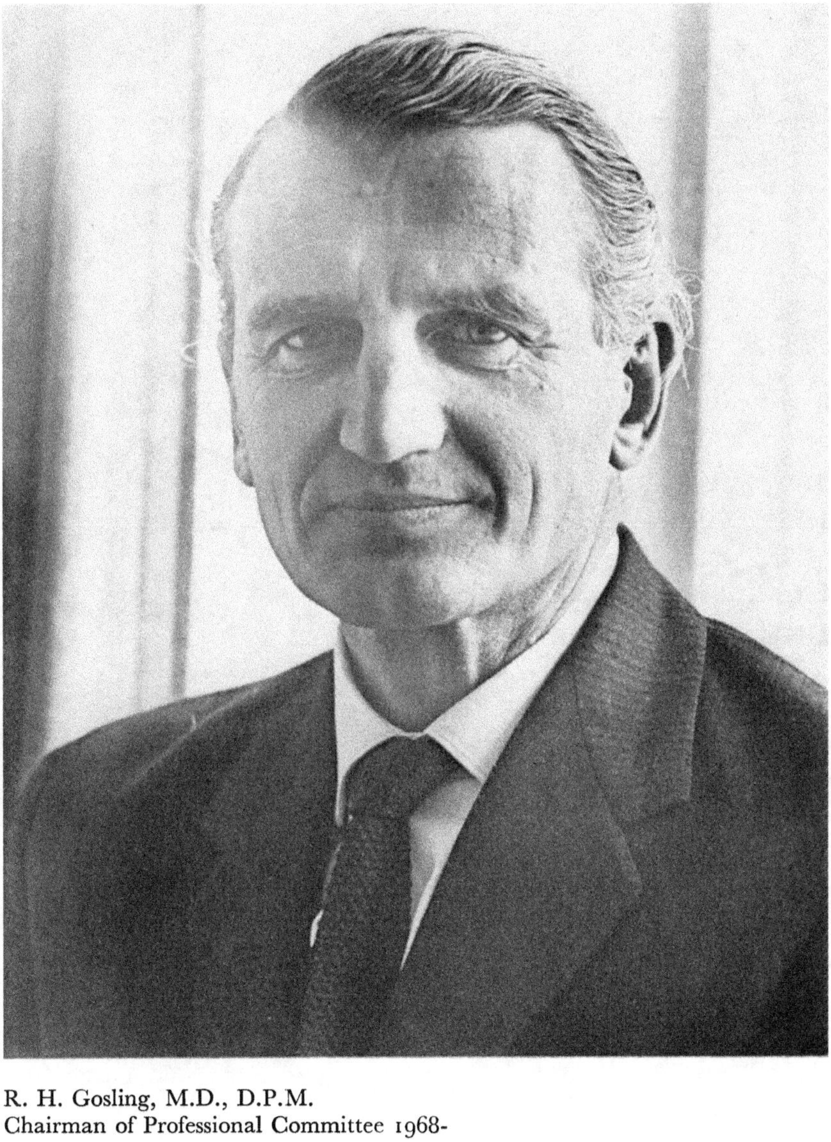

R. H. Gosling, M.D., D.P.M.
Chairman of Professional Committee 1968-

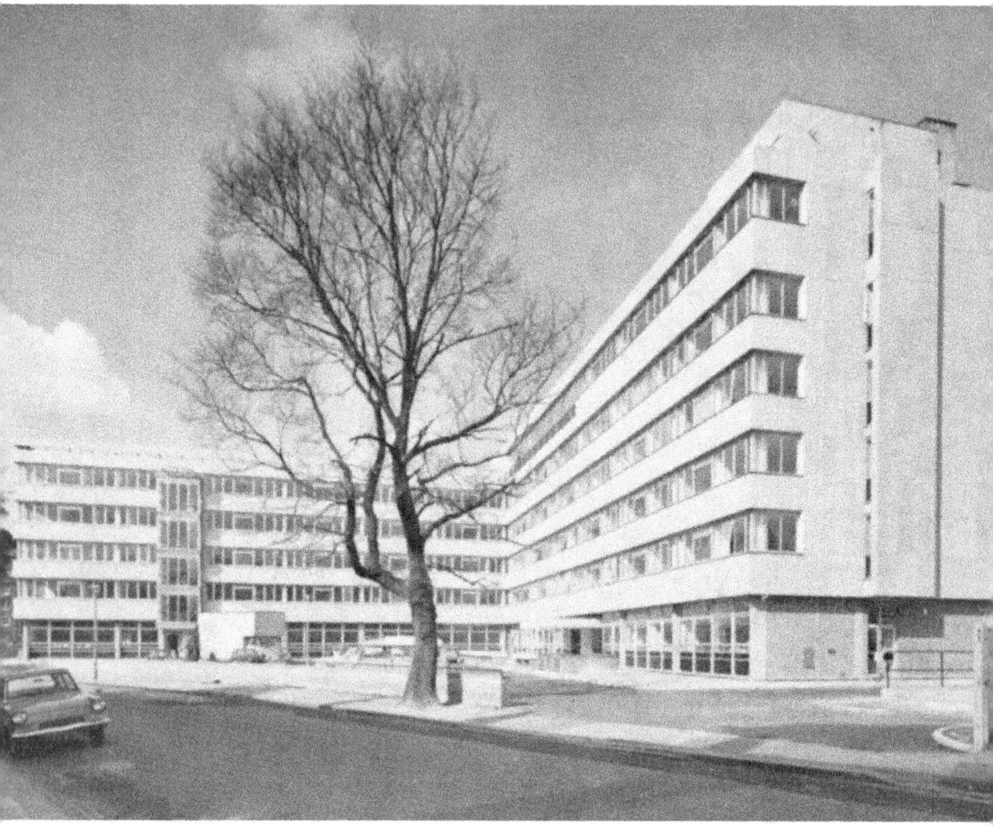

The Tavistock Centre

own administration under a real professional – Mr Sidney Gray, who has remained throughout as the Secretary of the rapidly expanding T.I.H.R. and is my co-author of ch. ix. Our friendship with him dates from the Army days, when he was in War Office selection boards and other related activities.

In 1947 the Professional Committee had done its best to create the optimal establishment for the Tavistock's staff for the appointed day. There were many who, as already mentioned, declined National Service and did not stay, and other who had preferred to work in other N.H.S. clinics or hospitals. So on the appointed day the following senior staff went into the Health Service: Medical Director, J. D. Sutherland; Deputy Director, John Bowlby. There were three other full-time consultants in the Adult Department. I returned after a brief and joyless tenure of the Leeds Chair to a full-time appointment in charge of one of the clinical units already mentioned, with John Kelnar in charge of the other unit. In addition, Henry Ezriel was newly appointed as consultant in charge of developing group methods. Major part-time appointments on the consultant staff were those of Mary Luff with six sessions, Leopold Stein (in charge of the speech unit) with five sessions, A. Geoffrey Thompson with eight sessions. The other part-time consultants were C. Boenheim, J. J. M. Jacobs, R. Evelyn Lucas, Erwin Popper, Amy M. Thoms, Alfred Torrie, A. T. M. Wilson and Eric Wittkower. F. T. Shadforth was somewhat more loosely attached, as he was about to become a consultant at Brighton. Our senior registrars were at this time: in the Adult Department, Elizabeth Loebl and R. E. D. Markillie, also a registrar with me at Leeds. There were two honorary psychiatrists not on the Health Service strength who were soon to leave us, W. R. Bion and Desmond Irwin, who gave as many sessions as possible. Bion did not wish to serve in the N.H.S., and returned to his basic work, psychoanalysis, in whose counsels he was to play a leading role. Our psychological staff consisted of Herbert Phillipson assisted by John Boreham and Gerald Staunton, all full-time. Our psychiatric social workers were Mrs Mary Williams, Mrs Marjorie Sprince and Miss Doris Tamplin. In the Children's Department there was but one consultant – namely, John Bowlby, full-time. He was assisted, however, by a large staff of senior registrars and registrars: P. J. R. Davis, H. Dugmore Hunter and Julian Katz (now in Australia), and at the more junior level by Elizabeth Kramer, Agnes M. Main, (wife of our good friend, Tom Main) and Jeannie Stirratt. The psychological staff of the Children's Department was also larger than that of the Adult Department. Headed by Miss Constance Simmins, there were five others: J. Bremner, Miss M. Flanders, Mrs B. Michaels, Mrs Yana Popper and Miss Doris Wills. We had also appointed two highly qualified child psychotherapists, non-medical, in the persons of Miss Theodora Alcock and Mrs E. Bick. There were four psychiatric social workers, headed by Noel Hunnybun, Miss Elizabeth Brown, Robert Tod, and last but not least James Robertson. He was employed under John Bowlby on a research grant from the Halley Stewart Trust, with which they began their now famous research into the effects on young children of separation from their mother. We also now had a salaried and full-time Librarian, Miss Daphne Seamark. In charge of the physical diagnostic services we retained Dr J. Barrie-Murray for adults and Dr Ronald MacKeith as paediatric consultant. Dr Marjorie Garrod remained medical officer in charge of records on a part-time basis.

Among the secretarial staff I should like to mention some further personalities who have rendered greatest service to the institution. Miss Marjorie Harborough was appointed as the head of the secretarial service and personal assistant to the Medical Director, in which capacity she is still at the Tavistock, with most lines of communication in her loyal and discreet keeping. Likewise we retained for many years the services of Miss V. E. Watts as the Clinical and Records Secretary, as already mentioned in an earlier chapter. In corresponding positions on the children's side we had Miss Dorothy Southern who remains Dr Bowlby's personal assistant, and Miss Lesley Braham, who retired only very recently, as Records Secretary. Mrs D. M. Longstaff, Secretary to the Children's Department, left us for the usual happy reason of remarriage sooner than the others mentioned. On the reception staff, among the most important of all the contact-making and image-building groups of a psychotherapeutic clinic, our Head Receptionist was Mrs F. Stanger, who joined us at Westfield College and remained with us for some fifteen years, one of the best-loved people on the Tavistock staff.

Our conversations with the Ministry and with our newly appointed Regional Psychiatrist, Dr Colman Kenton, led us to believe that we would soon be granted a somewhat larger establishment, especially for consultant child psychiatrists and for medical trainees, so that our quota of contributing psychotherapeutic specialists to the Service could be raised.

Apart from the intensive activities involved in the implementing of the new organization and establishing useful routines, record-keeping and all the other things by which a medical institution really lives, we were indeed still greatly concerned with how we could best fulfil these training aspirations within the new financial security. These aims were pursued along two lines. The first was in the Professional Committee, in which we were discussing such things as possible affiliations with a suitable mental hospital, analogous, perhaps, to our link with Hill End Hospital before the war, or alternatively initiating a teaching federation for the North-west Metropolitan Region which would be composed of the psychotherapeutic clinics plus one or two mental hospitals, a mental deficiency hospital, a neurological institute, such as Queen Square, also in our region, and perhaps some outside specialist teachers. The other line of action was through the now formally established Advisory Committee in Psychiatry for No. 5 Region, in which Sutherland and others had played a considerable part from the beginning, while J. R. Rees was the first psychiatric member of the Regional Board itself. Our region had perhaps the greatest concentration of specialized psychiatric talent in the country.

There was no obvious reason why we should not create an unofficial but none the less effective training scheme for young psychiatrists as well as psychologists and social workers in our region, which geographically extended as far as Bedfordshire and the borders of Oxfordshire. The scheme could not only offer a somewhat different theoretical framework for the study of mental illness and its treatment and prevention, but could also save many trainee psychiatrists the difficult trudge to the far south of London to the Maudsley courses. Several teaching-hospital psychiatrists, notably Noel Harris of the Middlesex Hospital and shortly afterwards J. D. W. Pearce and Kenneth Soddy (who had left us to take up appointments respectively at St Mary's and University College Hospital), were on the Regional Advisory Committee, providing the teaching-hospital link. The Ministry favoured our continuing in our special role. Dr Colman Kenton supported the 'federation' and would have promoted it with his Board. The Advisory Committee in Psychiatry within the next few years set up a sub-committee which created a teaching syllabus, years in advance of any existing programme, for the federation, which was to have its 'classrooms' and central office within the Tavistock. Yet this scheme never eventuated.

One cannot speak for other institutions, but it would seem that one of the possible difficulties in 'federating' might have been the fear of the smaller clinics of being swallowed by the powerful Tavistock. I refer here to the Marlborough Day Hospital (the Social Psychotherapy Centre), in which Dr Joshua Bierer applied his strongly held Adlerian concepts, the Child Guidance Training Centre founded by the Commonwealth Fund, with its proud record of pre-war days, and the Portman Clinic, sprung from the Institute for the Study and Treatment of Delinquency, also with a special tradition and field of its own. Then there was the Marylebone Hospital for Psychiatry and Child Guidance (which was the now-independent former psychiatric wing of the West End Hospital for Nervous Diseases) with its own powerful personalities, and, lastly, the small British Hospital for Nervous Disorders in the Camden Road, the oldest of us all, established before the First World War. In addition to the zealous guarding of identities, as was certainly the case with the Tavistock, nobody emerged to take the lead or, at any rate, the initiative in carrying this scheme through. It seemed to be 'up to' the Tavistock. But with our preoccupation with internal development and the demands of clinical duties, teaching and in most cases of part-time private practice, we did not act. This experience shows that a successful teaching scheme *must* be run by full-time personnel of the requisite calibre, appointed and paid for the purpose, and directed by an individual – a strong argument in favour of setting up professorial departments of psychiatry who are not under the obligation to give maximum clinical service to the maximum number of patients in need. To the Tavistock, the needs of treatment must always take priority over other considerations. I have stated my opinion elsewhere that persons of the psychotherapeutic cast of mind are as a rule not good organization men. The qualities most needed in clinically committed psychiatrists are rarely combined with high rating on system-building and policy-making.

When the late T. P. Rees,[1] some years after the exploration and discussions I am now describing, charged me as a Tavistock man with the words, 'You Tavi boys had a great chance after the war and you did not take it,' one is in a sense inclined to agree. Perhaps we were too concerned with the development on the one hand of our special institution, and on the other hand possibly also with the international aspects of our work: U.N.E.S.C.O., W.H.O. consultancies, the World Federation for Mental Health, the American and Continental links and similar 'global' activities. There was also a possible internal obstacle in many Tavistock staff members during those early years. Most were recent psychoanalytic graduates, and the psychoanalytic schooling was still very much to the fore. There was a typically analytic reserve and exclusiveness, perhaps a residue of the fears of compromise between the old psychiatry and psychoanalytic work. On the other side, some of our non-analytic friends may have had a matching ambivalent apprehension about letting a group who had proved their considerable abilities, but were first and foremost perceived as analysts, take the lead in a comprehensive training scheme for young psychiatrists which, with the coming of the new physical methods, might have seemed to them to be too one-sided and 'dangerous'. They did not perhaps want to 'sup with the Devil' either. Who knows but that if J.R. had remained Medical Director for some years more, his prestige, immense organizing drive and freedom from psychiatric dogmatisms might have not brought this plan to fruition, though he also had his 'global' visions at this time – larger than anyone else's! The regional

[1] Physician-Superintendent of Warlingham Park Hospital; not to be confused with our own J.R.

teaching federation might have considerably hastened the growth of a holistic, psychodynamic trend for a large number of young psychiatrists without neglecting the new physical methods in the right case. My experience during the short tenure of the Chair at Leeds showed me that it was virtually impossible to draw practising analysts away from the magnet of London, where they felt supported by their respective societies and the opportunities for private practice. Only London could have started at this time a psycho-dynamically oriented school of psychiatry of any weight and standing. Our failure has, I think, impoverished the sort of British psychological medicine as envisaged in the dreams of Crichton-Miller, Rees and others.

The preceding paragraph has described activities over some years, extending into the mid-1950s, of the Tavistock group in relation to education in our region. A much briefer encounter was an approach to Dr Horace Jules of the Central Middlesex Hospital with a tentative proposal for affiliation, because of the obvious advantages of being part of a large regional and community general hospital, where we felt we might be useful both on the clinical side and on the psychosomatic research side. An M.R.C. social medicine unit was at that hospital, under J. N. Morris. We were told that it might be a worthwhile thing, 'but we would not be allowed beds'. This was in one sense a rebuff, but it was also, as J.R. told us, the Board's official doctrine. It was at that time thought better to have hostels for psycho-neurotics and milder psychoses adjacent to community clinics, rather than to have psychiatric wards in general hospitals. This outcome is worth a passing mention, in view of the greatly changed attitudes and policies now current. At present the general hospitals, both teaching and regional, are being urged and helped to set up psychiatric departments, including wards with beds, in an attempt to offer earlier and more comprehensive psychiatric services for the local communities. This proposal also faded out.

So the Tavistock itself went ahead with its clinical training and research programmes. Quite early in its National Health Service career we appointed a training panel to consider all those aspects of education for mental health work which would have been our part of the regional scheme to implement.

Now it became the self-contained teaching activity of our 'school'.

The organization of clinical work so as to make the maximum contribution to teaching and experience for staff members in training bears some further description, as it was certainly a new departure from the large but inchoate staff structure of the pre-war Clinic. With the severely contracted numbers of staff, but with a core of consultants giving whole-time or maximum part-time service, the Adult Department decided, as mentioned, to organize its work in two clinical 'firms' or teams, each presided over by a full-time consultant, then John Kelnar and myself. There was a difference: we abandoned the idea of a separate 'diagnostic' unit formed in 1946. Each consultant had an 'assistant' psychiatrist, normally a senior registrar as these came into being, a psychologist and a P.S.W. Other members of the staff, sessional consultants, junior registrars and psychologists in training, were attached to one or other of these units.

The functions of these units *qua* clinical service have already been described, including the method of group reception, in order to bring to bear the fullest co-operation of the three disciplines on the diagnosis of each case. This assessment in depth by a team with full discussion before decisions formed the essence of the in-service teaching and training of junior members of the unit. These were case conferences in the full sense of the term, which other staff members attended. Here we would not only display and evaluate the psychological, social and psychodynamic factors in the individual case, but also discuss the suitability of various kinds of treatment and decide on the kind of disposal best suited to the case. The unit kept responsibility for each patient taken in by it and supervised progress. A third unit, Dr Leopold Stein's special speech department, was also given formal structure on the same lines, with a P.S.W. and the part-time services of a psychologist. Dr Stein's distinguished work in this field has already been alluded to. This former laryngologist, having transformed speech therapy, was a Jungian analyst with full consultant status in the N.H.S.

The group reception procedure, started in 1946, lived on, but in a limited form. Each unit had a group reception day at fortnightly intervals on which six patients from the consultation waiting list were asked to spend the day at the Clinic. Care was taken to convene a group tolerably matched by clinical condition, age and general background. The patients were received by a member of the unit, usually the clinical psychologist, when the purpose and procedure of group reception were explained and the aims and therapeutic resources of the Clinic outlined. It was pointed out that we wanted to understand their difficulties as they saw them, and thus asked them to fill in a quite elaborate questionnaire. This provided factual and socio-economic information, saving medical and P.S.W. time. After completing the questionnaire and a coffee break, they were asked to do intelligence and projective tests. The latter were at first a selection from Murray's T.A.T., sometimes the Rorschach in addition, and in later years Phillipson's Object Relations Test. The rationale for giving such tests was always explained. In general there was a great deal of trouble taken to tell and reassure the patients about our way of working. There followed also a brief group discussion of the six or so patients together with the whole clinical team. This was an adaptation of the War Office selection boards, an attempt to assess a person's social demeanour and capacity for communication in a social group. The psychiatrists then gave their long, individual, clinical interview in the afternoon. Most often the senior registrar would do these 'special' consultations in the light of all this background material. The cases so extensively investigated would form the material for case conferences the following day.

The group reception technique was initiated because of the supposed advantages for patients and staff. The patient had an early foretaste of a group which was likely to be the method of therapy for a good many; it was a demonstration to him that in working with other patients he could gain better and earlier understanding of his own difficulties and provide his doctor with information through which he could be helped more effectively in minimum time. It was also felt that it would enable patients to discover quite soon the resemblances of their own emotional difficulties to those of others, a discovery which often reduced fear and apprehension engendered by the feeling of being a 'unique freak'. But most important of all, the reception procedure was felt to set a pattern for the patient's future contact with the Clinic while under therapy. It illustrated to him the group approach and the importance of social relationships, because it would be in those terms that his difficulties would be mainly understood and treated.

From the training point of view, the method had some obvious advantages, in that all members of the team would have some first-hand experience of the patient they were discussing. Thus the consultant had at least had some group contact with patients who were subsequently seen in consultation by his junior and so on. There was a shared fund of data on actual living people on which realistic case conferences could be based.

It must not be thought that group reception was the only method of receiving new patients. This was our interprofessional teaching method. In addition there was the simpler, more time-honoured routine of the individual consultation by staff members of consultant rank or sometimes of more junior rank, who might request tests or social work. The unit was responsible for the follow-through and allotment of each case, and kept this responsibility for the patient throughout. The unit head exercised a general supervision over all the part-time staff.

An analogous participant method was to some extent also used in teaching group therapy based on Bion's staff group model. Groups, especially in the early days, presented rather a difficult departure to the individual therapist. But the very nature of groups permitted the presence of more than one doctor, of which the second could be a student, e.g. another staff member learning group techniques. Retrospective comparing of notes after sitting in with a colleague has proved extremely helpful in group-therapy training. At first this was done by the physical presence of more than one therapist, sometimes with several other observers sitting quietly in the background as well. Later a one-way screen was built, with sound recording in the observation chamber. For similar reasnos we soon began to acquire tape-recorders for the preservation of some group sessions or for full verbatim accounts of the whole process of some therapeutic groups. These were valuable for the study of the sometimes still novel material after the session, for the group therapist to think over them and especially to recheck his own utterances to the group, and, of course, for the teaching of less experienced colleagues. No recording or one-way screening was ever done except with the patients' knowledge and consent.

Our groups were of very considerable interest to the social psychologists of the Institute of Human Relations in their study of general group dynamics. This resulted, for example, in W. R. Bion's notable publications on this subject. His observations were on therapeutic groups. The methods just described, plus supervised experience on long analytic cases, were the earliest forms of post-war training, and much of it was nearer to mutual self-education than to dogmatic teaching. Our first trainees were rather experienced people who had been Majors or Lieut.-colonels in Army psychiatry. The trainee psychologists, on the other hand, were mostly young honours graduates. They were trained by our staff psychologists under Miss Simmins and Mr Phillipson in the various standard methods of intelligence and personality testing then in use. The Adult Department did not train psychiatric social worker students; our three psychiatric workers were fully experienced. They took part in therapy to perhaps an unusual degree for those days.

Therapeutic responsibility by our P.S.W.s began in our experiment with a therapeutic social Club. This was started in 1948 to meet an expressed need of many patients who found difficulty in taking part in normal social activities because of their symptoms of diffidence, shyness, etc. This Club was begun by a few enthusiastic patients and was built up with the help of Mrs Sprince and Mrs Williams, with Dr H. A. C. Mason as the first psychiatric adviser. On his resignation to go to St Thomas's Hospital Mary Luff took his place. By the end of the year Club membership had risen to seventy of our patients, with a weekly attendance of about forty. The Club was intended for those patients whom initially we could not take into any form of systematic therapy. They were therefore seen only in the manner of the usual out-patient clinic for perhaps half an hour a fortnight, and the Club provided a transitional 'therapeutic community'. Gradually, patients were able to take on more and more of the functions of running the Club for themselves. This in itself was a therapeutic achievement. The Tavistock Institute of Human Relations took a benevolent research interest in this

Club. As staff grew and more of them became proficient in systematic group-analytic therapy, so a new situation was created. After a year or two while patients attended both – a treatment group and the Club – it became clear that through the Club and through the personalized relationships and 'loose talk' with P.S.W.s and so on, a split in transference was apt to occur, a kind of leak which stultified some of the endeavours of of the group therapists. When no patient was without regular medical therapy, it was decided to abolish the social Club. This step led to some considerable upheavals and tensions in the staff relations between the P.S.W.'s and the doctors, as the former felt rather deprived of a therapeutic role, which they had greatly valued, and to some reduction in P.S.W. strength on the adult side. We used the resulting vacancy to appoint a research psychologist. Formal, extensive, domiciliary social work is less important when every patient is in regular treatment with a psychiatrist.

In the Children's Department the situation at the beginning of the National Health Service period was serious. Two psychiatrists of teaching status who would have become consultants in the N.H.S. with us left to take up other appointments: Kenneth Soddy went to University College Hospital and also became Director of the Child Guidance Training Centre; Gerald Caplan (now Professor at Harvard) left us to become an adviser in mental health to the new Government of Israel. Bowlby thus only had senior registrars initially to share the burden of his clinical and teaching work. Dugmore Hunter, however, functioned to all intents and purposes as a consultant before his imminent appointment to such a post. None the less, the clinical work there seemed to be carried on at a satisfactory level because of the high quality also of the non-medical staff.

The policy of both the Children's and the Adult Departments was one of deliberate reduction in the case-load in order to do justice to those whom we did see and endeavoured to help by treatment, and also to allow for reasonable time for reflection, training and research work for those of us who had made this way of service our new way of life and who were not in private practice. We returned, in fact, to H.C.M.'s desideratum of 'quality first'. John Bowlby especially was more rigorous in adhering to his policy of restricting new patients to the number which could be handled and treated promptly by his department so as to eliminate a waiting list altogether. There was a waiting list for consultations, but not for therapy once a child and his parents had been seen. He also gave priority to children under five, who were seen without delay, because he felt that far more could be done for a young child and his mother in a shorter time than could be done for older children with already ingrained difficulties. The diagnostic procedure was also rather more elaborate than that hitherto used in Britain, but Bowlby felt that the greatly improved co-operation obtained from parents and referring agencies, such as schools, etc., produced greater efficiency in assessment and treatment. Thus the hitherto neglected step of seeing fathers at the time of diagnosis was given particular attention. As in the Adult Department, great care was taken with the preliminaries of explaining why we took an elaborate history and gave preliminary intelligence tests before the psychiatric interview.

This model of extended programme of investigation permits thorough work, as well as uniformly adequate records for research and training for younger staff members. The preparation by interviewing of both parents at the start paid off by excellent co-operation in treatment. Treatment itself was usually on a once-a-week basis, although a few children attended twice weekly. Quite early on the technique of the joint interview with child and mother or both parents was also undertaken. The method of training was not unlike that in the Adult Department. There were two weekly case conferences in each unit of the department, attended by the full team of the disciplines; there were four seminars a week on various aspects of child psychiatry and psychopathology, and one general department conference on general and theoretical problems of child psychiatry. In addition, each student – that is to say, registrar, junior psychologist or junior P.S.W. – received at least one hour's private tuition each week. Distinguished visitors were invited to take department conferences. Anna Freud and Donald Winnicott were among such guest teachers.

Both departments did what they could in the way of extramural training. For example, at the adult case conference visiting senior psychiatrists and medical officers of health would attend by invitation. Similarly, in the Children's Department there would be a number of visitors at the case conference. Special seminars were held by Miss Hunnybun and John Bowlby for almoners and other senior social workers not primarily in the psychiatric field. The open case conference was at the same time our medium for introducing our ideas and methods to distinguished overseas visitors.

Research

In the Children's Department 1948 saw the birth of two systematic research projects, both concerned with the investigation of events in early life believed to give rise to maladjustment and psychiatric illness. The first was the start of the study of the effects on young children of temporary separation from their mothers which had already been mooted in 1947, soon after John Bowlby joined us. The project began in March 1948, when James Robertson took up his appointment as the Halley Stewart Research Fellow. He came to us from Anna Freud's Hampstead Clinic, where he had worked as a P.S.W. Others recruited were Mary Salter Ainsworth, Rudolph Schaffer and Dinah Rosenbluth. The projects were planned with the help of Eric Trist and Dugmore Hunter, but stemmed from Bowlby's pre-war studies on juvenile delinquency. Because some of the work was concerned with reactions of children in hospital and on return home, an advisory committee was appointed of distinguished paediatricians, other hospital doctors and members of the nursing and social work professions. All these made important contributions to the success of the study which was conducted in various institutions to which this committee provided the entree and the sanction. An early example was the film 'A Two-Year Old Goes to Hospital' shot and commented on by Robertson. The project aimed at the validation of certain hypotheses concerning the origins of maladjustment which (as Bowlby said in his report), if proved false would require reorientation of all clinical work.

In the Adult Department research in a formal sense started in 1949. Henry Ezriel, already in charge of group therapy development, obtained a major grant from the U.S. Foundation

Fund for Research in Psychiatry. Under the aegis of the Institute who administered these monies, and with Eric Trist's initial help in design, there began his extended work of the validation of psychoanalytic interpretation both in groups and in individual therapy. Bion's influence played a part in this study. This resulted in a number of important papers.

The second research line in the Adult Department was in the field of marriage, where in 1949 Mary Luff and I began a pilot study of methods of helping couples in marital difficulties and breakdowns. This work was based on techniques learnt from group therapy: the sitting in of two therapists in a group, checking each other's observations and insights. Only in this case it was a special group of two, the married pair. These clinical observations and concepts resulted in a number of publications by myself, and are fully described in the recent volume entitled *Marital Tensions* (1967).

A third line of enquiry whilst we had certain staff members with us was in psychosomatic studies. The consultant in charge of these was, of course, Eric Wittkower, already distinguished in this field. He now joined the Dermatological Department of St Bartholomew's Hospital, but also inspired and supervised a small project on allergy in the Tavistock itself by our then Senior Registrar, Ronald Markillie, and to some extent also by Michael Balint, who joined our staff just about that time, having been attached previously in an honorary capacity.

In all these developments we congratulated ourselves on having separately incorporated the Tavistock Institute of Human Relations, because we were now enabled to receive research grants which were to increase in scope and magnitude as the Clinic developed its training and research work. For we were soon to discover that the 'honeymoon' with our Hospital Management Committee had come to an end, partly as the result of bureaucratic rigidity not uncommon in lower-tier administrations, but also because of the economic stringencies of the period, a stringency which has never disappeared from Health Service provisions.

General Developments

The Clinic's new Professional Committee, now separate from

T.I.H.R., was composed, according to our new formula of representation, of both departments and all disciplines. Thus Sutherland and Bowlby were present as the Director and Deputy Director, Bowlby also representing the Children's Department, with Dugmore Hunter as soon as he became a consultant. Kelnar and myself represented the Adult Department consultants, Noel Hunnybun the P.S.W.s and Constance Simmins and Herbert Phillipson psychology in each department. The new Professional Committee devised its own constitution, and took powers 'to arrange all the necessary therapeutic, educational and research work, to recommend candidates for staff appointments, to appoint sub-committees, and select future additional staff'. We had hoped in a memorandum around that time to appoint sixteen full-time psychiatrists for the Adult Department and an equivalent smaller number for the Children's Department, but we have never achieved this number. We also hoped to train young psychiatrists, not only as psychotherapists in addition to their analytic training, but also to give them experience in all the other aspects of medical work concerned with mental health.

The minutes of the Professional Committee over 1948–50 mostly read rather drearily: we are much concerned with raising various people to the status that they were led to expect at the beginning, we discuss interminably the fixing of salary scales and hours of work, and often argue with the Hospital Management Committee on such trivia as the entitlement of staff members to take paid leave to attend professional conferences. Budgets had to be prepared a long way ahead; surpluses from budgets which had been saved by good administration and small economies were ploughed back into Management Committee finances and did not accrue to our benefit, and so on. This kind of bureaucratic battle in which Sutherland and Bowlby were directly involved as officers of the Clinic went on sometimes for months and years and absorbed a lot of time and energy away from 'higher' things. The old informal administrative methods were a thing of the past. We had been accustomed to the administrators being on the same side as ourselves! By 1949, as we had feared, Dudley Herbert resigned the Secretaryship, as he could not tolerate so much bureaucratic frustration. Our new Administrator, Miss Hinks, was rated an assistant secretary by Management Committee seniority. Though based in the Clinic, she was made responsible not only for administering us, but also the Child Guidance Training Centre and the Marlborough Day Hospital. To the Central Middlesex Hospital Management Committee, among whom individual members were well disposed towards us initially, we must have seemed a difficult and argumentative cuckoo in the tidy hospital nest. Our intelligent interest in budgets and administration and what might be called industrial human relations must have seemed unusual to the H.M.C. They could not understand why we did not need a vast expenditure on drugs and other medical equipment or want white coats, but always wanted staff, including secretaries. But it must also be granted that they were generous to the library, compared with other institutions. The H.M.C.'s figure was £500 a year, added to the provision by the Tavistock Institute, which shared this as many other costs. The greatest battles always raged over N.H.S. attempts to postpone increases in establishment already voted to us on the plea of budget cuts.

By 1949, however, the Regional Board agreed to an establishment of four registrars (two in each department) and four senior registrars (likewise two in each department), as well as two half-time senior hospital medical officers, with the consultant strength fixed as on the appointed day. We insisted on having S.H.M.O.s, not because we wanted to have permanent sub-consultant psychiatrists on our staff, but because of the dearth of consultant vacancies for people trained along our lines. We anticipated a need to hold promising, well-trained men until they could get consultant appointments elsewhere or in the Clinic itself. In addition, we were also granted an establishment of trainee clinical psychologists in each department. This was a very great help to the development of 'dynamic' clinical psychology under Miss Simmins and Mr Phillipson, as the country as a whole had few such trained people in the late 1940s. The year 1949 saw the resumption of general practitioner courses. We held a large lecture course with a view to catching those interested in more intensive training. It was from the 90 to 100 who attended that we recruited the first seminar groups that were to become a permanent part of the Tavistock's work in upgrading the psychiatric skills of general practitioners and other medical officers.

In 1949 the Royal Medico-Psychological Association recognized the Tavistock as a school for the Diploma in Psychological Medicine for Part One (psychology) and Part Two (psychopathology). In that year also first contact was made with a marriage-counselling agency of the Family Welfare Organization run by Mrs Enid Eicholz (not yet Mrs Michael Balint!), who wanted technical assistance with training and supervision for their social workers running this so-called Family Discussion Bureau. The year also saw the first discussions on how to launch serious training for senior social workers and for clinical psychologists beyond the confines of our own staff. The Home Office approached us about the same time for a joint training plan for probation officers, to which we responded with eagerness. Sutherland joined their Training Committee, while I began a long attachment to the probation school, teaching marital conciliation work, which had been laid upon the probation service by the Denning Report of 1947. John Bowlby in the same year was called as a consultant to the World Health Organization to prepare his now famous report: *Maternal Care and Mental Health.* He spent five months with them.

The correlation of work and development between the Clinic and Institute was fostered as much as possible by joint staff meetings devoted to discussion of ongoing projects and preoccupations. The training panel which had been formed by the Professional Committee was broadened to include both Clinic and Institute, with the task of deciding on the content and quality of all training given in the total institution, on ways of determining training priorities for mental health personnel, and also to consider our public relations in training matters. We also instituted a newsletter to keep the increasingly differentiated staffs of the building in touch with the whole. The panel early on instituted appraisal sessions for mental-health films.

At this point we could already be seen as three federated institutions, each with a programme and a planning executive of its own. Two of the three were Government-controlled; the third was private and controlled by substantially the same

Council that had run all of us before 1948. The image of a unified whole was strong, not only because of the joint committees and conferences, but also because of the aspiration of moving towards a teaching and research institute for mental health. The new Institute was the repository of the 'old Tavi' dream. In practice each of these three rather large units was moving towards a period of differentiation in order to find its proper roles in the new post-war world, rather than towards closer integration. It was perhaps illusory to think that the closely-knit body which the Army group had been and wanted to perpetuate for its diversified activities by psychiatrists, psychologists, social-work experts, social psychologists, anthropologists, economists, and so on could be maintained indefinitely when their work roles and their means of making a living were becoming so diverse. In fact, during this stage we developed some quite sharp differences and conflicts over priorities in accommodation, funds, staffing and the like. In consequence, we developed a highly Puritan morality in dealing with each other. This rigorous ethic also made us one of the most conscientious and law-abiding of all the National Health Service units. No unit must have an extra room or secretary but that a sister unit would have credit for a similar accession next time – and so on. Perhaps it was the effort of devising adequate defences against fratricide that made us constantly brood over perfecting our internal social structure and means of communication. Social techniques as man's biological invention for survival?

Differentiation and Integration

The next year or two in the development of the total institution are of some importance. On the Clinic side we had established a working relationship to the Health Service and to the Central Middlesex Management Committee, which was not always easy. This adaptation depended a great deal on our success in substituting informal exchanges with the individual officers and members of the H.M.C. for formalized bureaucratic paper requests for finance and establishment. Such working contacts with this particular Management Committee were accomplished with fluctuating fortunes. There were certain personalities on the Management Committee who had little sympathy or understanding for our work, who regarded us as rather a *de luxe* institution with a vast staff and a not very impressive patient load compared with some of the big general hospitals under their care. The image of 'psychoanalysis' in the pejorative sense haunted them. However, in general we were beginning to see success in our requests for posts – for trainees, for adequate secretarial help and so on. We were gradually winning our right to continue what the Ministry had agreed was our role. This process was more successful in the Children's Department because of its outstanding reputation, and also because child psychiatry was not weighed down by the old mental-hospital tradition and origins. It was not questioned so widely inside the profession. Progress was more halting in the Adult Department, where we had yet to find our fully-sanctioned role within the total mental-health services as they were coming to be perceived with the growth of physical methods of treatment.

We had established a 'routine' therapeutic institution in both departments, but we had yet to find the optimal way of translating our newly-won conceptual integration of the sociological and the intrapersonal ('object-relations') aspects of the behavioural sciences into a nationally accepted approach to research, teaching and operations. We aspired to a better model for 'mental-health' work than the older and separate skills of what I once called 'hack psychotherapy' for our clinical work, or the kind of industrial and institutional research which had been carried on in the past which ignored the psychodynamics of interpersonal and intergroup relations and resistances.

A rather important meeting of the training panel took place in May 1950, when we considered the whole position of this work on the British scene. While Bowlby was able to speak of the high reputation of the Tavistock Clinic and Institute in the estimation of foreign – especially United States and French – sociological and psychiatric bodies, I had to warn the training panel that, unless we could maintain and implement our pioneering contributions, the new developing teaching centres in London and in the provinces would probably largely displace us in doing what we had been doing. Perhaps I was over-optimistic about the rate at which the now multiplying professorial departments in the schools of medicine (Leeds, Manchester, Glasgow, Newcastle, etc.) would take over the teaching of psychological medicine on principles which we had so consistently advocated since 1920, and so implement Crichton-Miller's original aim.

We concluded that the work of the Clinic and Institute could be seen as working towards a closer fusion, but only after a period of development in their respective fields. We now wanted to produce a document clarifying our concepts and the evidence on which they rested, which justified this integrative trend in our group. We tried to make this a fairly practical quest and asked ourselves questions such as: (*a*) Is a given type of skill urgently required? (*b*) Do we wish to train personnel in such skills here? (*c*) Can we afford the time, manpower and expenditure on training for this purpose? (*d*) Are we doing the given training in the right way? (*e*) What are our public relations in regard to the region, universities and other professional groups? We soon reached agreement on most of the headings, except perhaps for differences which had become obvious in the training of psychiatrists and lay therapists. I again had to point out the possible political repercussions on our standing within psychiatry if we appeared to give preference and impart much higher skills in psychotherapy and interpersonal and family relations work to lay students, such as psychologists and social workers, than to psychiatrists trained mainly in other institutions. This point, which frequently worried me, was closely related to the work of the Education Committee of the Royal Medico-Psychological Association, of which at this time I was a member. There was in British psychiatry less prejudice against training lay psychotherapists for children than for adults. In any case the whole problem of the value (and economics) of psychotherapy was once again under very considerable nationwide scrutiny. The overall psychiatric trend was back towards priority for psychosis, and hence the new and rapidly developing physical methods to be given in psychiatric in-patient units. This put psychotherapeutic theory and training into the shade.

After much discussion, we did, however, decide to set up new professional training for these lay child psychotherapists on an experimental basis, emphasizing that we wanted to select in the first instance persons fit to become teachers and research workers rather than routine therapists. We felt that the lack of economic incentive in the National Health Service for psychologists and social workers (even as compared to the modest opportunities offered in local authority services) was likely to be remedied only by us pioneering a very thorough training by which the emerging profession of child psychotherapy could be established and eventually require the weight to change the conditions of its employment and of its standing in the mental-health world. An Association for Child Psychotherapy had just been formed on the initiative of some members of the Tavistock, Miss Freud's Hampstead Clinic and Dr Loewenfeld's Institute of Child Psychology. These centres became the bodies first recognized as having suitable training standards in this field. John Bowlby was for some years the first Chairman of the Association's Medical Advisory Committee, composed of a representative group of child psychiatrists and attended by people from the Ministries of Health and Education. Bowlby also presided from the beginning over its Training Committee. The syllabus at the Tavistock was very like that for child psychiatric registrars. It included a personal analysis, intensive casework under supervision, many theoretical and practical seminars, the study of normal infants in relation to their mothers, in play-groups and so forth, all of which appear in the syllabus of our training prospectus to this day. The earliest tutor in this field, apart from the P.S.W.s, psychologists and psychiatrists, was Mrs E. Bick, who later left us and was replaced by Mrs M. Harris, one of our original students, still with us as the senior teacher in this course.

Turning now to child psychiatry, agreement was much more easily reached by the training panel on the desirability of training doctors in this field. The question of providing superficial extra-mural experience at D.P.M. level was relegated to secondary importance. We discussed rather whether the training provided in a one-year course, which had so far been all that we had offered to psychiatrists, really qualified a doctor to call himself a specialist in child psychiatry, notwithstanding the fact that many child guidance clinics were run by doctors without even that much specialized training. The problems of what constituted a well-trained psychiatrist were reviewed, and there was some division of opinion about the wisdom and safety of training only to the level hitherto given to medical child guidance Fellows. It was felt that this amount of child psychiatry should be the *minimum* demanded of *every* psychiatrist, whereas a specialist child psychiatrist should be deemed to command not only all-round diagnostic skill, but at least the same therapeutic skill as the lay child psychotherapist. The aim of the Tavistock should certainly be towards the training of specialists in child psychiatry capable of the full range of activities in their field. We hoped that in this way we would have a strong impact on child psychiatry in the country. It was decided to prepare a memorandum which would clearly define the value of, and the differences between, the present so-called 'child guidance' work and the higher forms of specialism at which we were aiming for those who could call themselves fully-qualified child psychiatrists.

We next turned to the consideration of psychiatric social work training, which, it will be recalled, had hitherto been limited to a few months in the year for students seconded from the London School of Economics Mental Health Course. Here again we felt that the level to which P.S.W.s had so far been trained by us should be that which *every* social worker, not specialists in psychiatric casework, should reach. We were feeling our way towards a more advanced course for more senior or post-graduate training, and ceasing our under-graduate P.S.W. training, which had occupied a great deal of staff time so far. We hoped to substitute for it a new course under the leadership of Miss Hunnybun, with contributions not only from the clinicians, but also from the Institute of Human Relations. For this higher 'generic casework' training we would take both P.S.W.s and other qualified social workers in responsible posts. The decision was not taken at this meeting, but here was the germ of what has now become one of the major contributions of the Tavistock Clinic to the training of probation officers, P.S.W. tutors, senior almoners, child-care officers, and in some instances health visitors for their community roles as teachers of their own subjects in their own fields.

Similarly, we now began our differentiation between the work of what had hitherto been called educational psychologists and the emerging specialty of clinical psychologists. We agreed that we were probably the only Clinic in the country with a large and diverse enough case material to undertake such training upon lines of psychodynamic theory. We knew that there would be difficulties in devising establishments and financial opportunities for trainees in this emergent field, in view of the chronic freeze in N.H.S. expenditure, but we were prepared to consider even substitution of salaries saved from one department for use in another, and various other ways of attracting trainees and support for them in so far as they were not able to finance themselves. At any rate, this specialty in our view demanded very high priority. It was resolved to ask Sutherland to explore this question with the professors of psychology in the colleges of London University. The clinical psychology course was to be one of two years, with alternating experience in both the children's and the adult field, incorporating not only testing, but especially the meaning of testing in terms of personality development and psychopathology in closest association with the psychiatrists in our clinical units, to which such psychology students would be attached under the supervision of the senior psychologist of each department.

In the field of adult psychiatric or psychotherapeutic training for doctors there was less discussion, since the programme already described in earlier pages was essentially that which we had adopted and which consisted, as mentioned, of personal analysis of the trainee together with intensive individual and group-therapy experience under supervision, supplemented by seminars and attendance at staff meetings, etc. The panel now considered mainly a course of a more elementary kind which had been developed to meet the expressed demand of the psychiatric trainee group in our region. This course we called at this stage the Elementary Psychotherapy Course. A number of us provided part-time experience in the field of group observation, together with a didactic/therapeutic group for the students, in which they could experience in themselves some of the psychodynamic mechanisms seen in patient groups, and rounded off with theoretical discussion of the psychopathological issues involved. The course was slanted mainly at those whose main work would lie in the field of mental-hospital psychiatry with out-patient duties. At the beginning we had opened this experience also to P.S.W. and clinical psychology students, but the wisdom of this soon became questionable, and we decided to confine this part-time course to young psychiatrists in training at other institutions. This rich experience was to be concentrated into one afternoon and evening a week.

In this connection we also discussed the whole principle of extra-mural training and the priorities to be assigned to different groups of workers in the mental health field. We had given an embarrassingly successful and over-subscribed course for general practitioners on classical lecture/discussion lines. The feedback from it disclosed a vast need for more experience in the psychodynamic field on the part of general practitioners. In the light of this and similar popularity of all our teaching events open to outsiders, we decided that extra-mural teaching was an important part of our claim to recognition as an institute for mental health, even though the first priority always belonged to the internal training of specialists. The meeting favoured more intensive teaching in small groups or seminars to key people, rather than lectures to large numbers. The open conference or lecture course was felt to be worthwhile chiefly for the purpose of introducing the broad principles of our work to a considerable number of interested enquirers; it was to be looked upon as a 'trailer' for viewing the 'real film' at some future time. We noted a suggestion from T.I.H.R. for following up some of these open conferences or lecture courses with short summer schools for various professions. We adopted the idea of open conferences for all-comers, especially those from far away, not to be viewed as training, but merely as communication with them. We also adopted the idea of publishing henceforward an annual syllabus of training offered at the Tavistock, both for internal students (that is to say, registrars and junior staff members in established posts at the Clinic) and extra-murally. We finally laid down a scale of fees payable to the Hospital

Management Committee for teaching given by staff in Clinic time; and also for fees which might be charged for work done outside normal working hours, out of which teachers could be remunerated.

The training panel also adopted the syllabus for two rather highly specialized courses. The first was that for speech therapists under Dr Leopold Stein, which was in great demand and would be limited to five or six selected post-graduates each year. Secondly, we also adopted principles for specialized training in projective techniques for advanced students and for beginners under the direction of Miss Theodora Alcock, who had already been teaching our internal students and was internationally known in this field. This also became henceforth, with some modifications, a regular feature of the Tavistock's extra-mural work which passed more firmly under the aegis of the Institute, helped by the Clinic's psychological staff.

This, then, was the outline of what has become, with our Management Committee's consent, our teaching programme. The Tavistock in its new situation in the N.H.S. found itself in quite a difficult and challenging position. On the one hand there were the high expectations on the part of the mental-health professions in general for our training in our skills and approach. We were in constant demand for a seminar here, a lecture there. We had many native as well as foreign professional groups visit us, from midwives to Dutch forensic psychiatrists, for all of whom 'a show had to be laid on'. The learned societies too wanted to hear us. We were torn between the priorities of such different international and national demands within our budgetary and manpower limitations, which meant selection and regretful refusals. On the other hand, we were also under pressure by our administrators to confine ourselves to the narrower role of a 'treatment' clinic and turn in higher figures for patient attendances, rather than divert so much effort to activity appropriate to an academic institution. We were, however, clear, despite occasional pleadings, that we would continue the pattern of thorough therapy by those methods in which we were skilled, and not 'dilute' our effort by offering what we called a 'Class B' out-patient service. Dispensing drugs, short reassurance and suggestion, electroplexy and other physical methods could be done elsewhere, and, while relieving, did not deal with the patients' life situations or internal dynamics. These could be shown to have a high relapse rate, and we saw the failures and the pleas for 'real' help.

Within our own group there could be said to be two schools of thought in the training panel, of which I represented one, although not alone. My view was that we needed to cement our influence and good relationships, not only with psychiatry, but with many other institutions. In furtherance of this notion, I obtained leave in 1950 to work with Harvard University Social Relations Department and the Rand Corporation Social Science Division in the United States for six months in socio-psychiatric research on Soviet Russian behaviour, which resulted in a number of publications. I felt such secondments balanced our preoccupation with the internal integration of the Clinic's special work. For the same reason, several of us, including Ben S. Morris and myself, were frequently in Paris as consultants to the now growing U.N.E.S.C.O. Social Science Division, contributing especially to the so-called Tensions Project of that period. The wish to export our insights made me accept in 1951 the invitation to become the Chairman of the panel of medical advisers to the National Association for Mental Health, which had been constituted to replace their previous one-man medical directorship.

Our trend towards, perhaps unconsciously, favouring social work and clinical psychology at some expense to our relationship to psychiatry seemed fairly well marked to my mind. We were probably right in so far as the training in these disciplines was to assume very great importance in the future with the as yet scarcely visible shadow of the coming emphasis on community health services and the rest which belongs to the Mental Health Act of 1959, to the Younghusband Committee and other endeavours of the late 1950s and early 1960s. After all, we had been warned off training psychiatrists by Sir Francis Fraser. The staff as a whole were concentrated very much on differentiating themselves into skilled, applied psychoanalysts. The Psycho-Analytic Society was exerting a very considerable pull on the allegiances of many of our medical staff members as well as on our registrars and senior registrars because of the concurrent analytic training. None the less, our interprofessional Clinic-Institute integration of the social sciences with the newer object-relations theories of Klein and Fairbairn produced a distinctive Tavistock climate and orientation, which I gathered even led to some difficulties for some of our members in their relations to the Institute of Psychoanalysis.

In the rival pulls between our 'academic' functions and the disinclination of the N.H.S. to favour these, it was becoming clear that for our research and training activities we would have to rely more heavily on the Tavistock Institute. The latter was free to receive grants of any kind to be spent on clinical teaching and research. The first of such major donations (since the original Rockefeller grant of 1946–7) came in the sum of £3,000 from the International Children's Centre in Paris in October 1950 for furthering Bowlby's and Robertson's work on separation studies in the Children's Department. In the adult field research, if it could be so described, was largely of the workshop kind, in which we tried to analyse and consolidate our experience with groups, including selection of patients and results obtained. This is more properly described as development of therapeutic techniques. The only specific time allotted to research during this phase was the part-time employment of a promising psychologist on work towards personality measurement. This was Dr Joseph Sandler, who spent some creative years with us in the course of his developing career, which resulted, for example, in his psychodynamic personality inventory. Sandler's appointment was financed by a downward revision of the number of P.S.W.s required for the Adult Department after the closure of our patients' Club, as already recorded.

Here, then, is an account of our first few years in the Health Service. Our fight to secure our right to develop the kind of staff and activities we felt important had the effect of strengthening the awareness of our interdependence with our Institute. It was a time mainly of introversion of both the Institute and the Clinic, each trying to work out their own identities, in which the Children's Department was without doubt both happiest and quickest off the mark, perhaps because it had the clearest natural boundaries and also the largest support in public recognition of its field of therapy, teaching and research.

IX

The Tavistock Institute of Human Relations

by Sidney G. Gray

Origin in the Tavistock Clinic

The history of the Tavistock Institute of Human Relations begins with that of the Tavistock Clinic, as Henry Dicks has shown. There were always certain characteristics deeply rooted in the Clinic which made the birth of the Institute almost inevitable. Studies of the incidence and frequency of psychological illness had made clear that its treatment was time-consuming, difficult and uncertain once the illness had been fully established.

The policy of the Clinic had therefore become focused on four principles: First, to select appropriate cases for *treatment*, since it was at that time necessary to demonstrate that improvement and recovery were possible in a group of illnesses which, if not ignored, had by prevailing medical opinion been ascribed to purely genetic or physio-pathological causes. Secondly, to carry out *research* into aetiology as a means of devising, thirdly, methods of *prevention* in which, finally, *training* could be made available to a much wider range of professions and groups in the community than were reached by traditional medical education. For this reason, parents, teachers, magistrates, probation officers and other social workers, general practitioners, industrial medical officers and others were concerned.

The Emergence of the Institute from the War Experience

When the Second World War broke out, those who were then at the Tavistock Clinic knew from nearly twenty years' experience the social implications of their work and the wide range of social factors which tended to produce the conditions which the Clinic existed to treat. They had developed a viewpoint, therefore, which made them quick to recognize the needs and opportunities which mobilization created and took the initiative in bringing them to the attention of the Government. While new and economical forms of social therapy were developed to suit the opportunities and volume of work under service conditions, prevention included not only the examination, but where possible the change of the circumstances contributing to breakdown. Extension of this work included the planning and development of schemes of personnel selection for both officers and men and the establishment of new military institutions to carry them out; similarly, with regard to schemes of service training, of the civil resettlement of repatriated prisoners-of-war, and the development of therapeutic communities as points of transition for those who had suffered breakdown.

In these activities psychologists and psychiatrists became associated with a group of social scientists, particularly sociologists and anthropologists, whose skills complemented the resources of psychology and psychiatry. This enlarged group held that the combined approach to practical problems which they had helped to develop under service conditions was applicable also to the problems of a peacetime community. Since many of the psychiatric members of the group had been on the staff of the Tavistock Clinic, it was decided to establish from a base in that Clinic a small group to carry on interdisciplinary work. This development was chosen by the late Dr Alan Gregg, Director of the Medical Sciences Division of the Rockefeller Foundation – whose initiative had led also to the establishment of the Department of Social Relations at Harvard – for substantial support by his Foundation. (It was the Rockefeller Foundation which had supported the pre-war psychosomatic studies of A. T. M. Wilson.) Their grant, together with two anonymous donations, made it possible to found the Institute of Human Relations as a new activity deriving from social psychiatry under the aegis of the Council of the Tavistock Clinic. The aims of the new Institute, however, went beyond the boundaries of medicine. At the outset there existed a close relationship with the Research Centre for Group Dynamics – then at the Massachusetts Institute of Technology and later at the University of Michigan – and with its Director, the late Dr Kurt Lewin. A quarterly journal, *Human Relations*, which rapidly acquired a world-wide circulation and is now (1970) in its twenty-third volume, was established under the joint editorial responsibility of the Tavistock Institute and of the Research Centre for Group Dynamics.

Differentiation of the Institute from the Clinic

These developments were possible within the framework of the Clinic because it was run by a voluntary non-profit association (which still exists and is now known as the Tavistock Institute of Medical Psychology). The emergence as part of its activities of an Institute of Human Relations was seen as a natural development of the original aims of this body and presented no constitutional problem. Once a National Health Service Act was envisaged, it became evident that the therapeutic work of the Tavistock Clinic could logically become part of the Service, and the Council decided to prepare the Clinic for entry into it. Since it was equally clear that the research, training and development activities of the new Institute went beyond the scope of the Act, they also decided to incorporate, as a separate non-profit association, the Tavistock Institute of Human Relations. The Institute was incorporated in September 1947, and the Clinic entered the National Health Service in July 1948.

The seven members of the Council of the Clinic who signed as founder members the Memorandum and Articles of Association of the Tavistock Institute of Human Relations were: Dr L. F. Browne, Mr W. L. Farrer, Dr G. R. Hargreaves, Mr I. J. Pitman (now Sir James Pitman), Colonel R. S. Rait Kerr, Dr J. R. Rees and Lady Whyte. None were employees of the Council. These members formed the original Council of the Institute, though they soon added to their numbers. At the first Council meeting Colonel R. S. Rait Kerr was elected Chairman and for the first ten years he and Dr Leonard Browne alternated as Chairman and Deputy Chairman.

One of the first tasks which confronted the new Council was to work out a form of organization which would give the social scientists who were to be employed the greatest degree of participation in policy-making and financial management consistent with the maintenance of overall legal responsibility by the Council. With this object in view, the Council appointed a Standing Committee and the professional staff elected a Management Committee, and for some time the two bodies held joint meetings. The principle of the devolution of responsibility which was then embarked on as a wholly experimental measure has proved very successful; and the present-day structure of the Institute, with its five largely independent units, the staff of which report through their own sub-councils to the Council, owes much to the wisdom of those who laid the early foundations on which the Institute was built.

The first Management Committee of the Institute elected by a professional staff of twelve consisted of Ben Morris, Chairman (now Professor and Director of Bristol University Institute of Education), John Harvard-Watts (now Managing Director of Tavistock Publications Ltd.), Elliott Jaques (now Professor and Head of the School of Social Sciences, Brunel University), A. T. M. Wilson (now Professor of Organizational Behaviour at the London Graduate School of Business Studies), and the Secretary of the Institute.

In the elections a year later Eric Trist (now Professor of Organizational Theory at the Graduate School of Business Administration, University of California, Los Angeles) replaced Harvard-Watts, who had meanwhile become Chairman of the newly-formed Tavistock Publications Ltd.

The Management Committee met weekly and in the first two or three years the whole professional staff met almost as often. It was the practice to discuss major policy issues fully with the staff, and it was not at all unusual for a whole day, and sometimes two successive days, to be set aside for this purpose. Later, with the growth of staff and project commitments, such meetings became increasingly difficult to arrange. They were replaced by quarterly staff meetings, the main purpose of which was a review of current activities and exchange of information. The Management Committee, which continued to meet weekly, had as a result to take more direct responsibility in matters of policy.

The Work of the Institute

At first the new Institute was mainly concerned with discovering opportunities for its work and in giving organizations the chance to assess the competence of its staff to assist them with their problems. From the outset, the Institute's approach to research was problem-centred and involved a professional responsibility towards the 'client' organization.

In the first four years seventy projects were undertaken, ranging in size from a single discussion and report to work extending over three years. From 1948 onwards, however, the Institute became increasingly engaged in a programme of research initiated by the Human Factors Panel (under Sir George Schuster) of the Committee on Industrial Productivity which reported to the Lord President of the Council. There were two main projects: the first, led by Elliott Jaques, was an intensive study of the psychological and social forces affecting the group life, morale and productivity of a single industrial community; the second, led by A. T. M. Wilson, was a study of communications in industry which was undertaken with the collaboration of a number of firms together representing a wide range of industries. Concurrently, a training programme provided opportunity for young graduates from trade unions to receive research experience and training in a social-science approach to industrial problems. Although it was envisaged that they would return to the movement on completion of their training, none actually did so. For a time this programme of work for the Government represented, in staff time and finance, over half of the Institute's activities. Although most of the remaining work was widely spread, there was also emerging some programmed research for industrial clients.

The ending of the productivity research programme in 1951 was followed by a difficult transitional period in which staff had to be redeployed and other sources of finance sought. The most ready source was found in developing programmed research for one or two clients, which became focused on the adaptation for industrial purposes of selection and training methods earlier developed in a military setting.

Later on, studies were undertaken on the organization of work groups, e.g. in coal-mining, aimed towards the formulation of new principles of work organization. This led to a programme of research begun in 1954 under the direction of Eric Trist, which was financed initially by the Conditional Aid programme and later by the Department of Scientific and Industrial Research. A parallel research programme in India, led by A. K. Rice, made comparison possible between work in developed and underdeveloped countries. This work in particular demonstrated that it is possible to redesign a socio-technical system in manufacturing industry so as to satisfy simultaneously the technologist as well as the human needs and constraints.

By this time the Institute was well enough established in the consulting field so that more projects began to emerge which opened up the possibility of more structured research programmes, e.g. Eric Miller's study of the process of decision-making with Richard Thomas and Baldwin Ltd. during the building of their Spencer works.

This pattern has persisted, so that over much of the Institute's life there have been concurrently consulting research (specific projects carried out for particular clients), programmed research (also for clients, but in the form of a continuous programme), and sponsored research (priority being given to scientific purposes and finance derived from non-specific grants or from the Institute's own limited reserves).

In keeping with the tradition of the Tavistock Clinic, the Tavistock Institute of Human Relations has from the outset developed research and training alongside its professional services. Not only has the professional relationship been the means of establishing conditions for research: it has also provided the field experience which is an essential ingredient of the Institute's training methods. It is in this way that new staff have been introduced and equipped to share in the responsibility for the management of the Institute's affairs and the planning of its future development.

Inevitably, however, demands were made upon the Institute

to impart far more widely the principles underlying its approach to problems, its techniques, its experience. These took the form of invitations to staff to take part in meetings and conferences, national and international, for scientific and professional people and often for a wider interested public; to take part in broadcast programmes; and to visit universities overseas, particularly in the U.S.A. It was particularly difficult to meet this need during the early years when the Institute was preoccupied with its survival and development, though from the first some invitations in all these categories were accepted, particularly where the participation of Institute staff was felt to have greatest potential, as in the *planning* of special courses and conferences for other organizations.

It was not until 1957, however, that the Institute, jointly with the University of Leicester, launched the first full-scale experiment in Britain with the 'laboratory' method of training in group relations. The original concept of the Leicester Conference owed much to the experience of group psychotherapy pioneered by the Tavistock Clinic and reinforced by the contributions of social psychology and sociology. American experience, notably at the National Training Laboratory in Group Development at Bethel, Maine, had naturally an important influence, but the Leicester Conference was designed to meet the demand for a course of training which harnessed the new knowledge and understanding about groups, yet was rooted in British experience.

Since that first Conference in 1957, ten more have been jointly organized by the Institute and the University of Leicester. Many other conferences and courses have been run by the Institute alone, and still others by the Institute in collaboration with other bodies. In addition to these residential conferences, several courses have been run by the Institute, consisting of weekly events spread over six months. Much of this work is described in *Learning for Leadership* (Rice, 1965).

Tavistock Publications Ltd.

At the same time as the incorporation of the Institute was under discussion, much thought was also being given to the provision of outlets for publications. In those days a social science list was scarcely to be found in publishers' prospectuses. The problem of producing and marketing publications which were expected to result from the Institute's work was the subject of many lengthy discussions. Most of the staff then believed that the most satisfactory solution was to create a company with the specific purpose of publishing social science work. Those who favoured this plan felt that it would not only provide an automatic outlet for Tavistock books and papers, but would also meet the needs of others working in the social science field. In this way it was thought that a list could be established large enough to make an independent company viable. Others doubted the viability of such an organization and felt that it would be better for the Institute either to publish in its own name or to enter into a working relationship with one or two established publishers.

The staff view prevailed and Tavistock Publications Ltd. was incorporated on 28 October 1947, the Memorandum of Association having been signed by Mr J. Harvard-Watts – the Company's first Chairman and still the Managing Director – and Dr J. D. Sutherland, then recently appointed Medical Director of the Tavistock Clinic.

The Company took over publication on behalf of the Institute of the quarterly journal, *Human Relations*, but it was not until 1951 that the first full-length book, *The Changing Culture of a Factory*, by Elliott Jaques, was published. By that time the Company had entered into an association, which lasted for only two years, with Routledge & Kegan Paul Ltd. When the Company resumed independent operation in 1953 it had already built up an impressive list of forthcoming titles. Not all of these reached the stage of a finished manuscript, but the Company was able to publish a good many of them and to establish a high reputation in the field of social-science publishing.

Despite financial support from the Institute and individuals, the Company continued to experience the constraints imposed by the shortage of working capital, and efforts to remedy this situation were hampered by the fact that books did not come along fast enough to permit a scale of operation which would secure the future of the Company or financial investment in it.

The decision had to be taken, not without misgivings, to seek a merger with a larger company. As a result of negotiations with a number of interested publishers extending over many months, the Company's engagements were finally transferred in 1959 to Sweet & Maxwell Ltd., who have preserved the Tavistock imprint. This proved a very successful development, and Tavistock Publications Ltd., as a subsidiary of Associated Book Publishers Ltd., now publishes some forty books a year in the social sciences and related fields.

Emergence of the Clinic-linked Activities as a School of Family Psychiatry and Community Mental Health

From 1952 onwards the Institute began increasingly to be concerned with activities developing from the Clinic. Grants were received to enable the Institute to carry out programmes both of research and training in the mental health field. A major programme of research, led by John Bowlby, into the early social development of children and a number of smaller programmes were supported. Grants were made to assist training not only in the relevant specialties, but also in other professions where extensive preventive mental-health work is possible if new skills are imparted.

Among the generous supporters of this work were the World Health Organization, the International Children's Centre, the Josiah Macy, Jr., Foundation, the Field Foundation, the Ford Foundation, the Grant Foundation, the Old Dominion Foundation, and the Foundations' Fund for Research in Psychiatry. More recently, clinical research has also been supported by such British bodies as the Sir Halley Stewart Trust, the Mental Health Research Fund, the Medical Research Council, and the Mellanby and Southfield Trusts; and training by the Gulbenkian Foundation and the Joseph Rowntree Memorial Trust.

The launching of pilot services has also been an important feature of the work in this sphere. A notable example was the setting-up of an Adolescent Unit, based in the Clinic, where the attempt was made to develop a new psychological approach to the special problems of adolescents, hitherto only partially met by the methods and services available for adults and for children. This proved a successful development, leading to the establishment of an Adolescent Department of the Clinic, now largely staffed by National Health Service personnel.

The Institute of Marital Studies

One of the pilot services with which the Institute was concerned from the very beginning and which has now developed into a separate unit of the Institute is the Institute of Marital Studies, which for the first twenty years of its existence was known as the Family Discussion Bureau.

Public concern about the rising divorce rate led to the setting up in 1947 of the Denning Committee, which advocated the development of a State-sponsored marriage welfare service. In the event, the Government acted on the recommendation of the Harris Committee of 1948 to give support to three voluntary organizations which offered marriage counselling services and trained workers in this field. One of these organizations was the Family Welfare Association, whose earlier role had been largely taken over by the post-war social security and welfare services.

The Family Welfare Association, in collaboration with staff of the Tavistock Institute of Human Relations, created the Family Discussion Bureau to provide facilities both for those who sought help with their own marital problems and for those professional workers who were aware that marital difficulties played a part in many of the problems with which they were called upon to deal in the course of their work. The Family Discussion Bureau was always essentially a social casework agency, but with working links with the Tavistock Institute and Clinic, which provided consultation and the possibility of more direct psychiatric help in cases where the severity of the problem required medical treatment.

The widespread and growing need for help with marital problems led other organizations to develop branches throughout the country and to recruit more 'counsellors' to cope with the rising tide of referrals. The Family Discussion Bureau approached the problem in a different way. The experience of caseworkers soon made it clear that underlying marital difficulties were a significant factor in a wide range of problems, about which professional workers in widely varying fields were consulted. It was also clear that the greatest hope of resolving marital problems occurred when they were diagnosed and professional help was offered at an early stage. These were among the considerations which led the Family Discussion Bureau to concentrate on the provision of training facilities for the helping professions, while maintaining its own expertise at a high level.

In keeping with the Tavistock approach, research and training was based on the casework service, limited in size, which the Bureau maintained for couples, many of whom were referred to it by doctors and other professional workers, though there has always been a number of couples applying direct to the Bureau for help.

Because of the close association with the Tavistock, it was decided in 1956 that the Family Discussion Bureau should be transferred from the Family Welfare Association to the Tavistock Institute. It became one of the growing number of 'clinic-linked' activities of the Institute, and in 1967 it became an independent unit. It was decided in 1968 to adopt the new title of the Institute of Marital Studies as being more appropriate to the essential and growing importance of its training role. Its functions are complementary to those of the Clinic's N.H.S. operational marital unit.

The Institute for Operational Research

It was in keeping with the Institute's many-pronged approach to problems that it should extend its range of disciplines to include operational research. Equally, operational research workers had felt the need for closer collaboration with the social sciences. As a result of discussions between the Council of the Operational Research Society and the Council of the Tavistock Institute, it was decided to set up a new Institute for Operational Research as a unit of the Tavistock. The new Institute came into being on 1 May 1963 with the appointment of the first Director, Neil Jessop, whose untimely death in 1969 was a tragic loss to the Institute for Operational Research and to the Tavistock generally. In the first six years Neil Jessop has built up a strong, viable institution, with a permanent staff of twenty and a programme of work for some years ahead which will tax its resources to the full and make further expansion an urgent necessity. John Stringer, Neil Jessop's able Deputy Director for many years, has been appointed the new Director.

The Development of Internal Organization

During the first decade of the Institute's history, in which the general pattern of activities was being established, no new members were added to the professional Management Committee. Indeed, it had contracted through the loss of Ben Morris, who left in 1950 to become Director of the National Foundation for Educational Research, and of Elliott Jaques, who left at the end of 1951 to take up an appointment at the Glacier Metal Co. Ltd., where he had done a great deal of his research as a Tavistock member. A. T. M. Wilson became Chairman of the Management Committee, following the resignation of Morris, and he remained Chairman until he left the Institute in May 1958, when his place was taken by E. L. Trist. It was not until October 1956 that two additional members, H. Bridger and A. K. Rice, were appointed to the Committee.

Similarly, the Council had suffered attrition over the years, and by 1956 there were only seven members. The Council then proceeded to strengthen its own membership by several additions, the most notable of which were Sir Hugh Beaver (at that time President of the Federation of British Industries) and Professor E. H. Phelps Brown of the London School of Economics. Sir Hugh Beaver became Chairman of Council in 1957 and Dr Browne and Colonel Rait Kerr became Deputy Chairmen, offices which they held until their deaths in 1960 and 1961 respectively. Professor Phelps Brown succeeded them as Deputy Chairman.

There began for the Institute a process, extending over many years, of adaptation to the needs of a changed internal and external situation. The traditional sources of the Institute's income, and in particular grants from American foundations, were diminishing, and it was clear that new sources of support more firmly rooted in the United Kingdom must be sought. Important for these considerations was the Institute's position in relation to the university world. Although from the outset there had been collaborative relationships with university departments, and university staff had served on Council, the interdisciplinary nature of so much of the Institute's work had justified the Institute's remaining independent of the universities. Some aspects of its work more than others, however, could only hope for permanent financial support by becoming part of the university system; and in other fields the academic standing of the Institute was important if it was to compete for scarce resources.

One of the first steps which was taken under the leadership of Sir Hugh Beaver was the considerable enlargement of the Council to include distinguished representatives of science, the professions, industry and the community generally. At the same time it was recognized that, if this step was to succeed, there must also be major revision of the internal organization to take account of the widely disparate activities and the need for self-determination for those who were responsible for driving forward in their respective fields.

With the differentiation of the clinic-linked activities as a School of Family Psychiatry and Community Mental Health, and the Family Discussion Bureau as a separate unit, the original work of the Institute became the responsibility of a Committee on Human Resources, Organization and Social Change, composed of the senior professional staff and replacing the Management Committee. Following considerable expansion in the period 1962–6, the work of this Committee was taken over by two separate units, the Human Resources Centre and the Centre for Applied Social Research each with its own staff executive. Thus, with the Institute for Operational Research, there are now five virtually autonomous units within the Tavistock Institute of Human Relations. In addition to the operating units, there is a central administrative staff of seventeen, which provides services for the Council and various common services for the units. One of the responsibilities of the central administration is the maintenance jointly with the Tavistock Clinic, of a Library covering a wide range of the social sciences as well as of social and psychological medicine. It owns about 6,500 books, 6,000 offprints and pamphlets and 2,500 bound volumes of periodicals and receives approximately 200 journals annually. Library membership comprises over 300 staff, students and visiting scientists. The total cost of the Library, excluding accommodation, is at present of the order of £5,000 per annum, to which the National Health Service contributes about £2,000 per annum.

The major reorganization of the Institute, which had been guided over several years by Sir Hugh Beaver, received formal approval by the Council in November 1966, when Sir Hugh Beaver – only two months before his death – handed over Chairmanship to Professor E. H. Phelps Brown, who had worked with him as Deputy Chairman for five years.

No one could have been better fitted than Professor Phelps Brown for the task of guiding the Institute through the period of adaptation to its new organization and helping it to grasp the opportunities to which it was now better equipped to respond. Professor Phelps Brown had intimated at the outset that he was only in a position to accept office as Chairman for a period of two years, but during that time he did a great deal to ensure successful implementation of the new structure.

The Institute is now governed by a Council of forty members under the Chairmanship of Lord Fulton. Of these thirty-three have been appointed to sub-councils, of which there are five, each being responsible to Council for the work of one of the five units.

During the twenty-two years of its existence the Institute's whole-time professional and scientific staff has risen from twelve at the outset to about seventy at the present time. In addition, there have always been staff employed on short-term contracts or for a small proportion of their time or in a consulting capacity, and there have been many attachments from a few weeks to a year or more of scientific personnel from overseas.

The School of Family Psychiatry and Community Mental Health has a number of paid staff, though most are part-time. This is, however, no indication of the extent of its activities.

Some of the work, whether of training or research, is carried on by those partly, or even wholly, employed within the National Health Service (not all of them on the Tavistock staff); and the Institute's resources are used for the employment of professional and secretarial assistance, for the provision of accommodation and facilities of various kinds, and for the award of fellowship grants to enable students to undertake the specialized training which the Institute and Clinic together offer.

The growth in numbers of staff does not of itself indicate the considerable movement into the universities from the Institute. Of particular significance is the fact that twenty-four members of the staff have, on leaving the Institute, taken up university appointments; and two members of the present staff concurrently hold professorships, one in Rotterdam and one in California.

In addition to the advanced professional training provided at the Institute, eight graduate members of the staff have been awarded a Ph.D. degree for work carried out at the Institute.

The Sharing of Accommodation

When the Clinic first moved into its Beaumont Street premises in 1945 there was a good deal more space than was immediately required. There was, therefore, plenty of room for the new Institute of Human Relations when it was established in 1946. At that time it was possible to allocate to the Institute the top two floors of the building and naturally, since the Institute was part of the Clinic, it shared in many common facilities, such as the refectory in the basement, the Library on the second floor and rooms for lectures and seminars.

Under Section 6 of the National Health Service Act, 1946, premises forming part of a voluntary hospital or used for the purposes of a voluntary hospital became vested in the Minister of Health from the appointed day. Thus, on 6 July 1948 the lease of Nos 2–4, Beaumont Street, having forty-six years unexpired, ceased to belong to the Clinic. The Act, however, made provision for an apportionment of interests in premises used partly for the purposes of a hospital and partly for other purposes. The Institute, which by this time was separately incorporated, gave notice to the Minister of a claim for apportionment of the lease in respect of that part of the premises which it occupied. As the lease was originally in the name of the Clinic, the deed of apportionment, which, after long negotiation, was eventually concluded in 1955, involved the three parties concerned. Under this deed the Minister acknowledged that the Institute occupied, in terms of value rather than of area, approximately one-quarter of the building at the appointed day. The Minister acquired the Institute's quarter share for the sum of £5,000 and granted a new sub-lease to the Institute to run for the remainder of the term of the original lease.

In the course of the years during which these negotiations proceeded both the Clinic and Institute had expanded and a number of adjustments had been made. The Library had been transferred to the larger room on the top floor, and by means of partitioning a number of extra rooms were provided, both for the Clinic and the Institute.

Already by the mid-1950s the need for more space had become acute, particularly on the Clinic side. At about this time a Liaison Committee was established between the Institute and the North-west Metropolitan Regional Hospital Board, primarily to promote knowledge and understanding of the activities of the Clinic and Institute and their interrelation. The reports of these activities and of their need to expand brought early recognition from the Regional Hospital Board of the need for enlarged and improved accommodation. The Liaison Committee began the task of preparing proposals for the enlargement of the establishment of the Clinic and estimates of the future size of the staff of the Institute, together with schedules indicating in considerable detail the number and size of rooms required by both bodies. An important milestone in these negotiations was a meeting at the Ministry of Health in October 1957, at which the Ministry agreed in principle to the provision of a new building to accommodate both the Clinic *and the Institute*. This decision gave official recognition to the value which the Clinic and Institute derived from working in the closest proximity. It was not until February 1960 that the Minister of Health announced in the House of Commons that a new Tavistock Clinic building was to be erected as part of a hospital building programme; and in a separate communication to the Institute it was confirmed that accommodation for the Institute would be available in the new building. A project team was then set up by the Regional Hospital Board, on which the Institute was represented, whose task was to work out with the architects and engineers the detailed plans for the new building.

The National Health Service authorities had shown imagination and initiative in embarking upon this long-term project. Such a major undertaking could not be accomplished overnight, and in fact it was not until the spring of 1967 that the new Tavistock Centre – the present home of the Clinic and Institute – was opened by Her Royal Highness Princess Marina, Duchess of Kent.

Meanwhile, it was the turn of the Institute to take the initiative in providing some additional accommodation until the new premises could be built, so that the process of expansion could proceed. A number of steps had been taken. Premises in Weymouth Street had been acquired, principally for the research in child development; various premises were rented in the vicinity for the nursery school which provided the opportunity for students to observe normal children in a play-group situation; and the Family Discussion Bureau occupied rooms in Chandos Street. There was, however, a limit to the number of suitable rooms which could be added to the accommodation of the Clinic and Institute in this way. The decision was taken by the Institute in 1958, therefore, to purchase a fifty-year lease of No 3, Devonshire Street, which would provide accommodation for the main activities of the Institute and some larger rooms for the joint training activities of the Clinic and Institute and for the joint Library. This move released some space in Beaumont Street for clinical work, though the Institute retained the use of a few rooms for the Family Discussion Bureau, which was enabled to move from its rooms in Chandos Street.

The Institute moved into No 3, Devonshire Street, in July 1959, and at that time it was already beginning a phase of considerable expansion. In the following year two floors of an office building in nearby Hallam Street were leased, one of which was allocated for the new Adolescent Department of the Tavistock Clinic. For this latter development a grant to cover the rent was made by the King Edward VII Hospital Fund; and in 1964 another floor in the same building was acquired for the new Institute for Operational Research.

By the time the new Tavistock Centre was ready, the Institute had already expanded to a size which made the 8,750 sq. ft. of space allocated to it insufficient for its needs. It was decided, therefore, that the Institute for Operational Research would remain in Hallam Street, although it was possible to give up the other two floors and the rooms in Weymouth Street and to sell the lease of the house in Devonshire Street. Since then, following further expansion, the Institute for Operational Research has leased an extra floor in the Hallam Street building – the one previously occupied by the Adolescent Department of the Clinic.

The story of these moves is perhaps not without interest in itself, but more significantly it shows how, over the past quarter of a century, the Institute has continued to cherish its association with the Clinic and to value the close proximity which has made possible their many collaborative undertakings.

Financial Development

Some indication of the Institute's growth is conveyed by the financial dimensions of its activities. Average annual expenditure over the first five years (1946–50) was £23,000. For the five years 1963–7 the average was £230,000. This apparent tenfold growth, after adjustment for the fall in money values, is in fact only threefold, but it is significant.

What is perhaps more revealing of the financial trend is the change in the pattern of income. In the first five years 41% of income was received from British Government sources, 33% from U.S. foundations, 19% from industrial and commercial organizations, and 7% from British foundations and donors.

In the five years 1963–7, however, 50% of income was received from industrial and commercial organizations, 16% from British Government sources, 11% from training fees, 9%

from U.S. foundations, 7% from British foundations and donors, and 7% from sundry other sources.

The fall in the proportion of support from U.S. foundations was to be expected in the light of current American policy and because most of the grants had been given to promote new developments which were expected to find more permanent support in the local community.

The rise in support from British industrial and commercial bodies is encouraging, but the proportion may well be too high in relation to that of support from British Government sources, which has fallen, and from British foundations and donors, which remains the same. It is from these two latter sources that the Institute would hope to achieve a greater degree of support in the future.

Some Thoughts about the Future

A quarter of a century after the foundation of the Clinic major changes in the environment, notably the creation of the National Health Service, brought about a change in the constitutional position of the Clinic which was to be of tremendous importance for its future development. Now, another quarter of a century on, the Institute is confronted with changes in its own complex environment which will undoubtedly influence the direction of its development.

The recent reorganization of the Institute has been a valuable preparation for these changes. The differentiation within the Institute of five units with distinctive characteristics has made possible the identification of their distinctive environments.

The future of the School of Family Psychiatry and Community Mental Health will be influenced by whatever governmental action is taken as a result of the recommendations of the Royal Commission on Medical Education (1968), the Committee on Local Authority and Allied Personal Social Services (1968), the Green Paper on the Reorganization of the N.H.S. (1968), and the Royal Commission on Local Government in England (1969). To give but a single instance of this, the Royal Commission on Medical Education recommends that responsibility for the financing of professional training should be accepted in future by the National Health Service rather than, as at present, by the University Grants Committee. Since the School is predominantly concerned with professional rather than academic training, this recommendation, if implemented, would profoundly affect its planning. Hitherto the School had no alternative but to think in terms of becoming part of a university system, though the difficulties were considerable, not least because of the essential professional and interdisciplinary character of its work. Now the possibility may be opened up for the School jointly with the Clinic to take an important place in a National Health Service whose boundaries may be extended to include responsibility for professional training. The outcome remains uncertain, but what is certain is that changes will take place beyond the control of the School which will greatly affect the nature and extent of its influence in years to come.

The Institute of Marital Studies cannot but feel the effects of any changes resulting from the recommendations of the Committee on Local Government and Allied Personal Social Services. More specifically, it will be affected by changes in the divorce law recently implemented. New emphasis is likely to be placed upon exploring the possibility of reconciliation before the Courts grant a decree. Apart from this, the more permissive character of the proposed legislation will place a greater responsibility upon individuals concerned who, more than hitherto, may be expected to turn to the already overburdened agencies which exist to help in such cases. The importance of the role of the Institute of Marital Studies in training a wide range of professional workers to cope with these problems will be highlighted, and the Institute will need to prepare itself to respond to the demands and the opportunities which will doubtless emerge.

There have been changes too in the environmental influences affecting the development of the other units of the Institute. In the previous section we have referred to the fall in the proportion of income derived from governmental sources over the first twenty years, but there are signs that this trend may be reversed. An increase in Government expenditure in the social sciences was recommended by the Committee on Social Studies

(1965). The response of the Government was to set up a Social Science Research Council, which has already made available a great deal more money – though many feel that it is not enough – for social-science research and training. Although the Human Resources Centre, the Centre for Applied Social Research and the Institute for Operational Research have received funds from the Social Science Research Council for some projects, this is far from being a major source of financial support for the work of these units. The Committee on Social Studies recognized the value of research institutes outside universities, and drew attention to the fact that most of these institutes did not receive a regular recurrent grant from Government sources and that other sponsors were reluctant to give general grants. Thus the research institutes outside universities often had difficulty in securing sufficient money to cover their administrative expenses, for planning projects, or for the publication of results. The Committee concluded that institutes of proved worth should be able to seek public funds for longer-term programmes of research which would not need to be approved project by project. The Social Science Research Council accepted the principle of programmatic, as distinct from merely project, support. It is noteworthy, however, that although applications for such support have been invited from and submitted by the Human Resources Centre, the Centre for Applied Social Research and the Institute for Operational Research, none has been granted. This situation may change, and it is hoped that it will. Meanwhile, substantial sums for long-term programmes of research are being given not to the research institutes outside universities but to the universities themselves.

There have been parallel developments, however, which have had more positive results for units of the Tavistock Institute. In recent years individual Government departments have been able to make more funds available for research from their own budgets, and this trend appears to be continuing. There has been an increase also in the number of longer-term studies supported by industrial sponsors.

Mention has been made of some of the environmental factors which will affect the future of the various units of the Institute. There are equally important internal factors to be considered.

The Institute has reached the point where its spheres of activity and influence are more clearly differentiated than in the past. What further internal changes are likely to take place in the next decade? In the past few years the units have been to some extent preoccupied with discovering and establishing their own identities, and the organizational structure has been redesigned to permit a great measure of independence between them. If this trend were to continue, it would be logical to suppose that in a few years the units would become separate legal entities with little or no connection with the parent body. Although such a possibility has been discussed, all units value their relationship to the Tavistock Institute as a whole and would wish to maintain it, whatever form future organization may take. It may well be, therefore, that the next phase will be one in which the emphasis will be upon the *interdependence* of units and the replenishment of the parent Institute which facilitates it.

It is evident that the Tavistock Institute of Human Relations represents something more than the aggregate of the units which it contains. It provides a framework within which scientific interchange can take place, and in which new activities and priorities can be planned and set in motion. It provides a stable, nurturing environment in which creative individuals are free to pursue their special interests.

It is this function, sometimes referred to by the staff as a *matrix* function, which justifies the continued existence of the Tavistock Institute. Whilst it remains, and it may need to be strengthened and replenished, as some units may move out and others move in without threatening the stability or the freedom of those that remain. Above all, through the cross-fertilization of ideas between its components and the Clinic which the Institute encourages, new concepts can emerge, new models be planned and new institutions launched to meet the changing needs of the community.

X

Further Differentiation and Integration

Mr Gray's outline of the development of the Tavistock Institute of Human Relations shows that the later history of the Tavistock Clinic, though a part of the National Health Service, is almost impossible to write without constant reference to the relationship between those two bodies. It may be tempting to compare this link to the two parts of a medical school in which the Institute or school is something distinct from the parent hospital in which the school may be situated. Yet this obvious analogy would be very superficial. In the case of a British medical school and its associated hospital both parts are maintained from the national Exchequer: the hospital from the National Health Service, the College or school from the University Grants Committee. In the case of the Tavistock Clinic and the Tavistock Institute of Human Relations it is only the former that is financed by the Treasury; the Institute of Human Relations remains a private corporation, registered as a charity. As Sidney Gray has shown, Treasury money has only come to the Institute as grants or fees for specific work undertaken for one or another of the Government departments, such as the National Coal Board, the now defunct Department of Scientific and Industrial Research, and latterly from the Medical Research Council for some of John Bowlby's research into child development.

The unity of the Clinic and Institute in our case rests on an informal consensus and will to co-operate in a common cause, as Sidney Gray also shows. The unifying factor is the experience of, and ability to spell out, the close links in theory and practice of 'depth psychology' with social, cultural and group phenomena in the wider problem of psychiatric aetiology and community mental health. This consensus resides in the society we call the Tavistock Association, the formal embodiment of what we called 'the invisible college'. To it the core of both sides belongs by voluntary membership (originally by a small entrance fee, later abolished) to which people are elected, by no means restricted to staff or Council of the Tavistock. The Association is the body which elects the Council of the Institute of Human Relations. All or nearly all the permanent staff of the Tavistock Clinic are members in their private capacities, whether they combine part-time service in the Institute of Human Relations with that of their N.H.S. appointment in the Clinic or not. Thus there has not only been a broad consensus about aims and fundamental concepts, but a full representation of all disciplines in the spectrum of Tavistock staff. The sub-title of our journal, *Human Relations*, contained the phrase, 'towards the integration of the Social Sciences' of which medical psychology is regarded as one.

Before the formal separation of the National Health Service component from the private component, this overlap was naturally more complete. We find the leading early figures of the Institute working in the Clinic: A. T. M. Wilson was a pre-war physician on the staff of the Clinic, and E. L. Trist contributed a good deal to clinical psychology in the immediate post-war years. Likewise, J. D. Sutherland, our third Medical Director, was for a long time predominantly an 'Institute man'. When the division had to come, in 1947, there was a polarization into those who decided to become mainly Institute and those who decided to become mainly Clinic staff. Thus Sutherland, whilst maintaining a close informal link at Committee and scientific levels with the Institute, was in fact whole-time in the Clinic. A. T. M. Wilson went the other way, maintaining but one National Health Service session in the Clinic, and becoming a social scientist and Chairman of the Management Committee of the Institute. It could be said that the Institute, mainly staffed by social psychologists and other behavioural scientists, was not allowed to forget its psycho-biological roots by the part-time or spare-time services of some of the psychiatrists and psychoanalysts on our staff. The Clinic was enriched by the sociological know-how from the mainly non-medical members of the Institute staff. Thus whilst there was this integration at conceptual and co-operative levels, there was also a differentiation into mainly social science and mainly clinical activities.

This chapter will deal in not too great detail with the period almost right up to the present. The nearer to the present we get the more difficult it is to write 'history', because the personalities who are making this history are still with us and the more risky it is to evaluate the significance of any given action or event in its historical significance. It would be tedious to be too detailed about what is already current knowledge about the ongoing activities of the Tavistock for the last fifteen years or so.

Possibly the most significant event which took place in 1954 and may be said to mark a stage in both the differentiation and integration of the two institutions was the convening of what called itself a 'meeting of representatives and members of the Association of the Tavistock Institute of Human Relations working in No 2, Beaumont Street'. This group met on 15 April, and there were present Dr A. T. M. Wilson and Mr E. L. Trist, representing 'those working on the fourth and fifth floors', Dr Henry Ezriel, 'representing those working on the third and second floors', and Dr John Bowlby, 'representing those working on the first and second floors'. This loosely-described foundation meeting of a new body had the purpose of facilitating liaison between Clinic and Institute. The anatomy of spatial distribution seemed the best way to distinguish us: the top two floors were 'the Institute', the third and part of the second floor were the 'Adult Department' and the remainder of the second floor and the first floor the 'Children's Department'. On that unwittingly momentous occasion Sutherland and Dugmore Hunter even sent their apologies! The agenda of this meeting was to thrash out nothing more high-minded than the procedure by which individuals should apply for research grants, how these research grants should be administered, and to produce some co-ordination, lest departments of individuals quarrelled over money or cross-applied to the same foundations for funds which only one of them could get. The issue was quite hot because there were two contenders who had independently hoped to approach the same American foundation for disparate projects. Thus it was a question of haggling over slices of cake and methods of avoiding internecine strife. The meeting was called urgently because Tommy Wilson was about to visit the United States in order to seek support with various foundations for research for the total Tavistock organization, and he insisted on being briefed. The difficulties and misunderstandings which had arisen in the past over such matters were briefly reviewed and attributed simply to the absence of appropriate co-ordinating machinery. We were determined not to have it again. We agreed that since the work carried out at No 2, Beaumont Street, was perceived by outsiders as a whole and since it was agreed that this was desirable, we now wished to have a committee to regulate these matters. We spent a great deal of time as usual on devising the structure and representation of this committee according to the best patterns of social science. It was felt that the membership group should not only contain those working in the three major divisions of the total institution, but also might have professional persons not working in Beaumont Street. This was the most important early reference to the Tavistock Group or Association as the sanctioning body for the whole building, hence for this committee. It was a big step in integration through creating a structure linking Clinic and Institute, not merely for electing a Council for one half of it.

At first this new committee could only have provisional status, but it hoped that such decisions as it took would later be binding on itself after being formally constituted by resolution of the Institute's Council. They also invited Mr Gray to take over the Secretaryship of this committee, as he was already the Secretary of the Institute Council. The earliest purpose, then, of this new body was to arbitrate and to reduce tensions between the contenders for research funds. At this stage the contenders were still feeling that this meeting, Institute-inspired, was presenting a threat to the independence of research. Before they would agree to its ruling they wanted proper constitutional authority from the Council. What in effect was being discussed here was the future of the support policy for research and teaching in the Clinic through the mediating function of the Institute, which, unlike the regional hospital, was in a position to receive donations and grants and parcel them out to whoever they wished.

That meeting was thus the birth of an organism which was to become the main administrator as well as sponsor for various grants on behalf of a number of persons and teams within the total institution. It would endeavour to collect and allocate rationally for research or for teaching programmes such grants as were given to the total institution. It would also hope to guide and, where appropriate, support the initiative of individuals in the use of their personal research grants, fellowships, subventions, etc., and decide the awards of bursaries to those who could not otherwise have afforded to take training courses. Part of such help were the necessary ancillary services, such as secretarial help, duplicating, recording machines and publications.

At this early meeting of the body which was to become the so-called Research and Training Committee[1] the controversy was not only over the right to exercise institutional supervision over the distribution and priorities of funds. At least one of the contestants at that stage was very worried lest there would be through this Committee – if it came into being – technical control over the actual work done by individuals. At a second meeting at which this issue was still thrashed out Sutherland and Bowlby, speaking as members of the then Council of the Institute, carried the proposal that it would be the overall responsibility of the Committee, and of the Council working through it, to see that funds entrusted to the Association were properly administered and applied for purposes for which they were given, and also to maintain an overall responsibility for the public relations aspect of the Association. But there was to be no technical control over how a person carried out his research work, provided always that he was working on the subject for which the grant was received, and produced some kind of results at the end.

In addition to those safeguards for the freedom of research, once budgeted for and started, the R.T.C. also adopted a third clause in its constitution — namely, that

in future any project, before being submitted to a foundation,

[1] Hereinafter abbreviated to R.T.C.

> should have included an agreed sum, to be added to the actual cost of the project as such and to represent the estimated cost of the administrative services which would be centrally provided by the Tavistock Association in connection with the project.

This meant not only that the R.T.C. would, so to speak, 'vet' applications for research grants before they went out, and give them their blessings, but would also see that the administrative costs of the Institute's service would be covered. In other words, we saw here the birth of another important structure linking the two bodies – namely, the so-called central administrative function, or Central Services, as they were called. This was to be provided by the Institute not only for the Institute's common purposes, but also as a 'College Office' for the Clinic's teaching and research activities, over and above its N.H.S. obligations to junior staff. Out of central administration came that part of the joint services, such as the fund-holding and disbursing, the office of the Secretary, and a large part of the Library and lecture-room services, etc., which, it will be recalled, were shared between the N.H.S. and the Tavistock Institute.

Two circumstances made the establishment of proper machinery for the co-ordination of independent funds flowing into the Tavistock Clinic a necessity. The first and welcome one was the very considerable interest which our work had aroused on the international scene, and to a lesser extent even in Britain. It has, I think, already been mentioned that, for example, Bowlby's and James Robertson's research was financed by British (Halley-Stewart) money. There had been other awards from British sources. But it must also be said that, by comparison with British funds flowing into *research*, other than in fees earned of various clients by the Institute, it was for a long time the United States that was providing the bulk of moneys to be used on major research in the more strictly clinical sphere. This welcome encouragement for the Clinic, however, made it important that we should be seen to behave responsibly.

Wilson could now take with him the information on how we proposed to deal with grants from potential donors. The other circumstance which necessitated the Clinic's concern about the financing of our teaching and research has already been mentioned. This was the absence of funds or of encouragement of Government money for our teaching and research functions, confirmed and sanctioned though the latter were by the Ministry of Health. The allocations for research at the disposal of regional boards were almost derisory. In any case, research and teaching were paid for out of University Grants Committee or Medical Research Council moneys to post-graduate and research institutions, which we were not designated to be. Because we had anticipated just this, we had deliberately created the Institute as a portion of ourselves to retain liberty of movement. We now decided to transfer our 'academic' functions very largely to the Institute of Human Relations through the new R.T.C., from which were later to grow other bodies and expressions of this college/hospital relationship to which I have already alluded.

Health Service establishments were now frozen; it was difficult even to get an extra 'half-time' social worker. Minor improvements, it is true, occurred over the middle 1950s: thus we had one trainee P.S.W. added to our establishment, a new-style post equivalent to a registrar. Our intra-mural training remained stabilized in numbers because these were the numbers for which there were posts. If we wanted extra numbers, they would either have to bring their own money from elsewhere as fellowships, and we could appoint them as honorary or super-numerary staff members, or we would have to pay them fellowship grants. It was for this latter purpose as much as for research that we wanted the free moneys in the keeping of the Institute. Thus, much of what has been accomplished over the last fifteen to twenty years in teaching and research in the Tavistock has been due to the strong and large doses of United States fertilizer poured into the rather poor soil of a regional hospital not supposed to grow such expensive plants.

The Finance of Training and Instruction

To perceive the Institute of Human Relations as a division of the Tavistock Group solely concerned with industrial and other social projects and consultancies would be erroneous. True, as Sidney Gray has shown, its work and standing in these has grown steadily. As already explained at the beginning of this chapter, the Tavistock Institute, based as it is on the membership of the whole Association, has always seen itself primarily as the integrative body which, because industrial and similar group projects could not yet be conceived as lying in the preventive psychiatric field, had to remain outside the Health Service. But from *within* it regarded itself as the heir of the 'old' Tavistock's distinctive concepts and skills, and of its aspirations towards becoming a school and post-post-graduate institute for community psychiatry and mental health, from infant development to institutional development. As such it was in harmony with its aims, as incorporated in its Charter, to take on the development of teaching and education in psychological medicine and the basic behavioural sciences relevant to it.

We have already listed the various foundations through whose generous donations and awards of grants this has been made possible. I want here to specify a little more precisely how the quality of some of our internal courses, as well as the great development of extra-mural teaching, has benefited from this infusion of funds over and above National Health Service provisions. At the same time it must also be acknowledged with varying degrees of gratitude according to whether the National Health Services were grudging or generous in this respect, that the physical base of these teaching operations and research was chiefly that of the Health Service clinic. It not only made it possible for us to see our patients, but also provided the rooms, lighting, heating and other amenities in which the work could be carried out. This goes without saying for the teaching which was carried out in accord with the National Health Service provisions for the training of the new generations in every hospital, teaching or regional. This was implied in the provision for four registrars and four senior registrars in psychiatry, the gradual increase in trainee clinical psychologists in N.H.S. posts in the two major divisions of the Clinic, and a trainee P.S.W. post – all from Treasury funds, and whose training was done in Clinic time. Its programme has already been sufficiently described. It appears annually in the training prospectus of the Clinic and Institute available to all those who care to read it.

Secondly, there was the kind of teaching which was done outside National Health Service time. Among such courses the Course on Projective Techniques (Rorschach, etc.) by a mixed team of the Institute and Clinic staffs was self-balancing. But the grants from various funds, – especially, when it came, the Old Dominion grant – were of crucial importance in non-N.H.S. courses, which could not have been done without such money. Among the most notable of these, and perhaps earliest in the field, was the Senior Social Casework Course to which some allusion has already been made. We believe it to be far-reaching in its benefits to the maturing skills of a number of social services in the country. Its aim was to train, on a one-year basis, a number of senior personnel to a point at which they could act as tutors to other workers in their own fields. Independent funds meant not only that we could subsidize some of these senior students who would otherwise have had to forego parts of their salaries. We could also employ essential outside lecturers and tutors to enrich the course. Similarly, the creation of the new profession of non-medical child psychotherapist became to a not inconsiderable extent dependent on the existence of such moneys. The new profession, which, I repeat, was to no small degree sponsored by the Tavistock in conjunction with Miss Anna Freud's Hampstead child therapy clinic, has now achieved its own complete professionalization through an Association. A third major development of our extra-mural services was the Introductory Psychotherapy Course, which began after the Second World War as the 'Elementary' Psychotherapy Course. As outlined in ch. vii, this was one of the major teaching events for registrars and other young psychiatrists, not excluding consultants, in the North-west Metropolitan Region and places much further afield. It aims at providing some insight and experience of the basic psychodynamic doctor/patient relationship and so repair to a slight degree the woeful deficiencies of most psychiatric training in this respect. The course now extends over two years; over fifteen years old, it is always over-subscribed, and regrettably having to turn away would-be participants in order not to prejudice the quality of the learning experience for the students themselves, given our limited consultant manpower.

Another extra-mural development of very considerable and international importance has been the teaching of general practitioners associated with the name of Michael Balint, a distinguished psychoanalyst, whose books on the subject are well-known. As mentioned, it began in the early 1950s, in the wake of a large 'ordinary' general practitioner lecture course at the insistence of a batch of doctors who wanted more intensive training. Some of these doctors stayed to become forerunners of the general practitioner psychotherapists who by now have published books and have in other ways greatly contributed to the enrichment of the content of general practice as advocated by the new Royal College of General Practice. These courses were begun at the time when general practice was at a very low ebb. It was the time of the Collins Report of 1950, when the demise of the general practitioner was gloomily forecast. Not only Balint, but I also saw in this a challenge, I published a paper entitled 'Education for General Practice – the Psycho-social Factors' in the *Lancet* of 1950. It was soon after this that this development was begun, which soon became Balint's major contribution to the work of the Tavistock Clinic and, I venture to think, to the future of general practice in this country.

Balint's model has certainly been followed not only by a number of other physicians of the Tavistock Clinic helping him and learning his skills, but also in various other related fields, notably among social workers. For example, the Family Discussion Bureau which Michael Balint helped to found with his wife, Enid, had similar training for its role; more latterly the doctors of the special marital counselling clinics within the Family Planning Association have also been trained either by Balint himself or others using his methods in this special technique, which he has raised to a very important skill within the 'helping professions'. When I was again Training Secretary of the Tavistock I received a letter from a general practitioner in Norwich who asked me whether they couldn't have a 'Tavistock' at Norwich. This turned out on further correspondence to be an allusion to one of the Balint seminars which he wanted held there. The doctor in question had no idea that the Tavistock Clinic did anything else! On the other hand, there was a time when 'the Tavistock' to a large number of people simply meant John Bowlby's separation research!

Still under the heading of training, allusion has already been made to our developing contact with the probation services as part of our extra-mural teaching, which was being constantly enlarged. In this connection, it is relevant to reiterate Sidney Gray's point that in 1956 the Family Discussion Bureau, originally a part of the Family Welfare Association, finally became a unit of the Tavistock Institute of Human Relations and functioned from then on as a special marriage casework service within No 2, Beaumont Street, moving in from a separate building. It was felt important that this agency, part social service, part crypto-psychiatric, should be under the same roof as the developing marital unit of the Clinic which I had pioneered with Mary Luff. Certain staff were employed by both in the typical Clinic/Institute sharing manner. It was through the coming of the Family Discussion Bureau, then led by Mrs Lily Pincus, that we were able to offer a fruitful intra-mural teaching programme for probation officers, who were to become in-service tutors to their colleagues for the expanding matrimonial services in the magistrates' courts. The introductory teaching of marital diagnosis and counselling had been my responsibility at the Probation Officer Training School since 1949.

Perhaps the most strenuous of all the forms of extra-mural teaching by the Tavistock staff was the sending of tutors, in Health Service time, to outlying hospitals where the staffs wished to learn more about the handling of psychoneuroses and related skill for their growing out-patient work. A Tavistock consultant from the Adult Department would go out for a half-day of intensive seminars, not otherwise available to these psychiatrists – often brought together from several hospitals. The usual method was akin to our own Introductory Psychotherapy Course: the basis of such teaching was the students' own cases brought for discussion and interpretative comment by the tutor, followed by a more generalized case discussion in groups in which varying degrees of theory might be injected as the contact proceeded. The Children's Department also undertook an increasing number of such missions. One of the more notable ones was a long tutorial relationship of certain maternity and child welfare teams of the London County Council with a consultant and a senior P.S.W. in which a somewhat similar teaching technique by case discussion with tutorial comment was instituted. Another project was the piloting of a new scheme for the borough of West Ham under the aegis of its Medical Officer of Health by a consultant/P.S.W. team from the Adult Department, which resulted in the setting-up of a comprehensive mental health service, now under the direction of Dr Jack Kahn. Innumerable lectures and seminars were given by all of us to B.M.A. groups, and to staffs of local public health departments. Programmes of close in-service training with many classes 'off or on the premises' were developed, in which not only our two departments but certain members of the Institute took part, latterly the F.D.B. staff. One of the leading promoters of these developments was the Medical Officer of Health for Middlesex, assisted by his Social Work Adviser, Mr Eugene Heimler.

Clinic staff as part-time members of the Institute of Human Relations participated in the significant development, already mentioned by Sidney Gray. This was a joint project with the University of Leicester – the now well-known Group Relations Conferences, originally referred to as Leicester Conferences. Pierre Turquet was especially concerned on the medico-psychological staff of these. Here some of the skills of group dynamics and the understanding of what happened in groups, including some experience of the personal stresses, were taught to industrial managers, production engineers and other professional groups in an effort to improve the quality and insight in industrial and work-group life in general. Allusion has already been made to the great demand made upon our teaching which led the Clinic, especially the Children's Department, to institute open case conferences to which interested visitors would be admitted upon scrutiny of their professional qualifications. A semi-internal, semi-external case conference of this kind was that in the writer's own Marital Unit, which held a weekly discussion of interesting marriage difficulties seen by either trainees or senior staff of the Marital Research Unit in the building. By and large at this time it was the Marital Unit under my direction which did the internal teaching of registrars in marital techniques. The F.D.B. did most of the external teaching and social casework training in techniques and approaches to marital counselling for use within the framework of the caseworkers' own institutional settings, such as maternal and child welfare clinics or other community casework centres and agencies. It will be appreciated that this volume of teaching could only be provided by the financial aid available to us by the generosity of such foundations as the Grant Foundation and the Old Dominion Trust of the United States. It enabled us to 'buy' staff time which would otherwise have gone into private practice. I have already mentioned the important principle that any fees charged to the various external students for courses in Clinic time were returned to the Hospital Management Committee. Those training fees which were earned outside Clinic time went into the coffers of the Tavistock Institute Training Funds to be offset against the grants. Tutors received fees according to a scale laid down for the particular event, related to the complexity of the task and the seniority of the lecturer. All staff members of the Clinic, medical and non-medical, and sometimes senior registrars as well, were almost continuously involved in one or more of these teaching activities.

The Growth and Financing of Research

Since the generous Rockefeller grant which made possible the development of the Institute, other grants have greatly helped to stimulate and fertilize research and development in our field of interest. In this development as in that of teaching, it would again be a mistake to underrate the positive support and contribution of the Health Service authorities themselves, who were almost entirely sympathetic after 1955 (as will be seen in a later section of this chapter) as far as their statutory obligations permitted. It may be said that by choosing the strange way out of being both a regional clinic and yet possessing an independent training and research institute as our non-statutory twin, we seemed in some respects to have had the best of both worlds. But without question we suffered sometimes from considerable administrative stress in trying to reconcile ourselves and our employing National Health Service authority to this conflict of roles. In this respect, however, our later administrators were wise enough to see that what we were doing by way of training and also by way of trying to discover about the causes of the conditions we were called upon to treat was just as important a contribution to the National Health Service as if we had settled down in a static, unimaginative way to carry out routine treatments.

Omitting those in themselves fascinating and outstanding research projects which were done exclusively by the sociological and socio-psychiatric teams of the Institute of Human Relations (for example, in personnel selection or in group dynamics and morale in industry, to mention but two outstanding fields with obvious mental health components), our research strategy was well described by Sutherland and Bowlby in the early 1960s when they defined three main research areas linked to the clinical work of the Tavistock. One of these was that of *psychodiagnostic* and *therapeutic procedures*. Here they named the study of therapeutic process carried out by the doctor on the basis of his experience in treating patients. The special research resources required precise recording and the study of verbatim records of what actually takes place in individual or group therapeutic sessions. The second area they described as the *detection and assessment of pathological family process*. On this they said, there was much evidence that the difficulties for which adult patients seek help and for which child patients are referred are closely linked to tensions within the family. Increasing attention at both diagnostic and therapeutic stages to interaction between members of families is therefore the object of study. As in the case of interaction between individual patient and doctor, so in the study and treatment of pathological family process, the first requirement was the devising of methods for recording and describing relevant data in a reliable way. The steps were (*a*) the development of reliable methods of observing and recording data on interaction and (*b*) the study of particular kinds of family interaction that seemed to contribute to particular forms of psychiatric illness. Thirdly, they described the area of the *pathological sequelae of loss*, their causation, prevention and treatment. Here the memorandum stressed the prevailing uncertainty about many aetiological factors producing psychiatric illness, but also the pretty reliably established fact that the loss of significant persons occurring either in childhood or in adult life could play an important part in causing psychiatric stress or illness. This should lead to the systematic study of a class of aetiological events and their effects, and of methods by which ill effects might be prevented. The events which they said were at present under study in the Tavistock were (*a*) the loss of a parent in childhood due to temporary separation and (*b*) the loss by death of a spouse in adult life.

This statement summarized most of the major research projects which had been running for some years. Bowlby's work in his child development research unit has already been alluded to; its findings have been widely published. They include two films and two books on children in hospital by James Robertson, and a book reporting in detail the findings of a systematic study of brief separations by Christoph Heinicke and Ilse Westheimer. This work has not only changed the routine in children's hospitals, but has greatly influenced child-care techniques generally. The second phase of studying the effects of loss was begun somewhat later, when a fellowship from the Mental Health Research Fund enabled Dr Colin Parkes from the Maudsley Hospital to join the group. His work on bereavement in its relation to mental illness was carried out mainly with widows. Parkes' work (related to other investigations on the same theme which had also received publication in the *British Journal of Psychiatry*, as well as by Geoffrey Gorer in his well-known book)[1] has since been extended to the study of reactions to the loss of a limb. John Bowlby has himself been studying the implications of all these findings for psychoanalytic theory and practice and has been attempting a reformulation in such key areas as instinct theory, the child's tie to his mother, separation anxiety and problems of mourning, healthy and pathological. A series of papers published in

[1] Gorer, G., '*Death, Grief and Mourning*', London; Cresset (1965).

1958–63 is now being superseded by a two-volume work on *Attachment and Loss*, the first volume of which is recently published. Bowlby applies to these problems principles derived from ethology and control theory as well as from psychoanalysis.

Another venture of Bowlby's group was to convene a series of four interdisciplinary seminars on mother-child interaction. Held at two-year intervals with the help of the Ciba Foundation, their proceedings have been published in four volumes, edited by Brian Foss.

Work in other centres on problems of separation and loss that has derived directly from the Tavistock group is that of two of its former members, Mary Salter Ainsworth (now Professor of Psychology at Johns Hopkins University) and H. Rudolph Schaffer (now Reader in Psychology at the University of Strathclyde); and also the studies of rhesus monkeys begun at Cambridge in 1957 by Robert Hinde (now Royal Society Professor of Animal Behaviour in Cambridge University).

The other area of research, on the nature of the psychotherapeutic process, includes, first, the ongoing work of Henry Ezriel, the earliest Tavistock recipient of a Foundation Fund grant. As mentioned in ch. vii, he aimed at validation of psychoanalytic hypotheses by carefully controlled transference interpretations, for which he predicted the expected effects if such interpretations were what psychoanalysis claimed. Henry Ezriel is still pondering on the final presentation of this extensive labour. Another field – the detection of pathological family process – envisaged in the above summary was mainly that of Ronald Laing, who also obtained a Foundation Fund grant on completing his senior registrarship and his psychoanalytic training with us after his original psychiatric training at Glasgow. Laing's work in pathological family process not only consisted of vivid observation of schizophrenic families, but also laid the foundations of a new method of recording interaction. This resulted in a book by Phillipson, Lee and himself, listed in our appendix. A long clinical study in family process was the marital research work carried out in my own unit. The aim was to construct a conceptual framework as well as a clinical therapeutic model for diagnosing and helping seriously disturbed marriages and parent relations. This work was mostly done on patients (married couples) with staff and resources of the Clinic itself. A third piece of research on the family, with important bearings on mental health, was that done by Elizabeth Bott, an anthropologist, on normal 'happily functioning' English families. Bott's work gave us a baseline or norm in dynamics and role-playing to which to compare pathological families. Elizabeth Bott (Mrs Spillius) was an Institute staff member.

A somewhat later development in Bowlby's research programme, with a major bearing on the validation of certain psychoanalytic theories about the infant's development of social bonds was Anthony Ambrose's work on the earliest social responses in babies. This research was one of the earliest to attract Medical Research Council money to the Tavistock, a step which was followed by John Bowlby himself becoming a part-time member of the M.R.C.'s external scientific staff – a most notable achievement for psychodynamic theory and for his work. Lastly, Dr Dorothy Heard, then our 'newest' consultant in the Department for Children and Parents, took further the methodology of study of interactional behaviour in families, concentrating especially on methods of recording and testing various interaction sequences which would subsequently be used in operational description of family processes.

From quite a different source came the origins of another important research project which is to the credit of the Tavistock Clinic. This began as a 'workshop' by staff members on an interest basis, convened in the first instance by Michael Balint and myself, concerned with the dearth of verifiable and communicable methods of brief psychotherapy on individuals. We had concentrated so much on group work that I at any rate felt that it was time we studied individual psychotherapy of a compass which would make it feasible in busy hospital out-patient conditions. It was this workshop which was attended, among others, by David Malan, and stimulated him to begin his research, resulting in a book entitled *A Study of Brief Psychotherapy* and other publications dealing with the follow-up of both treated and untreated patients. David Malan was for a time in receipt of a modest research grant, but much of his work was carried on as a by-product of treating patients in the Tavistock.

In a previous chapter I mentioned the deferred aspiration towards devising reliable methods of assessing psychodiagnostic and therapeutic procedures as a whole. This work, which was always at the back of our minds, and especially that of Sutherland and Phillipson, has now begun its development. It is concerned with devising a short battery of tests that would expose in scoreable terms the main kinds of conflict in an individual and assess the degree to which the conflict areas are impeding the satisfactory function of the personality. This very important research area for the future of psychotherapy will lead, it is hoped, to a means of devising reliable methods for testing patients at the beginning of treatment, during its course and again at the end of treatment, by which the results of the psychotherapy and possibly other treatment would be assessed with a greater degree of realism and of depth than is at present possible. It is the lack of such methods and the complexities of devising them that has led to much justifiable criticism of psychotherapy by hostile or even well-meaning critics who have found that 'there is nothing to show' that psychotherapy does anything for people.

Other researches, of a less formal character, have consisted chiefly in the evaluation of such things as the results of group therapy within the Clinic itself, not unlike the paper published before the war on the results of 500 cases of psychotherapy, the work of writing up the concepts and practices governing the general practitioner groups by Balint, Gosling and others, and many similar kinds of work. The point of this section is to show that a very great deal of exploration and methodology in fundamental areas of psychopathology and personality development has been and is still going on in the Tavistock Clinic, and to emphasize the crucial role of the Institute as the treasury and base behind the clinicians in the Health Service.

Relations to the National Health Service

Over the first eight years or so the relationships with our own Management Committee fluctuated a great deal, as already mentioned. In 1956, to achieve a change of management, the Tavistock Clinic was transferred from the Central Middlesex to the Paddington Group, which already administered our sister foundations, the Child Guidance Training Centre and the Portman Clinic, *inter alia.* The steps by which the change was brought about were initiated by the concern of the Mental Health Committee of our Regional Hospital Board under the Chairmanship of Mr Kenneth Robinson (subsequently the Minister of Health for some years in Mr Wilson's Government) about the difficulties which the three clinics had had in securing the right conditions for their development. Mr Kenneth Robinson was known for his interest in wider developments of mental health and was among those sponsoring the devolution of the mental hospital, in favour of its supersession by psychiatric units in general hospitals. His sympathies also lay with the kind of community psychiatry which the Tavistock stood for. I have little doubt that Mr Robinson's influence, as well as that of the Senior Administrative Medical Officer of the Region, Dr Macauley, and of the Chairman of No. 5 Board, the Hon. John Fremantle (later Lord Cottesloe), brought about this change.

Paddington Group was accustomed to administering the Portman and the Child Guidance Training Centre and found us no more trouble. In the Chairman of this Hospital Management Committee, Alderman Sir Frederick Lawrence, and his Deputy, Mrs Bolton, who also presided over our House Committee, and in Councillor Mrs M. R. Forbes, J.P., who later succeeded Sir Frederick as Chairman, as well as in the chief officers of the Management Committee, notably the Group Secretary, Mr Jolly, and Mr Harding, the Establishment Officer, we acquired good and helpful friends. All sorts of minor as well as some quite major requirements were met, and our feelings of appreciation were very real. We could not achieve all the things we wanted. There was, especially, a rigid ceiling on psychiatric posts in the London area, due to Ministry policy dictated by the pressures to divert psychiatric manpower into the understaffed provinces.

With the Regional Board, too, we had friendly links at two levels. First, there was the general participation by Tavistock staff members in the Regional Advisory Committee for Psychiatry, of which I was Chairman for some eight years. In this capacity I also sat on the Mental Health Committee of the Regional Board. A notable change, however, occurred when Lord Cottesloe ceased being Chairman about the same time that Dr Macauley retired and was replaced by a new Senior Administrative Medical Officer. The climate of opinion in the country as a whole had changed in the direction of organic psychiatry, and this inevitably affected the counsels of our Board. Hand in hand with this, a kind of administrative centralism became noticeable. Before long the Mental Health Committee was administratively reduced to a small sub-committee of the General Purposes Committee and lost most of its expert personnel, whilst the Psychiatric Advisory Committee also was considerably reduced in scope. This Committee had to complain frequently that we were not consulted, but faced with *faits accomplis*.

Our second contact with the Regional Board, already touched on in chs. viii and ix, was the quadripartite joint committee formed in 1955 to regulate the complex cost-sharing arrangements of the Tavistock Institute with its N.H.S. Clinic. It was presided over by Lord Cottesloe, and had on it representatives of the Board, the Hospital Management Committee, the Tavistock Institute and the Clinic. Here originated the first proposals for a new and adequate building, for us beginning with the prospecting for various sites. Sir Frederick Lawrence favoured a building site in the immediate vicinity of Beaumont Street, either in Beaumont Street itself, where a number of houses were scheduled for demolition and rebuilding, another by the side of St Marylebone Church, and a third on the Regent's Park Nash terraces, also scheduled for rebuilding. None of these locations proved to be available by reason of a veto on planning permission for a medical institution. However, the discussions between our two bodies and the Liaison Committee bore good fruit. We could now communicate our hopes and needs fully. It was clear that at this level the Regional Board, now well informed about what we were doing and hoping to achieve, were convinced of the necessity for a proper building permitting the development of both the Clinic and the Institute.

In the meantime we had to use temporary expedients for expanding our premises, such as leasing the splendid house at No 3, Devonshire Street, and other extensions already described by Sidney Gray. These developments were made possible mainly through the Institute's independent funds, as well as by its exemplary budgeting and 'housekeeping', which can be justly credited to the labours of Sidney Gray.

But while our relationships with the National Health Service authorities were now very good, it was not so with our regional post-graduate training scheme as a whole, about which I wrote in ch. viii. The Tavistock's own part was played without there ever being the complementary larger scheme contributed by the other hospitals and institutions such as had been envisaged by the earlier work of the Education Sub-committee of the Regional Advisory Committee in Psychiatry. It has to be recorded that this region, so rich in psychiatric institutions and specialists of every kind, was recently adjudged by an R.M.P.A. survey one of the most backward in respect of a co-ordinated post-graduate training scheme. Somehow, the impetus of the early post-war years was lost. By default it was left to the various hospitals individually to provide what training they could or would in general psychiatry as well as in the more special subjects such as mental deficiency or whatever, all of which we had planned on quite a comprehensive and academic pattern.

One other important Government liaison already alluded to requires a progress note here. This was our growing good relationship with the Home Office Probation Division. Not only did Tavistock members contribute greatly to the training and orientation of probation officers in the marital field, but Sutherland was invited to join the Advisory Committee on Probation Training. Very shortly after this the Family Discussion Bureau became involved in intensive training courses while Pierre Turquet and Herbert Phillipson also took courses on 'Balint'-like lines for probation officers in the wider context, not only that of family and marital work.

Relationships to Psychiatry and the Profession

Whilst the Tavistock was thus developing its internal and

external teaching and research activities, it also had to define its boundaries with the wider psychiatric field, which was gradually reverting closer to pre-war attitudes than it had been immediately after the Second World War. The causes or contributing factors to this drifting-apart after the war effort were complex. They resided to some extent in the continued power of the post-graduate Institute of Psychiatry in London to sway leading psychiatric appointments, such as the new professorships, towards the 'organic' approach; in the real advance made through the invention and successful application of new pharmacological substances to the control of disturbed behaviour which seemed to point to such a physiological aetiology for mental disorders; hence for the greater promise of personnel drawn from within the schools of classical psychiatry to man positions of power and responsibility on the councils of the profession. Sir Francis Fraser, during our wartime interview, had certainly warned us that all academic status would go to the schools under the aegis, in London, of the Post-graduate Medical Federation, and in the provinces of the universities. The likes of us, it will be recalled, were to be permitted to do 'little general practitioner courses and that kind of thing', but we were not to be a teaching school. This was to some extent belied by our actual achievements, but the status and role of a university school continued to elude the Tavistock. There were plenty of reasons why the psychoanalytic and allied schools should continue to enjoy less than full academic and scientific status. Many of the resistances which I have already described and which are endemic in the profession against psychoanalytic concepts in psychiatry continued to operate.

It must, however, also be said that our handling of the situation was by no means brilliant. I have already alluded to the introversion and lack of talent for 'putting ourselves on the map'. Perhaps we concentrated too exclusively on building a model mental health institution within the Tavistock, to the relative neglect of professional public relations. To this John Bowlby and I were exceptions. He, like myself, spent much time and effort in giving papers at scientific meetings, sitting on policy committees, and so on. But of the group as a whole it could be said that, while we in fact created a redoubtable body of theory and practice, we were not good at manning key posts and taking part in the sometimes dreary job of convincing our own professions and public opinion about the worth of what we were doing. As a group we stood perhaps too much on the ground that the truth would in the long run prevail, and that if we only published enough and produced good enough results and good enough skills in the helping professions, both inside and outside psychiatry, etc., then recognition must surely come. It may even be that the reluctance to enter too ardently or vigorously into the battle between two kinds of psychiatry broadly divided into 'organicist' and 'psychodynamist' was right. One can spend too much time in ideological polemics in the struggle against major resistances. Our manpower was needed for the positive build-up of an institution and a school which would stand when the various fashions in psychotropic drugs and other physical methods had worn thin, and it had been shown that personality growth cannot result from suppression or even abolition of symptoms.

In the meantime, however, the senior appointments and the new chairs in psychiatry went steadily to the pupils of Mapother's school and to other classical psychiatrists versed in the new physical methods who, in varying degrees, continued to hold or developed further their critical attitudes towards the psychodynamic viewpoint in psychiatry. The newly-formed Mental Health Research Fund, perhaps the nearest equivalent to the American Foundations Fund for Research in Psychiatry, was also initially manned by the same personnel as filled the teaching appointments in academic psychiatry in Britain. Applicants from 'our side', whether Tavistock or those from other hospitals and institutions, had difficulty in formulating their projects in a way that commanded M.H.R.F. respect. Whatever may be the historical evaluation of Professor Eysenck's own work in behavioural psychology and Pavlovian methods, his sustained polemics under the umbrella of the Maudsley against the lack of scientific validity of psychoanalytic psychotherapy had, one may be sure, a fairly serious result on the standing of the Tavistock's work.

It would be a mistake to describe these polarities in the post-war psychiatric scene as if they were absolute. There were many psychiatrists and there were also many medical officers of public health and many lay administrators within Government and local authorities who could see the value of the kind of work we were doing for the broader mental-health scene. We had good friends within psychiatry. By 1956 two of our members were invited to join the Scientific Committee of the Mental Health Research Fund, and our R.T.C. debated seriously whether this addition of one or two people of our way of thinking was in fact useful to our cause in psychiatry. In the end it was decided that Bowlby and Trist should join, but only after making their position quite clear: that they felt that the 'organicist' trend just described was very unsatisfactory for the broader development of psychological medicine in general.

Both in that year and again two years later the R.T.C. specifically resolved, after exhaustive re-discussions, to uphold its decision to work towards a wider institution for the teaching and advancement of an integrated theory and practice of psychotherapy and mental health for individuals and institutions. We reaffirmed our stand against the trend of the newly optimistic and over-confident majority in Britain who felt that the cure for every mental ill by suitable pharmacological products was just round the corner and that major biochemical or genetic breakthroughs into the aetiology of schizophrenia, depression and the like were imminent. Not that our decision was made in any doctrinaire spirit. In fact, in the late 1950s it looked for a time as if an eminent pharmacological research worker, dissatisfied with conditions in his university, would join the Tavistock if we could provide suitable facilities. The aim would have been an integration of research into pharmacodynamic and psychodynamic studies of personality. At the level of the Liaison Committee between the Regional Board, the Clinic and the Institute, an in-patient unit and laboratories for such a research purpose were mooted. We did not want an in-patient unit merely for the sake of treating a few psychotics equally well cared for elsewhere. But we were eagerly prepared to have beds for a special unit pioneering a new service or research interest not provided elsewhere.

As regards the status of our subject within psychiatry, a

notable post-war development was the establishment within the R.M.P.A. of a new section for psychotherapy and social psychiatry to advance the achievements and psychiatric philosophy of the wartime period. Here some of our members spoke, served on committees and in due time became officers. Together with colleagues from the Cassel Hospital and others interested, we were able to play some part in furthering this degree of integration into the main body of psychiatry of activities which had hitherto mainly centred on the Medical Section of the British Psychological Society. This meant that, somewhat timidly, the psychodynamic viewpoint also found its way on to one or two of the policy-making committees of the R.M.P.A., the professional body under whose umbrella all branches of psychiatry were united. It is a fact of my observation that psychotherapists and analysts are less able to be good committee members. They do not, in the nature of their commitment to patients, care to attend meetings during therapeutic working hours. This alone puts the 'organicists' in a stronger position in this respect. I believe, however, that a deeper incompatibility between these two roles is also involved, and to this extent the psychodynamicists will always be somewhat handicapped in the 'corridors of power' by comparison with the psychiatrists whose methods do not include intensive personal involvement with their patients. Whilst not purporting to make this volume a history of British psychiatry in general, it can be said that even to the present day the Section of Psychotherapy is in a somewhat isolated position within the R.M.P.A., as are the Sections of Child Psychiatry and Mental Deficiency, when seeking to influence the great mass of 'general psychiatrists' – which in practice means psychiatric hospital staff. Just as medicine in the olden days regarded psychiatry (as a whole) as a marginal discipline, so psychiatrists themselves tend to regard psychotherapy and child psychiatry, and by implication those institutions which specialize in them, as somewhat peripheral. None the less, of some 3,500 members of the R.M.P.A., 1,200 are at least nominally members of the Psychotherapy and Social Psychiatry Section, although not even a tenth of that number attend its monthly meetings, where papers of the kind that would be central to the interests of the Tavistock Association are apt to be read and discussed.

If, then, our relationship to psychiatry in general was in some ways not a great deal better than before the Second World War, despite the immediate post-war efflorescence of interest in our affairs, the relationship to psychoanalysis as an organized body had changed a good deal. As the consultant staff recruited before the war (of whom I may be said to be one of the last survivals on the post-Second World War staff) gradually retired by superannuation, it was replaced exclusively by men and women who were 'card-carrying' psychoanalysts. This inevitably meant that the Tavistock to the outside world acquired the soubriquet of a 'psychoanalytic clinic'. We came to be regarded as something of a satellite to the Psychoanalytic Institute. In some ways there was a grain of truth in this description in the earlier years. During the late 1940s and early 1950s one sometimes felt that to our 'Young Turks' almost anybody who was an analyst was better than anyone who was not, if not quite irrespective of other qualities, then nearly so. Thus there was in the recruitment of new staff a built-in bias in favour of appointing people who were analysts, even though otherwise not well-known and in some instances perhaps not so well-qualified in general psychiatry as some of their rival applicants, of whom there was no dearth. But when this has been said and the loyalty of the psychoanalysts among our staff to their own teachers and school taken into account, there still remained an essential spirit of sturdy independence which has grown with the years. That independence was always essentially quite real. The Tavistock has had and continued to have a climate of its own which, without offence to the psychoanalysts, could be called a more realistic and at the same time a more community-centred attitude to the work. This is partly a function of having to deal with massive patient numbers and a responsibility for helping far more and less selected patients. At the Institute of Psychoanalysis and its associated Clinic the selection of patients was completely in the hands of the Training Committee, who needed only to pick suitable cases for their students. Both in the pre-war Tavistock and now there has been a much greater call to devise methods and forms of help which, whilst leaning on psychoanalytic concepts, were none the less free and creative applications of principles. The description of our research work is in itself an illustration of the way in which our wide contacts in psychopathology and in sociology had had their effect in making us somewhat critical of the 'sectarian' or dogmatic features of the psychoanalytic movement, and this independence could not help breaking through. Thus already in 1955, arising from our constant scrutiny of the training of medical and ancillary personnel in skills required for psychotherapy and community mental health, the R.T.C. formally minuted its dissatisfaction with training analysis as the sole method of teaching registrars the elements of psychodynamics and inter-personal relations. I quote from the minutes of the R.T.C., 4 February 1955:

> Dr Dicks referred to the need to develop methods and training facilities generally for short-term psychotherapy. It was recognized that the Tavistock role in this matter would be that of providing advanced training for tutors and key operators. It was felt that the advanced course in Social Casework provided a good example of work already being done in this direction, and foreshadowed the possibility, under improved financial and other conditions, of the development of a school for social work tutors and key operators . . . some comparison was then made between the position in children's work and that in the corresponding *adult work*. There was felt to be a similar need for a school of Public Health psychiatrists, that this would underline the need for operations on which teaching could be based. Considering the present training afforded for registrars it was felt that the turnover needed to be considerably increased. . . . It was also necessary to provide for the personal analyses of young psychiatrists, who needed the most thorough possible grounding in this field, and here the position was contrasted with the training of child psychiatrists and psychotherapists. Independent facilities of a high standard existed for the training of child psychotherapists . . . without the necessity of undertaking a training analysis at the Institute of Psychoanalysis. This led to a discussion of the

> present dependence upon the training given at the Institute of Psychoanalysis for the acquisition of analytical skills and insights. Dr Sutherland felt that this situation should not continue indefinitely and reported a view expressed that if psychoanalytic training was an essential in any branch of the Health Service, then the Health Service should itself provide it. The general view of the meeting was however that provision of comparable training under the auspices of the Clinic would raise difficulties of considerable magnitude. . . . The statement was made that from the Tavistock viewpoint the training provided by the Institute of Psychoanalysis was limited, and that the real task of the Association [i.e. the Tavistock – H.V.D.] was to provide training which was different from, but complementary to, the training given by the Institute of Psychoanalysis. Some suggestions were made as to steps which could be taken in the development of this special form of training, such as the holding of theoretical seminars in social psychiatry and other relevant subjects.

These difficulties were in fact openly discussed by several of our members, notably Sutherland and Bowlby (themselves past or present office-holders of the Psycho-Analytic Society) with the senior officers of the Institute of Psychoanalysis. This exchange resulted in a most amicable decision that it would be proper to have our registrars undergo training analyses within the organization of the Clinic now made possible by the Old Dominion and other grants. In fact, the Health Service itself also agreed that we should make two appointments to the consultant staff for the specific purpose of acting as psychoanalytic trainers for our own registrars, and in due course Drs Charles Rycroft and Fanny Wride were appointed to undertake this role, as well as the related tasks of taking some theoretical seminars and supervisions for our registrars. The independence achieved provided a point of departure in principle and also eliminated clashes in time-tabling between our training and clinical schedules and the demands made on the registrars' time by the Institute of Psychoanalysis. Moreover, the training of a psychoanalyst is very limited *per se*, and we had to complement it by the already indicated experience and teaching in brief psychotherapy, counselling, work with groups, families, marriages and all the rest, as well as by the special skills for the registrars in the Department for Children and Parents. The final development of this training is described in the latest training prospectus. This shows that our training syllabus, whilst based on and delivered by exponents of psychoanalysis, is none the less a course *sui generis* geared to the community and national health functions of future specialists who are expected to contribute at least part of their skills to the national effort.

In the course of the years we have had the interesting further development that, whilst practically all the medical staff members have been or were in the course of becoming psychoanalysts, a large proportion of our social workers had had (Jungian) analysis at the Society for Analytical Psychology. This development began with my close collaborator on the Marital Unit, Mrs Mary Williams, the first of the P.S.W.s in the Adult Department to be appointed after the war, and continued with others, including some of the P.S.W.s who formed the core staff of the Family Discussion Bureau. In fact, it may be said that whilst a number of the senior staff of the Tavistock in the recent past have occupied important positions in the psychoanalytic movement, they also have, to the credit of both the Psychoanalytic Institute and the Tavistock, maintained a great deal of independence. Thus Sutherland, though Editor of the *International Journal of Psychoanalysis*, was always critical of the one-sided training and the doctrinaire narrowness of the psychoanalytic movement proper and its lack of interest in scientific validation and critical examination of its own procedures and training methods. Bowlby, also in high office for a considerable time in the British Psychoanalytic Society, has quite clearly shown his scientific criticism of unalloyed psychoanalytic views in his writing and by the need to base his researches increasingly on the solid observational data of child study and comparative ethology. But as with psychiatry and the heritage of Mapother, so in psychoanalysis and the heritage of 'Old Vienna', the change in generations is clearly bringing about greater rapprochement and also very considerably greater self-criticism on both sides. None the less, it is interesting to record the recurrence the second time round of the Tavistock's situation between the upper and the nether millstones of orthodox organically based psychiatry and orthodox dogmatic psychoanalysis.

Something should also be said about the history of the Tavistock's relationships with the wider mental-health movement, embodied in those voluntary societies of which the most active is the National Association for Mental Health. This body, it will be recalled, was formed shortly after the Second World War by a fusion of three previously independent committees called the National Council for Mental Hygiene, the Child Guidance Council and the Mental After-care Association. The first two were organizations with which the old Tavistock had been greatly concerned. With Dr Doris Odlum, Dr Helen Boyle and Sir Maurice Craig, J. R. Rees and Crichton-Miller had been powerful figures in the promotion of their activities, which aimed at creating informed public opinion and concern which could drive towards reforms in the direction of mental-health provision and training within medicine and the social service professions. In the early years after the Second World War the Tavistock viewpoint and its personnel were in very considerable demand within that Association. First, Kenneth Soddy, closely associated with the child-guidance aspect of psychodynamic psychiatry, and later Alfred Torrie, one of our consultants, became successively Medical Directors of the Association. After the post of Medical Director was abolished when the next incumbent, Coleman Kenton, went to the Regional Hospital Board, a Medical Advisory Panel was formed instead, of which I found myself Chairman for some years. Earlier, the International Congress for Mental Health in 1948 had involved some of our members to a considerable extent, as already mentioned, including myself as a member of the interprofessional International Preparatory Commission. That International Congress founded the World Federation for Mental Health. This body was the new creation and main field of innovation work of J. R. Rees after he had resigned his Directorship of the Tavistock. The role of both the national and the international body was, of course, that of popularization and dissemination of existing knowledge, techniques, models of organization and the like. Subsequently J.R., who had been accustomed to look upon the members of the Tavistock staff as 'his boys', both pre-war and during his Army days, found that the new Tavistock was not so ready to share his enthusiasm for these diffuse activities. Once again we meet the problem of our old friends, the 'psychopathological snobs'. The Tavistock, with its new and more rigorous scientific approach to the whole development of a science of human relations, etc., was in a sense no more reluctant than, for example, the new professors of psychiatry in involving itself with a great deal of public education and promotional activity in these fields. There was considerable pressure from J.R. to do much more than in fact we did, either on a national or an international level, for the mental health movement. We held that for our specialized clinic it was more important to secure our own base in order to advance knowledge than to go about from congress to congress contributing snippets of knowledge to variously prepared or unprepared groups of human beings. This is a crudely over-simplified way of describing the prevailing attitude of our staff. This led to a paradox. Much of what was talked about in the councils of the national and international mental-health movement was derived from the theories and practice originally worked out by such teams as the Tavistock. For example, the themes of parent-child relations, the effect of school on children, various forms of stress in industry and living in a technological age, etc., had been our staple for years. None the less, it was rare for Tavistock staff to play any major part in the movement, and we acquired the reputation of absentees. I think this was almost certainly a justifiable saving of professional energy and time. Thinking back to my own involvements, it was frequently a most disheartening experience to sit through meetings at which one felt one could not make any kind of impact, unless one was 'in' by giving the major part of one's effort to the cause. On the international scene there was the further complication that meetings were held literally all over the world. Anyone who had committed himself to be elected a member of the Executive Board or undertaken to speak frequently at the annual meetings of the World Federation would have been very greatly out of pocket as well as hampered in doing his own primary job. These were posts which could only be held by full-time professors or persons not tied to actual clinical responsibility for their patients in the sense in which the Tavistock and psychoanalysts interpret that commitment. None the less, I stayed in my very part-time role as a member of the Advisory Panel for the N.A.M.H. for some years, being replaced at my own request by the late Dr T. P. Rees, then recently retired from Warlingham Park Hospital. I then accepted nomination as the representative of the Tavistock Institute on the United Kingdom Co-operating Committee for the World Federation for Mental Health, and found myself in the Chair of that body for some further six or seven years!

But if in general our role in the national and international mental health movement was at best lukewarm, individuals made their contributions by speaking and consultancies. At official level, W.H.O. not only used John Bowlby as a consultant laying the scientific foundations for the considerable attention now paid to mother-and-child relationships. Others also had consultancies and took part in W.H.O. and W.F.M.H. activities.

Not the least of our contributions was the selection of Ronald Hargreaves, one of our brightest stars, as head of the Mental Health Section of W.H.O. from its inception to the late 1950s, when at last he wanted to return home. When Hargreaves had expressed such a wish and had not yet settled on a venue for his future activities in the United Kingdom, the R.T.C. very seriously considered setting up a special department or project for him, broadly speaking in the field of public health, in which he now had almost unrivalled experience as a psychiatrist, not only with W.H.O., but also as late Chief Medical Officer of the Unilever Corporation, a firm as large as many smaller nations. In this connection we were prepared to set Hargreaves up in the activity he might choose – not necessarily at the Tavistock. We would have been glad for the Tavistock attitude, as reflected in this outstanding man's mind, to be represented, for example, by a post in a university. In the event, Hargreaves accepted my former Chair at Leeds as successor to Douglas MacCalman. We had hoped for a senior post for him in London, such as the Chair in Industrial Mental Health long ago held by Millais Culpin at the School of Hygiene and Tropical Medicine and never filled again.

Nor did it seem necessary for the whole Tavistock staff to be deployed in the activities of the non-Governmental or voluntary mental health organizations. There was certainly no shortage of working liaison with our American and Canadian colleagues. Whilst the majority of these were in the field of social science, most of the scholars who came to spend sabbatical years or shorter periods with us also contributed greatly to the general development of our theoretical concepts and our therapeutic techniques. Among those who spent years or months with us were Professor Nevitt Sanford of Stanford, Professor Irving Janis, then of Yale, Professors Theodor Newcomb and Dan Miller of the University of Michigan at Ann Arbor, who made particularly important contributions in the analysis of the theory of interaction, Dr M. Schwarz of 'Stanton and Schwarz' fame, and Professor H. Coffey – to name but a few of the distinguished band of social scientists and psychologists who valuably helped us whilst also acquiring some of the Tavistock point of view. Here again it must be mentioned how irksome was our absence of teaching status. Some of these distinguished scholars came on Fulbright grants. Fulbright grants were tenable only at universities. These people always had to have a sponsoring university which nominally regularized their attachment to the Tavistock, where they did all their work.

Not all our visitors were pleased with what they saw. In 1959 we had a visit from Dr David Shakow from the Foundations Fund for Research in Psychiatry, who expressed his concern that there was not enough training of our psychiatric staffs in research methods. This was corrected in the following year, again thanks to the possession of free moneys, by appointing Dr Marie Jahoda to conduct research seminars. These were attended by all clinical research staff and by a number of visitors from other institutions, including Dr Robert Hinde, the Cambridge ethologist.

Nor were Americans alone in wanting to have such contact. There were many visitors also from Holland, Belgium and France, both at clinical and at behavioural science research levels. A rather special case was that of Professor Alexander Mitscherlich, who, together with his also medically qualified wife, both analysts, and several of his staff, at various times spent sabbatical years with us in preparation for the opening of the new Sigmund Freud Institute at Frankfurt, Germany, which Mitscherlich was to direct. This is a University clinic combining some of the features of an institute of psychoanalysis with those of the Tavistock Clinic. We were honoured and glad that this team of post-war Germans who were going to introduce new psychodynamic and applied psychoanalytic techniques to both clinical work and to the study of post-war German social problems should have chosen us as part of their training ground. This Institute now flourishes, trains young psychiatrists in psychoanalysis and psychodynamic research on lines of the Tavistock Clinic. An earlier much briefer contact in search of an adequate model for Germany was Professor Bitter, who founded a psychotherapeutic teaching clinic in Stuttgart. It was also rare for the Tavistock to be without at least one or two associates from Latin America. Among the most rewarding of such attachments was that of Dr Guillermo Teruel and his wife, who were concerned to develop marital treatment services in their country, Venezuela. Teruel's work with groups and his contribution to the theory and practice of both the Marital Unit of the Tavistock Clinic and of the Family Discussion Bureau were very impressive.

Around 1960 these family studies had got to the point where members of the Tavistock were in very considerable demand for papers and demonstrations, especially of their work with families. Laing was spending periods at Bethesda and other American centres of psychiatric research; Mrs Lily Pincus (the senior caseworker of the Family Discussion Bureau) and I were temporary consultants on an international W.H.O. seminar on family mental health in Athens in 1962. In 1961 a team comprising Mrs Alison Lyons, Mrs Mary Welch and Mr Douglas Woodhouse with myself gave a seminar on marital work at the World Mental Health Congress in Paris. Sutherland was Visiting Professor at the Menninger Clinic, Topeka, as well as helping to set up a Community Mental Health Service at Ahmedabad, India, working alongside A. K. Rice (see ch. ix). John Bowlby, in addition to his five months with W.H.O. in 1950, spent 1957–8 at the Centre for Advanced Study in the Behavioural Sciences in California, and in 1968 was Visiting

Professor in Psychiatry at nearby Stanford University. Michael Balint also was in great demand overseas for teaching his views and techniques on training. Dugmore Hunter made a fruitful contact with the mental-health services for adolescents in Finland.

New Developments in the Early 1960s

(*a*) *The Adolescent Unit*

It has already been recorded that the Liaison Committee with the Regional Board had decided on a new building, and this plan had been sanctioned for the Ministry's building programme in 1960. Because of the promise of expanded facilities and consequently a prospect of more staff, we went ahead with a project which had been dear to the hearts of Dugmore Hunter and Derek Miller. The finance was, needless to say, provided by Institute funds. Both had taken a leading part in the design specifications for adolescent centres for our region entrusted to its Advisory Committee for Psychiatry. They had formed a unit for work with adolescents. The Professional Committee gave them full backing, but at first they had to make do with a few rather shabby rooms rented for them in Hallam Street (see ch. ix). They had to rely on part-time services of psychologists and P.S.W.s on loan from the other departments. We had written the provision for staff and space for a fully-functioning Adolescent Department into our new building plans. Meantime, the new unit functioned with very considerable energy, making its contribution to tackling the mounting problem of disturbed and anarchic youth. Originally the unit had been oriented towards the other kind of adolescent – namely, the gifted, neurotically inhibited student – but the pressure of events brought it about that we were also getting the behaviourally disturbed, acting-out delinquent. Derek Miller had returned to England for family reasons after he had already been settled at the Menninger Clinic, Topeka, where he gained much experience in the treatment of adolescents. He now hoped to contribute this expertise with disturbed young persons to the British scene through the medium of the Tavistock, where he had to run through the stages of registrar and senior registrar whilst also completing his own didactic analysis. Dugmore Hunter had for a long time been hoping to switch from his role in the Department for Children and Parents to this new field. The new unit was envisaged as a service not only for individuals, but also to the families of disturbed adolescents. The other social settings, such as schools, employment, or the transition from school to work or school to university soon involved the unit in very live relationships with a variety of relevant agencies, from universities and technical colleges to remand homes and Borstals. This was a very considerable addition to the scope of our clinical services. Though there had always been liaisons with schools, etc., in the Department for Children and Parents, we were now carrying out a further process of differentiation in dealing with another critical area of the human life-span as a specialism. One of the latest creative innovations which can be credited to the Tavistock is the residential centre for disturbed adolescents at Southfields, Hendon, largely the work of Derek Miller, begun in the planning stage within the Psychiatric Advisory committee at No 5 Regional Hospital Board.

(b) Marital Services

The second innovation was the consolidation of some pilot work with disturbed marriages by Mary Luff and myself, begun in 1949, into a Clinic unit for the treatment of disturbed marriages by joint as well as individual techniques. It has been described in previous sections. The unit had functioned as a research team, but this had to be abandoned for lack of adequate funds. The constant discussions on how to re-shape the same programme to suit the orientations of various grant-giving foundations became such a tiresome exercise that we decided in favour of a more operational programme as part of the regular treatment services to our clients. By about 1964 we had already seen some 2,000 couples and treated some 35% of them. The work of teaching marital diagnosis and therapy to registrars and to some selected social workers, as well as open case conferences to interested members of the medical and allied professions, followed as part of our unit system of functioning, from the late 1950s onwards until my own retirement in 1965, when Pierre Turquet took charge.

The Family Discussion Bureau, holding essentially similar concepts and using not dissimilar approaches to these problems, continued to function as a social casework agency not so overtly psychiatric, sponsored by the Institute. Its role developed into that of in-service training of a number of social workers from various community agencies, including the Probation Service. The techniques of the joint interview, as part of interpersonal work with the family, were gaining acceptance and skilled handling not only as research interests, but also in the routines of the two marriage treatment units as well as of the Adolescent Unit. In the Children's Department the joint interview had been used for a long time, unsung. The technique had great influence in the U.S.A., as shown by an article by John Edison Bell. Not only was the Children's Department re-christened the Department for Children and Parents as far back as 1953, itself a significant change, but the use of joint techniques where several workers interviewed either various combinations of a family of which one or more members were their patients as a method of therapy became almost standard practice.

(*c*) *Institute Changes*

Perhaps one of the innovations of the early 1960s was more imposed upon than desired by the Clinic as such. This was essentially an event of differentiation and search for proper identities of two major units within the Tavistock Institute proper. Sidney Gray has covered the Institute aspect of it. One, under Eric Trist and Harold Bridger, was called the Human Resources Centre, and the other, under A. K. Rice and Cyril Sofer, was called the Center for Applied Social Research. A new unit, the Centre for Operational Research, had also come into the Institute. This meant that the old R.T.C., which linked the activities of the Institute and the Clinic, had become somewhat obsolete. It functioned for some time longer until it was superseded by the Common Purposes Committee. The so-called 'Clinic-linked activities' of the Institute, largely those described in this chapter, now required a further differentiation of structure. In 1961 there was created a new co-ordinating body which was called the 'Q' Committee, (soon to be re-named Committee for Family Psychiatry and Community Mental

Health). With the emergence of 'Q' and the fission into H.R.C. and C.A.S.R. within the social science part of the Institute, there was some anxiety about the hitherto unified total institution drifting apart into component parts. With new people in both Clinic and Institute, there was bound to be some erosion of the unifying matrix of the wartime 'invisible college' that cemented the clinical and the social science parts of the institution. It was at this point that the Association was once more perceived as the matrix. It was, after all, the Association which was collectively striving for an integrated science and practice of mental health and human relations, in the community as in individuals. So the supersession of the old R.T.C. by three or four different management committees under the Council, though further differentiating, must not be allowed to disintegrate the organization. The Common Purposes Committee was an expression of this desire. The members of the Clinic staff were not threatened in their job securities. But they were greatly involved in the anxious and long discussions in a further effort at co-ordination or integration of the total institution against possible splitting. This was not a split in ideology or an abrogation of the basic psychodynamic viewpoint which was shared also by our newer staff members who had not been with us in the war. It was simply the difficulty of maintaining an integrate when there was so much work differentiation and so many diverse interests and primary tasks. Although, as will be seen in the next chapter, the problem was solved for the time being, the dialogue on the unifying matrix is ongoing history without an end-point and may well become part of the content of our history in the next fifty years.

In addition to the Common Purposes Committee, we also formed a Staff Board, composed of all the senior staff of all parts of the organization. The Board spent a great deal of time on the redefinition of the common purpose and the reshaping of the total structure. Once again there emerged the unifying goal of a school (never very far absent from us) – a school which would teach all the relevant subjects and skills of our range of activities with the aim of increasing understanding of personal and social change and stress in human development to those concerned with its rational management.

In 1959 there was a sudden unforeseen development. The Tavistock Institute of Medical Psychology, already mentioned as the residual entity of the old Council, retained to receive donations and legacies, was suddenly the recipient of a windfall of some £37,000, under the will of the late Hugh Eric Robertson. It was perhaps my finest hour, as years earlier I had pleaded for the preservation of this purely nominal shadowy corporation, which subsisted from year to year with a small Council on a budget of some £10 or £12 with a few welcome guineas coming in from faithful subscribers. Suddenly we were important, we were a sizeable charitable Foundation (with a capital F), right inside the heart of the Tavistock. The validity of this gift was established by the Scottish Courts and in due course we were in business, with an enlarged Council, able to help those parts of the Tavistock's work not likely to attract other donations. A full list of grants made in the nine or ten years since the fund was received is scarcely required. But here was a body able to further the charitable intentions based on the Charter of the old incorporated Tavistock Clinic of 1929. The acquisition of this sizeable fund for cushioning moves, giving temporary loans, underwriting projects, or financing pilot phases of research has been of the greatest benefit to the organization, especially with the coming of the move from Beaumont Street and Devonshire Street to our new building.

The sudden springing to life of this new/old body had another pleasant side as well. It was a reunion of people who had worked together under quite other conditions. Thus we welcomed to the Council of T.I.M.P. Mr Dudley Herbert, our former Secretary, Professor Ben S. Morris, one-time Chairman of the Management Committee of the Tavistock Institute, and Sir Leslie Farrer, the last Chairman of the 'voluntary' Tavistock Council. Lady Whyte, one of the staunchest wartime members of the Tavistock Clinic's Council, who had chaired the T.I.M.P. in its darkest days, remained for a time our Chairman in our new affluence. We were reassured also by the presence of two old friends, Mr David Ross and Mr Sidney Berlanny, who could speak with authority on finance and investments.

It now remains to mention other significant personalia. In

1954 Mary Hemingway Rees, the wife of J.R. and an original member of staff, died, greatly mourned. Her friends in the World Federation of Mental Health set up a memorial lecture fund called after her to perpetuate her deep interest in relationships between religion and mental health. This lecture is given biennially at meetings of the World Federation of Mental Health. It was my privilege to give the first of these lectures at Vienna in 1958, in which I paid tribute to Molly Rees's lovable personality. Some of her contemporaries also left us: Amy Thoms and Leopold Stein retired. The latter, after much further pioneering in Birmingham, died in July 1969. Curt Boenheim emigrated (to the U.S.A.), J. J. M. Jacobs was lost to us by premature and tragic death. Ronald Hargreaves, though not strictly a staff member since 1946, but of our heart's blood, died in 1962, also far too young. Wittkower went to McGill, to our impoverishment and to the enrichment of Canadian psychiatry. In 1958 his erstwhile research colleague and a creator of the Institute, A. T. M. Wilson, left the staff, after long tenure and outstanding services to our 'integrate', to become special adviser in the social sciences to the Unilever Corporation. He did much for the reputation of the Clinic long before he became an 'Institute man'.

Reference has already been made to the deaths of Colonel Rait-Kerr, the first Chairman of the Council of the Institute, and of his Deputy, Dr Leonard Browne. Leonard, a near-original staff member of the old Clinic, was one of the important unifying personalities between psychological medicine and public mental-health policy.

Some important recruits from the Maudsley Hospital joined our staff: Robert H. Gosling, David H. Malan and J. L. Wilson. Hyla Holden and Dorothy Heard also were newcomers during this period, and Marion Mackenzie achieved full consultant status after languishing under the disadvantage of a frozen establishment for far too long. Some others of our staff still labour under these disadvantages. Balint, that creative and vivid personality, retired in 1961. His work, however, was carried on. Joseph Sandler left us to join Professor Denis Hill at the Middlesex Hospital. In 1960, Miss Daphne Seamark, who had created the post-war Tavistock Library, retired. She was replaced by Miss Ann Sutherland, who has amply maintained that important and expanding service.

We were lucky after a period of transitory incumbents to acquire Mrs Ida Hunt as our Administrative Officer, with the rank of Assistant Secretary to the Hospital Management Committee. Mrs Hunt has made the Tavistock and its two sister clinics her real concern and has remained one of our best-appreciated administrators, not excluding our pre-N.H.S. phase. Administrative skill sits lightly on her flexible and friendly personality.

XI

History Becomes the Present

Our negotiations with the Ministry of Health through the Liaison Committee of the Institute, the Clinic and the Board were crowned with success. In the 1960 five-year budget of the Ministry for capital expenditure a new building for the Tavistock was sanctioned and put into execution. Before that time the Institute had asked a firm of architects to prepare contingency plans and a model for a new Tavistock building. This model was quite unofficial, though very attractive. To our dismay, it was later shown at the Summer Exhibition of the Royal Academy! There is no evidence that the design influenced our real architect. But the Regional Board officers could be forgiven if they felt annoyed.

Not long after this we had a visit from the then Minister of Health, Mr Enoch Powell, who spent a whole morning with us and went into our work and over our cramped premises very thoroughly. He talked with many members of the staff of Clinic and Institute, attended two case conferences and asked many highly pertinent questions. At the end he seemed at ease with us and made the humorous remark, 'So it seems that you are missionaries after all'. He had certainly perceived that we were a highly integrated group with a purpose and strong ethical conviction about the role of psychological medicine and social psychology in the public weal. At any rate, it was not long after his visit that the site of the bombed Marie Curie Hospital at the corner of Belsize Lane and Fitzjohns Avenue in South Hampstead was offered and accepted by us as our new location, and building operations soon began.

There were many meetings with the Board's architect, Mr F. A. C. Maunder, who, with his assistant architects, designed the building and who consulted with the consumers – namely, ourselves and the Hospital Management Committee – on the details and layout. The foundation-stone was laid, when the building was already rising, on 14 October 1965 by J. R. Rees. This stone can be seen in the entrance hall of the new building, suitably inscribed. This was a small but charming ceremony at which J.R. made an excellent speech at the age of seventy-five. We had previously celebrated his seventieth birthday with a reception and cocktail party, at which we presented him with what we hoped would be pleasant gifts with affectionate sentiments from both the Clinic and the Institute of which he was a Council member. His death, in April 1969, after some months of ill-health, came to his old colleagues with a sense of overwhelming loss. He was the master-builder of nearly all that we had achieved.

The Institute part of the organization had had considerable misgivings about moving the bulk of their activities from the handsome and prestigeful, Embassy-like building at No 3, Devonshire Street, to what the late Sir Hugh Beaver had described as the 'country'. None the less, in the end they decided that they would move in after considerable negotiations with the Ministry of Health and the Regional Board on an equitable financial arrangement. Sir Hugh, as Chairman of the Institute's Council, played an important role in these talks. There was sufficient drive left in our quest for integration and continuing close association between the Health Service and the non-Health Service part of the Tavistock effort, and this motivation won over the convenience of separate handsome premises in W.1 for the Institute. Only the new unit for Operational Research has remained outside the Belsize Lane building. The growth of the Institute since the building was first planned made it impossible to fit all its units in.

Contrary to a pessimistic forecast by the Ministry officials themselves, the new building was completed before schedule around New Year, 1967, and well under the ten years they had prophesied. The organizations moved in during the Easter recess of 1967 and opened the doors of their new home unofficially for work in the week after Easter. The five-storey building standing in considerable grounds was soon christened by our witty friend Geoffrey Gorer 'the Freud Hilton'! A tribute is certainly in place to Mr F. A. C. Maunder and his architectural staff for producing such an imaginative design in a period when glass and concrete boxes are the rule. He was assisted and advised by consulting engineers, Messrs Tintern, Jones & Partners, in association with Mr R. C. Hodge, the Regional Engineer; consulting structural engineers were Messrs Andrews, Kent and Stone and the quantity surveyors Messrs Young & Brown. The general building contractors were Pitchers Ltd, whose boards were seen on the site during the building. There were also various sub-contractors, Benham & Sons Ltd on the mechanical side and Electrical Installations Ltd on the electrical side. The latter was important to us with our more elaborate recording and one-way viewing systems in the new building, and a filming unit with special construction also installed.

This handsome and spacious building, which more than doubled our total accommodation, was opened at a most pleasant ceremony on 4 May 1967 by Her Royal Highness, Princess Marina, our Patron. The Chair was taken by Mr Maurice Hackett, O.B.E., Chairman of our Regional Hospital Board. On her entry Her Royal Highness was presented with a bouquet by little Louisa Gosling, the daughter of Robert and Veronica Gosling. Her Royal Highness, after a speech of welcome by Mr Hackett, gave an address in which she briefly retraced the history of the Clinic and Institute, much as has been done *in extenso* in the present volume. After paying tribute to H.C.M., J.R. and Jock Sutherland, the Princess went on:

> Although in recent years the two bodies [the Clinic and Institute] have had to work in different buildings, they have maintained throughout this period the closest scientific collaboration. It is this unique association of the Clinic *and* the Institute which has made 'The Tavistock' the internationally recognized centre it is, attracting professional workers and social scientists from all over the world.
>
> Many developments have changed the Clinic's original pattern of work. People in trouble seek help from diverse sources, and so, in addition to its own treatment services, the

Clinic has devoted a large part of its effort to working with the various professions concerned: the clergy, doctors, and social workers of all kinds. Collaboration between psychological clinics and schools has gone on for many years, but much more of this is needed, especially with those engaged with the education of adolescents and the young adult. In this latter direction the Adolescent Unit of the Clinic, which started a few years ago with very limited resources, space and staff, has made significant, indeed remarkable progress; and its services are in great demand.

When it was decided to situate the Child Guidance Training Centre in this new building, a great addition was made to the existing resources. With its long experience of training professional staff for the mental health services for children, alongside those of 'the Tavistock', there has now been formed the largest training centre of its kind in the United Kingdom. Both units will have an opportunity to pool their experiences, so that this very important work will be developed to the best advantage for the needs of the country.

I need hardly comment on the urgent necessity for the advancement of the human sciences, for more specialist staff, and more centres in which research can be undertaken. The creation of this new Tavistock Centre is a recognition by the Health Service authorities of the great importance of these needs. By facilitating such a wide range of work under the same roof with opportunities to exchange ideas and to share in complex tasks, the staff have been given an inspiring setting. Your past record in meeting challenges led the authorities to give you this chance.

But in the last resort it has always seemed to me that the only way to bridge the gulf and try to reach the hurt mind or a disturbed human being is by the selfless giving of heart, mind and time, and even though this very specialized vocation must often be discouraging in the seeming slowness of response, it must also be infinitely rewarding when that response is made. So for you all I have nothing but the highest praise, and I am confident too that you will make full and purposeful use of this splendid centre in the years to come.

It is therefore with the greatest pleasure that I declare open the Tavistock Centre.

After this speech Mrs M. R. Forbes, C.B.E., D.TECH.(Hon.), J.P., Chairman of the Paddington Group Hospital Management Committee, accepted the building from the Chairman of the Regional Board into the care of our old friends, the Paddington H.M.C. The Duchess then toured the new building and, lastly, unveiled a commemorative plaque in the main entrance before departing. Needless to say, a number of parties and receptions were held at which the whole psychiatric and social science world and our many friends in medicine, business, industry, psychology and the 'helping professions' were entertained and shown with considerable pride our new and, one may unaffectedly say, splendid home. It was our great pleasure that members of the Crichton-Miller family as well as many other friends were with us.

The sudden translation from our accustomed 'face-to-face', tight accommodation in Beaumont Street to a palatial building, for all the world resembling a large insurance office or other industrial headquarters, was not without its repercussions on the staff. Many people expressed the feeling that something might easily be lost unless we were very careful. Not only was it now difficult to maintain interdepartmental relationships by meetings in a small space between colleagues, but the whole efficient and impersonal atmosphere with long passages and lifts and distances between offices and consulting-rooms seemed to carry a certain threat of being caught in a large organization which it was difficult to recognize as the tight little friendly Tavistock Group of pre-war days. Not a few staff members also regretted the loss of our faithful Mr Arthur Wicks, the chef-cum-caretaker at Beaumont Street, who had had a very personal interest and concern to feed us well, even if limited by his National Health Service budgets for canteen services. The new refectory, though spacious and gleaming with modernity, does not in fact cook anything! All the food is mass pre-cooked and merely doled out from hot-plates, packaged in expendable containers, plastic cups and the like. This seems rather disconcerting and somehow injurious to the intimacy of the very important feeding function of the Institution,[1] totally at variance with the early post-war aspiration that the catering unit should be also a sociatric project contributing to the integration of the whole institution. I privately wonder why the staff do not rebel at this. But against this sort of disadvantage must be set the real sense of dignity, spaciousness and suitable working accommodation as well as common rooms, lecture halls and library which the staff have gained. I retired some eighteen months before the new building was opened. Coming in as a quasi-visitor, I could see that somehow most people seemed to be dressed more smartly and to walk about with an air to match the new surroundings. There are always a lot of flowers, and with its good colour schemes it is a cheerful building to be in.

From the excerpt of Her Royal Highness's speech it will be seen that the Tavistock was not to occupy the entire building, as had originally been contemplated. The history of the National Health Service has been punctuated by the conflicting and contradictory motives of generosity, the best possible provisions of space, establishments, etc., and the equally powerful and usually decisive need for economy when it comes to the execution of plans made some years before they can be implemented. In this instance we found that the Regional Board, faced with the necessity of rehousing the Child Guidance Training Centre, which has already been mentioned in earlier parts of this book, decided to give it one floor of the building and have it share some of the common ground-floor accommodation and refectory. There was considerable difficulty over this, since, as already mentioned, the other institutions doing similar work to the Tavistock's had been jealous about guarding their independence and their identities. Here seemed to be a real threat that the Child Guidance Training Centre, with its long tradition of service and teaching, might be 'swallowed' by the Tavistock. There was, I think, some difficulty in convincing some of the senior staff of the Child Guidance Training Centre that this housing move was none of our doing. In fact, the Professional Committee and the joint Clinic/Institute com-

[1] Cf. Goldring's *The Broilerhouse Society*.

mittees felt quite severely disappointed in not getting the full facilities of the building to allow for the inevitable expansion, if not of the Clinic, then at least of the Institute and of the joint teaching projects which had been growing apace. However, we could do nothing about it, and it was at least with some relief that we found that the third of the possible occupants of the Tavistock Centre, as the building was officially known – namely, the Portman Clinic – was not to move in. The other evidence of the conflict between generosity and economy was the fact that the medical establishments which we had asked for especially for the expansion of the Adolescent Unit, as mentioned by Her Royal Highness, had not been granted. It is remarkable, as seen from the vantage-point of a member of the Regional Mental Health Committee and other national committees, how often the Treasury will grant vast sums for new expensive buildings, but then refuse to sanction the necessary increase in manpower to utilize the accommodation. The Tavistock is not alone in suffering from this curious dichotomy between bricks and mortar and bodies to work.

We knew for some years that the Ministry of Health had been greatly concerned at the undue concentration of psychiatric manpower in the Metropolis, and had put a very severe limit to new psychiatric posts anywhere in the London area, so as to try to channel the rather meagre supply of psychiatrists into the provinces, where, it is true, they are more urgently needed. However, since the Tavistock could be regarded as a kind of 'model' (not necessarily of performance, but of design), it seemed rather short-sighted not to let at least its rather novel Adolescent Unit have the manpower asked for. Instead, staff for it had to be diverted from the existing larger units, the Adult Department and the Department for Children and Parents. Such an enlarged establishment had been – I will not use the word 'promised' – confidently foreseen in the plans for the move, not only because the appearance of juvenile delinquency and alienation was preoccupying the country and its authorities, but also because our new adolescent services had already made their impact uuder the energetic leadership of Derek Miller. None the less, the Adolescent Unit has managed to extend fruitful co-operation and in some instances joint appointments with the juvenile penal and reformatory services. The newly-established Young People's Consultation Centre, which had been located in Hampstead, was now put inside the Adolescent Unit at Belsize Lane. This service is maintained on a twenty-four-hour 'walk-in' basis and is proving its worth.

The Young People's Consultation Centre had been set up originally by a Dutch charity, the Bernard Van Leer Foundation. It was while Dr W. G. Joffe was its medical head that this proposal was implemented. At one time one of our senior registrars, Joffe was now on the staff of the Academic Department of Psychiatry at the Middlesex Hospital. The move of bringing it into the Tavistock Adolescent Unit suited both sides. The Centre required an adequate technical base of psychologists, social workers and so on; for us its finance opened a way round the starving of the Adolescent Unit of staff, as just mentioned. The original financing of the Adolescent Department had been almost entirely done by the Tavistock Institute, and this could now be shared. The Department's link with the new in-patient centre, Southfields, has already been referred to. Joint staffing arrangements are in being.

The attitude of the N.H.S. authorities in particular towards the Tavistock Clinic establishment might possibly be excused if we look at the attendance figures – for example, for 1961. At this date there were a total of 642 new patients seen in the calendar year (450 in the Adult, 113 in the Department for Children and Parents, 79 in the Adolescent Unit). The total attendances seemed imposing, 21,253 (of which 17,963 were in the Adult Department). However, when one analysed the attendance of patients per medical half-day, it only worked out at 2·45 patients per doctor session. This is something with which bureaucrats would have difficulty. These figures are small. What they fail to show is the chosen policy, sanctioned by the Ministry, of not allowing ourselves to be swamped by patients, but instead supporting by consultant seminars an unprecedented number of people in general practice, the social services and public health, enabling them to deal collectively with thousands of early cases, children or adults, marital and other interaction problems in their own fields, thus increasing skill and expertise in the helping professions and saving a large number of specialist referrals. In a subsequent paragraph, where I deal with extra-mural training, I quote the most recent available figures for this educational and consultative effort of the Clinic. While this new role of the psychotherapeutic clinic as a supporting base for community mental health work was fully endorsed at high levels in the Ministry, the consequential fall in attendance figures can give support to derisive description of the Tavistock as a *de luxe* outfit by comparison with the turnover of the rest of the psychiatric profession, where from eight to ten attendances, consisting of rapid classification and a prescription, was the pattern. But at any rate the internal Tavistock ethic held: it continued loaned sessions from the other two departments and also invoking the support of the Institute for temporary staff and financing of the Adolescent Department.

It remains to mention briefly some staff changes in the more recent past. In 1961 Michael Balint retired, although he continued his teaching group work in other centres, notably at University College Hospital, with the Family Planning Association and elsewhere, lecturing and disseminating his ideas and techniques on teaching mental-health and psychiatric skills to the medical and social-work professions. In 1965 I myself retired after what seemed a very long service – in fact, my life's work – with the Tavistock, with most kindly celebrations and every expression of affection from my colleagues and good friends. The point should be made that with neither of these retirements was new blood introduced into the life of the Clinic. The sessions vacated were filled by the allotment of more sessions to existing staff members, especially consultants, to take up a larger part of their working life. It is surprising that David Malan, already internationally known for his work with brief psychotherapy, was only then appointed a consultant.

On the non-medical professional staff Mrs Elizabeth Irvine, for many years our distinguished Psychiatric Social Work Tutor in succession to Miss Hunnybun, was appointed Reader in Social Work in the University of York. Miss Elizabeth Brown, who had been her second-in-command, was now appointed the Chief P.S.W. Tutor to the Department for Children and Parents. Mrs Yana Popper, who had followed Miss Simmins as the head of the psychological services in that department, also retired after many years of much appreciated work. Her place was taken by Miss Irene Caspari, who is currently the Chief Psychologist to the Children's Department. Also in 1968 John Bowlby relinquished the formal headship of the Department for Children and Parents, which he had so creatively reorganized and shaped over twenty-two years, in order to devote more time to the research and training activities of the growing School, of which he had been Chairman from the beginning. In his stead the Department elected Dr Marion Mackenzie as the Chairman of the Department for Children and Parents. Dr Mackenzie was associated with the Tavistock even before the war whilst still in general practice and has been one of the clinical and administrative stalwarts of our children's services.

Around the time of John Bowlby's retirement from headship of the clinical services, his department issued an interesting internal document on the scientific principles and working philosophy of that department. A brief summary may be of relevance, in view of the current developments towards community and family psychiatry in the country. The document declared that its aims were, first, to promote the health of families and children growing up within a community; secondly, to gain a better understanding of the conditions making for healthy growth; thirdly, to devise more varied and better techniques for bringing those conditions into being; lastly, to train professional personnel for those functions. Its clinical policy was to be limited by area in order to give a model total service of the above kind in a community. It stated its theoretical base as being on the lines of broadly psychoanalytic theory, with especial reference to Melanie Klein's, John Bowlby's and Gerald Caplan's work, also leaning on the later work of Ronald Laing in interpersonal perception and attribution. The Department recognized that the individuals working in it had individual differences, and sometimes a conflict of working theories, and that this conflict and controversy was a respected part of a growing subject rather than suppressed for the sake of uniformity. The statement of these theoretical bases emphasized not only intrapersonal factors but also human environments and interaction as playing their part in the creation of either good mental health or mental ill-health in the child. The document further stated that its working philosophy was not merely to sit in a clinic and receive sick children, but to extend its roots into the community, especially schools, in collaboration with the educational world, where much clinical work could be done at a much earlier stage by the staff actually going out and dealing with incipient trouble in the places where children were actually living and having their social being. It was also made clear that work should always be done with families, and never with the child patient in isolation. The therapeutic goals and ambitions were flexible in so far as the most insightful families were likely to yield better results with intensive work, whereas the least insightful, most limited and disturbed families might never consent to come to a highly specialized institution, but would have to receive treatment outside, mainly by social agencies in consultative relation with the Department. Lastly, the document also reiterated its belief in the cross-fertilization between clinical work and research. The clinician fed into research problems requiring solution, whereas research findings would be fed back into improved clinical insights and techniques resulting from new or better-validated theories and hypotheses. This last point reiterates the important principle of *problem-centred* research, characteristic of the Tavistock as a whole. This point of view has been further elaborated in a longer document submitted by the Institute to the Social Research Council, to which I will return.

In the internal Clinic sphere the professional staff undertook to reorganize and review the functions and modes of appointment of its own Professional Committee. Sutherland had for a long time felt that a 'Medical Director' was an archaic misnomer, since he had never seen himself as other than the Chairman of the Professional Committee, a post which within the Health Service usually brings with it the conduct of external relations between the Institution's professional staff and such agencies as the Health Service authorities and outside organizations. The prolonged discussions – as usual, very intensive and thorough – resulted in a system by which the Chairman was elected by the entire professional staff voting an individual into the office and maintaining him in office for five years before re-election, with indefinite tenure. In other words, we would always have an elected Leader who could go on being the leader as long as the staff wanted him. For the rest of the representation, the departments and professions within the Clinic voted on much the same lines as previously, but the Committee would have a constitution somewhat more professional and structured. The representatives would now serve for three years, but would automatically have to represent all the clinical units as well as professions of each department, with the addition of the new Adolescent Department. The real power now seemed transferred to a collectivity known as the 'Staff Meeting'. This meeting has become a greater reality than hitherto in the life of the Clinic and discusses broad issues of policy, as well as having at all times access to the Professional Committee minutes.

The dropping of the title 'Medical Director' was by no means welcome to the authorities, who seemed to like knowing with whom they were negotiating. It was resurrected somewhat equivocally mainly in relation to 'foreign affairs'. Within the Committee greater formalization has also occurred with the growth of departments. It was felt suitable that motions or decisions of the Committee should be formally proposed and seconded and voted upon rather than left, as over all the preceding forty years, to democratic and anonymous consensus. Also the Professional Committee decided to have a Secretary appointed from its own midst. Mrs Elsie Osborne, Clinical Psychologist in the Department for Children and Parents, became the first elected holder of this post.

In the educational activities, in so far as they were part of the Health Service arrangements, no major changes have occurred. But it was felt necessary to strengthen the integration of courses and eliminate duplication. This has meant more training events shared by the psychiatric registrars, supernumerary or honorary trainee doctors (on their own bursaries), and by the psychologists and social workers in training. An additional long, four-year training for one clinical psychologist per annum has also been instituted for the nurturing of exceptionally promising people. The registrars, though rooted in one department, are now also expected to do some part of their work in another department for wider horizons. Moreover, as in universities, every trainee, whether on the Health Service strength or attached overseas personnel has been allotted a tutor from among the small number of core staff of the Clinic to route them most profitably through various training experiences in the light of their background and already achieved expertise, to avoid training becoming too stereotyped. In the Department for Children and Parents this has obtained from the beginning of Bowlby's Chairmanship; the larger Adult Department has now achieved it too.

Perhaps a word on a timely innovation, created in 1968 – a Trainee's Committee. Long before the junior hospital doctors' 'revolt' broke surface and long before the various troubles of students everywhere, we had already decided that the junior staff should have the right to criticize the training at the Clinic. They now not only have real contact through a tutor with what they need to do, but also have a very substantial voice in two meetings per term with the Staff Training Executive, devoted to evaluating the training and to propose improvements.

Extra-mural training done (as always) in conjunction with the Institute of Human Relations has grown very greatly. After Balint's retirement, the general practitioner seminars have been continued by four consultants under the headship of Robert Gosling, serving some fifty general practitioners at any given time. There are regular seminars for medical officers of health, chiefly in the Children's Department. The Introductory Psychotherapy Course for psychiatrists has flourished with more applications than places available. Three kinds of probation officer courses are held regularly, not only in the area of marriage counselling, but also for generally extending insights and knowledge of psychopathology and human relations. A course of seminars for dermatologists, much of whose work is so closely linked to psychosomatic method, has been given by Dr T. W. Goldblatt; another is going on for Borstal assistant governors and prison officers; and another course of a different kind for medical officers of health and health visitors in the field of community psychiatry. There have been external courses for educational psychologists working in other child psychiatric clinics; the staffs of schools for maladjusted children have also had opportunities of attending seminars. For all these varied activities a co-ordinating committee for training and liaison with community mental health services was formed under the chairmanship of Dr Marion Mackenzie some years ago. A particularly interesting and valuable summer school has been held for some years by Professor Gerald Caplan (many years ago one of our registrars) of Harvard University on his crisis theory in relation to mental health action.

The bald numbers for training courses mentioned above, and also referred to earlier in connection with the relatively low patient attendance figures for the quinquennium 1963–7 read:

(*a*) *Internal Training:* 281 professional workers, of whom 106 were full-time; psychiatrists, 67; clinical and educational psychologists, 97; social case workers (including P.S.W.s), 78; child psychotherapists, 35; public health medical officers and paediatricians, 4.

(*b*) *External Training (part-time, seminars, etc.):* 357 professional workers, of whom there were: psychiatrists, 59; psychologists, 34; general practitioners, 47; public health medical officers, 94; other public health staff, 90; teachers, 40; probation officers, 14; social workers, 19; university and college tutors, 10.

The growth factor in this function is shown in the report of the School for the most recent years.

(*a*) *Internal Training* (1968–9)

	(*i*) *N.H.S. post trainees*	(*ii*) *Associate trainees*	*Total*
Psychiatrists	18	8	26
Clinical psychologists	9	11	20
Educational psychologists	7	6	13
Child psychotherapists	12	18	30
Social case workers	13	13	26
	59	56	115

These trainees came from twenty countries.

(*b*) *Extra-mural and part-time Courses and Consultative Seminars:* psychiatrists, 53; psychologists, 56; general practitioners, 34; public health medical officers, 26; other public health staff, 76; teachers, 50; probation officers, 26; social workers, 60; university and college tutors, 18; psychotherapists, 8; town-planning officer, 1; giving a total of 408 external students for one academic year (1967–8).

These teaching and consultative services were distributed between the staffs of the Clinic, the Institute of Marital Studies and other Institute staff as well as some 'outside' teachers, usually members of the Association. New courses started in 1968 include one for teachers on problems of relationships in schools, on co-operation of senior educational psychologists with remedial teachers, and a redesigned course in Rorschach and other projective techniques. This work demands not only the actual delivery of teaching, but also staff 'workshops' and evaluations of methods. An international conference for G.P. seminar leaders, for example, was held under Tavistock auspices in April 1968.

Mention should also be made of the help provided by Dr Colin Parkes and Mr Michael Foster (of the Institute's Human Resources Centre) during the first eighteen months after the Aberfan colliery tip disaster on principles of social psychiatry and community mental health. During this emergency, Professor Mary Essex, a former associate in the Department of Children and Parents, now in Cardiff, also rendered signal service to Aberfan survivors.

I mentioned in ch. x the creation of 'Q', a 'Management Committee for the Clinic-linked Units', co-ordinating joint Clinic-Institute training and research activities, with executive powers delegated to it by a Staff Board, linking all units of the enterprise. More recently still, the Council of the Institute created a number of sub-councils. Of these that for the School (formerly the Committee) of Family Psychiatry and Community Mental Health now takes formal responsibility for the development of the School. The teaching and research group form a Staff Committee of the School, of which John Bowlby is Chairman. A sub-committee for research is chaired by Colin Parkes, and another for training also by Bowlby.

Ronald Laing's research under T.I.H.R. continued until 1967. He is now no longer Tavistock-based. It has resulted in a number of books on family interaction and interpersonal perception, with emphasis on a psychodynamic theory of schizophrenic behaviour. He has also created a new model residential unit at Kingsley Hall, London, E.3.

The research work under John Bowlby recently received a further substantial grant for Mr and Mrs Robertson's studies of brief separation effects on children from the Grant Foundation. Three further film studies are now published: two of children in foster care, one of a child in a residential nursery. Bowlby's own work, with M.R.C. support, continues on the implications of the studies on loss and separation for theories of personality and psychopathology. A research component is also being explored, as I write, for the work in the Adolescent Department, while in the Adult Department the clinical psychologists, until recently under the leadership of Sutherland, are working towards solving the complex problem of adequate validation measures for the effects of psychotherapy on personality change which are beginning to see publication.

In its external relations the Tavistock has been affected by the undoubted change in general atmosphere in which, despite great progress with the physical methods of treatment for psychoses, the need for community psychiatry and hence for an adequate theory of interpersonal relations and human environment has become more insistent. The highly successful Psychotherapy Congress of 1964 owed not a little to the influence of the psychoanalytically oriented institutions and individuals of the Tavistock, the Cassel Hospital and elsewhere. T. F. Main, Robert Gosling, Malcolm Pines and S. T. Hayward of Shenley Hospital played very important parts in its organization.

In 1966 the International Association for Child Psychiatry and Allied Professions held its large Sixth Congress at Edinburgh. This was the culmination of John Bowlby's four years' Presidency, and he as well as Mrs Elizabeth Irvine played important parts in the Congress. Similarly, the World Federation for Mental Health at its Twentieth Anniversary Congress in London (1968) drew on a considerable number of Tavistock personnel to man its technical seminars and special sessions. A major contribution was made by the Family Discussion Bureau to the subject of marital diagnosis and therapy. We are clearly ready to emerge on the scene much more than ten years ago!

As a further sign of change in psychiatric climate, I was in 1967 inducted as President of the Royal Medico-Psychological Association. A personal honour and recognition was one aspect, since I had done a good deal of work in connection with the R.M.P.A.'s moves to becoming a college. But such an event, following upon the Presidency of another analyst, Professor Erwin Stengel of Sheffield, could not have been conceived during earlier phases of British psychiatry. It should be said that I was not the first 'Tavistock person' to reach this honour. Some years previously our colleague from the 1920s, Dr Isabel Wilson, C.B.E., had been President – moreover, as the first woman – but her eminence was not achieved through the Tavistock, but through her subsequent work as a Senior Commissioner of the Ministry's Mental Health Service. The fact that the whole 1967 Annual Meeting of the R.M.P.A. was expected to be devoted to the exposition of the psychodynamic viewpoint indicated psychiatrists' interest in the Tavistock and its works. At the plenary scientific meeting both Sutherland and T. F. Main of the Cassel made clinically oriented contributions, whereas Elliott Jaques and Hugh Murray, respectively past and present senior staff members of the Institute of Human Relations, spoke on more sociological aspects of mental-health work in the industrial field. The seminars which are usually held in connection with major R.M.P.A. meetings were taken by Tavistock members. The R.M.P.A. was also entertained by the Tavistock and the Paddington Hospital Management Committee at a very handsome reception. In my Presidential Address I stressed the necessity, first propounded by Crichton-Miller, for a more integrated or holistic vision of psychological medicine in which the psychodynamic psychotherapeutic viewpoint was the cornerstone of all psychiatrists' skills. The human being should be the centre of attention rather than any organ system or any impersonal laboratory approach to our subject. It was highly significant in the light of past history that the new Professor of Psychiatry at the Institute of Psychiatry at the Maudsley Hospital, Sir Denis Hill, made what was the most brilliant contribution in opening the discussion. His appointment, and that of Professor G. M. Carstairs to Edinburgh, can be said to herald a new era in British psychiatry in which the kind of views and techniques steadfastly promoted and practised by the Tavistock and the Cassel Hospital will find recognition among the second generation of professors.

Another way in which the changed climate has lately been felt is the greater ease and speed with which our senior registrars from the Adult Department at the end of their training period have obtained consultant posts, not in special psychotherapeutic clinics, but in the psychiatric services in general. This is in marked contrast to the 1940s and 1950s, when there were often long waits and many excellent men eventually had to go into full-time private practice against their inclinations. This is due to a number of posts created for the specialists in psychotherapy with consultant rank in both teaching hospitals and in a number of psychiatric hospitals which include the teaching of junior staff and organizing this side of the hospital's work. There had never been great difficulty for the senior registrars in the Children's Department in obtaining permanent posts.

Latterly the problem of whether the Tavistock should grant any kind of diploma has once again been aired after having been always turned down. This has special relevance to the long and advanced course of training for clinical psychologists at the Tavistock Clinic, in consequence of which they are in great demand; but they have no paper qualifications to show for their achievements, which, it appears, are looked for by prospective employers.

After the move into new premises, the event which was to dominate 1968 was the announced intention by J. D. Sutherland to resign in order to take up a university teaching appointment in the Department of Psychiatry of Edinburgh University before his due retiring age. He gave long notice so that the staff could fully discuss the issues that would arise from his going, including perhaps even the structure of the Clinic. Sutherland's expressed motive was that since his sixtieth birthday he had felt that his position should be held by a person who could take responsibility for at least ten years – the time limit for planning in a place like the Tavistock. There were now a group of consultants of the age 'we' were just after the Second World War. Obituaries should not be written about the still living and active, but an appreciation lies too near to my feelings to avoid. To someone like myself who welcomed Jock Sutherland's arrival as a 'new boy' only as recently as 1946, it was a shock to realize that he had in fact held the chief executive medical position in the Tavistock far longer than his two predecessors (H.C.M. fourteen years, and J.R. thirteen years). For twenty-one years the Tavistock had been under his tolerant and gentle direction, characterized by the absence of any tinge of authoritarian leadership or scientific dogmatism. Some might even have considered that he did not provide enough leadership, but after all he came into a rather adult group of many strong and quite senior personalities, all of whom had held responsibility for a long time. The regrets and genuine reactions of sorrow at his going and the immense warmth and generosity of the tributes in praise as well as in farewell gifts to him and his gracious wife, Molly, spoke eloquently of the esteem in which he is held, despite, or because of, his conscious resolution not to act as a 'boss', or as a promoter, or as a blower of trumpets, or an overseller of what we had to offer. Jock, like Crichton-Miller, had the Edinburgh attitude to his subject, and it is pleasant to record that when the aged and ailing H.C.M. met him at the beginning of his tenure of office he was extremely pleased at Jock's election to succeed J.R., towards whom, one gathered, H.C.M. had been somewhat ambivalent, although he esteemed his immense working capacity, energies and enthusiasm. It is certainly significant of the change of which I have written just now that Professor Carstairs should have invited Jock to become one of his senior colleagues in the teaching of psychotherapy, psychopathology and the elements of community psychiatry in the University Department at Edinburgh. Some of his good friends are not surprised that he wished to hand on the extremely hard administrative burdens of the Medical Direction or Chairman of the Tavistock Group to a younger man. It is equally natural that he should wish to return to his native city and to the place where his first teacher and analyst, the late W. R. D. Fairbairn, for long ploughed a lonely but fruitful furrow. We are now seeing the gradual acceptance of

Fairbairn's original new formulations of a consistently *psychological* theory for psychoanalysis. One always felt that Sutherland's affection for this great gentleman was an abiding loyalty, and Edinburgh will be greatly enriched by all that Fairbairn's pupil has already achieved and distilled from his years at the Tavistock. Despite his dislike of organization, it is surprising in retrospect to see how much travelling and how much committee work Jock did, as it were, despite himself. He was invited to advise on the reorganization of the Menninger Clinic in Topeka; he had been to India to organize and advise on mental health services for a great industrial settlement; he was instrumental in advising on and piloting the community mental health scheme for the then borough of West Ham. He had much to do with the Home Office committee for the training of probation officers, with the Family Planning Association, and with the Family Discussion Bureau in its more technical aspects. He had also been Chairman of the Medical Section of the British Psychological Society, and more recently of the Psychotherapy Section of the Royal Medico-Psychological Association, in addition to being Editor first of the *British Journal of Medical Psychology* and then of the *International Journal of Psychoanalysis*.

Jock was the model of the new integrated 'Tavistock man'. As already mentioned, he embodies within himself the disciplines of academic psychology, social psychology, psychiatry, psychoanalysis and all the special skills and experiences which he had accumulated over the years from the Army and War Office selection boards and his constant membership, usually in the chair, of various joint committees and projects of the Institute and the Clinic. He may with truth be said to have been the keystone articulating the unity of these two increasingly differentiated bodies. He was always a rational and scientifically minded critic of dogmatism in any form, whether from the organicist side or from the more 'devotee' psychoanalytic side. He created an atmosphere in which diverse talents could pursue research work, a function he expressed by his notion of a 'matrix' in which promising people could be nurtured. He had supported many men in their research assignments: Henry Ezriel, Ronald Laing, Joseph Sandler, David Malan and H. S.

Gill. His was a wise and 'remote control' kind of nourishing leadership, hoping for people's self-direction. It was nice for us and a fitting coda to his career at the Tavistock that Her Majesty bestowed upon him in 1968 the dignity of a Commander of the Order of the British Empire (C.B.E.). It was fortunate for the Tavistock that he left us Miss Marjorie Harborough, his personal assistant for the whole period, in whose capable hands and brain so many threads of policies and plans have received clear arrangement and safe keeping. She remains one of the central figures in the life of the Tavistock, much admired and appreciated by all parts of the house.

It was perhaps not unnatural that there should have been considerable discussion, not without some heat at times, on the future structure after Sutherland's departure. There was no 'palace revolution' or conflict: the Medical Director himself gave due notice that he would retire and thus gave an opportunity for long and mainly rational discussion of what should happen. As is the custom in the Tavistock, the vote was free for the entire senior staff of the Health Service component of the organization. In the end it was Dr Robert H. Gosling who won the unanimous vote of all his colleagues under the new title of Chairman of the Professional Committee, and began his duties on the expiry of Sutherland's tenure on 1 August 1968. A consultant in the Adult Department with special interest in group therapy and in the training seminars for general practitioners and other professional personnel concerned with the helping services, he had taken Balint's place as the organizer of these extra-mural events, to which he also added considerable experience in collaborating with the Institute in some of their Group Relations Conferences, at which the same kind of techniques were used in the training and orientation of managerial and similar personnel in industry and the like. One can probably assert that his psychiatric training began as an undergraduate when he came under the influence of Dr Carl Binger, then the senior teaching psychiatrist at Cornell Medical School, New York. Robert Gosling has known ill-health as a young man and has triumphantly overcome it. He was trained formally chiefly at the Maudsley Hospital, from which jokingly he described himself as 'a refugee'. He qualified as a psychoanalyst whilst in a trainee appointment at the Tavistock, and had no difficulty in obtaining a consultant post and the M.D. of his University at Birmingham. History ceases when at the time of writing one is dealing with a very recent appointment, but already Robert Gosling has a notable career of service, not only to the Tavistock, but also to other causes, to his credit. One of his great successes, as mentioned, was the organization of the 1964 International Congress in Psychotherapy. He is a member of the Education Committee of the Royal Medico-Psychological Association. Contrary to a frequently held stereotype about the Tavistock staff, Gosling is a very pukka physician and well-trained general psychiatrist in addition to his chosen field. Whether he will succeed in dodging the appellation of Medical Director, which he intends and which his colleagues by their new policy are expecting, remains to be seen. It is very likely that the outside world, including the Health Service authorities, will still wish to see the head of the Professional Committee so designated. His place on that Committee is now not by virtue of being representative of any one department, but the elected Chairman of the whole Institution, overriding departmental loyalties. The head of the Adult Unit as of 1968 is Dr Pierre Turquet, while Derek Miller[1] and Marion Mackenzie respectively are the Chairmen of the Departments for Adolescents and for Children and Parents.

While these changes at the top have been going on in the personnel of the Clinic, the Institute, with its increasing size and diversification of projects and research interests, has also made changes over the 1947–68 period. The first step in this direction was greatly to enlarge the Governing Council of T.I.H.R. and then to differentiate out the new structures, called sub-councils, responsible for what had become virtually separate units or, one may say, 'institutes within the Institute'. By 1968 there were five such sub-councils in operation, one of which, in the area of the Clinic's work, has already been mentioned. It forms the nucleus from which a possible school of psychodynamic psychiatry, or of mental health, etc., might be developed on the analogy of a medical school functioning alongside a teaching

[1] As I correct the proof I learn that Derek Miller has accepted a Chair in Clinical Psychiatry at Ann Arbor, Mich.

hospital. The second sub-council closest to the work of the Clinic is that running the Family Discussion Bureau, which, as I write, has been re-christened the Institute for Marital Studies. The third, fourth and fifth sub-councils take care respectively of the units concerned with the more specifically extra-medical aspects. The first is called the Human Resources Centre presided over by Fred Emery until June 1969, since Eric Trist's appointment to a professorial chair in the University of California at Los Angeles.

Here I want to pause to pay tribute also to Eric Trist, who came and went about the same time as Jock Sutherland. The Interim Planning Committee certainly knew what they were doing when they 'co-opted 'these two men, still in uniform, to our councils and so into leading positions in our group.

Eric is one of those massive, slow-moving intellects whose role during and after Operation 'Phoenix' has been, as I see it, that of our chief theoretician and scientific conscience. A product both of the English and the psychology schools of Cambridge in a year which abounded in future professors, he came to us via the Research and Training Centre of War Office selection boards. He had experienced a period at the Yale Institute of Human Relations and had been in social psychological studies at St Andrews. I regarded him always with awe as a polymath in our field. Passionately devoted to the integration of the psychodynamic and sociodynamic disciplines, Eric's hidden hand can be traced in the design and conceptualizing stages of nearly all post-1946 research work at the Tavistock Clinic, whether in the field of personality development, psychometry or validation of psychoanalytic hypotheses. His contribution also to the planning of our education of clinical psychologists – and above all to the goal-setting and cohesion of the total institution – have been crucial. It has been a great experience to watch this originally introverted thinker and 'backroom' scholar blossom into the recent professional head of the Institute, and so into one of the more important social scientists of the Western world. Much of the rigorous thinking-through embodied in some of the policy documents I have cited was his. His son Alan is on the Institute's staff, and Eric himself retains a formal working link with the place he did so much to shape in the twenty or more years when he was one of its pillars, embodying in his person the new empirical, deeply caring 'Tavistock man', at home in the whole spectrum of the growing sciences of human behaviour. I predict that, notwithstanding all he has already contributed (see publications in Appendix III), his best is still to come. Already he has nourished a whole series of pupils and successors – Hugh Murray, Fred Emery, Gurth Higgin, Hans van Beinum and many others.

The second unit is the Centre for Applied Social Research, led by Dr E. J. Miller, while the newest one, the Institute for Operational Research, was headed by Mr Neil Jessop until his premature death in 1969. The five sub-councils are composed of members of the main Council who have special interest in particular aspects of the work. Some members of Council serve on more than one of the sub-councils.

In the N.H.S. administration also a change took place when the main unit of the Paddington Group Hospital Management Committee, the large Paddington General Hospital, became associated with St Mary's Hospital in a teaching group. The Paddington H.M.C. was now transformed into the St Charles Hospital Management Committee. In this new grouping the Tavistock has become one of the largest units in size of staff. Some years previously our valued friend and excellent administrator, Mr H. R. Jolly, was transferred to higher spheres and was replaced by an equally good friend, Mr R. S. Pollard, as the Group Secretary who actually saw us into the new building. The relationship to our Management Committee has continued to be excellent and mutually co-operative. At the time of writing, it seems likely that this Management Group will have its own psychiatric advisory committee to deal adequately with its mental-health clinics – of which it has three in addition to the Tavistock.

Even before the change in leadership by the impending withdrawal of Sutherland and Bowlby from the two chief posts in the Clinic,[1] the consulting staff of the Tavistock had been earnestly concerned with reviewing all aspects of its work

[1] John Bowlby, of course, remains on the active staff, as shown in earlier sections in this chapter; he is also still Deputy Chairman of the Professional Committee of the Clinic.

through a series of informal staff discussions by the 'young' consultants. This group, convened by Derek Miller, started work in 1966 and met on numerous occasions to deal with the co-ordination of all three departments in clinical services to patients; in administrative changes to make these more efficient; in improving communications between the now large units in the building. There had always been a felt need for a forum for such interchange and institutional self-scrutiny, the shape of which has not been easy to fashion, in view of the busy lives people lead. Equally the areas of research and training have been once more under serious scrutiny. The meetings seemed to disclose a conflict between the 'clinicians' who wanted to maximize our service to sick people and those who were more concerned with research into the rightness of our hypotheses and who wanted to validate what we were doing before going on doing more work somewhat uncritically in the old way. The latter, 'scientific', trend would, of course, mean the diversion of considerable staff time into armchair work in devising follow-up methods, into comparing and checking selection procedures for various methods of treatment and the consequential results of these methods. One could detect a certain (not uncommon) tendency to delegate actual therapy down the line from the consultants to the trainees. This led inevitably towards a greater participation of the clinical psychologists in some types of work with patients. Thus the initial assessment procedure became points of departure for the test situation being used therapeutically. A more obvious delegation of therapeutic 'counselling' or 'case work' also devolved on the enlarged staff of psychiatric social workers, especially as already exemplified in the family area: in the Department for Children and Parents and in the expanding field of marital work in the Clinic itself and in the Family Discussion Bureau. In these areas usage throughout Britain has long sanctioned the deployment of social workers with special expertise based on training. As a sidelight on the Tavistock's consistent help to social work and its standing, timorous psychiatrists are now attributing the 'up-start' claims of social workers reflected in the Seebohm Report (1968) to our pernicious influence on them!

What other trends are emerging from these meetings? The

Department for Children and Parents, as mentioned, has emphasized the need to extend and assess its work with the whole family; secondly, to enter into community work, including the school service in the Borough in which the Tavistock is located; thirdly, to contribute to the development of 'person-centred' paediatric services; fourthly, the need to widen services and training to embrace the complete field of child psychiatry, including the provision of an in-patient unit. This latter trend is particularly interesting in view of the hitherto resolute decision, many times taken, not to provide in-patient services on various rational grounds. The Adolescent Department stressed, as well as 'walk-in' emergency services for certain disturbed patients, an extension into the complete field of adolescent psychiatry, including possible in-patient facilities and hostels in conjunction with the health services of the local authority. In the Adult Department the greatest need seemed to be for systematic clinical comparison and evaluation of treatments with the advocacy of the desirability of a 'servo' unit for such systematic studies. The Adult Department also wanted to develop its counselling services and associated training for social workers in the sense mentioned above. It wanted to intensify its Introductory Psychotherapy Course for external psychiatric registrars and also to review and possibly extend its clinical and research work into the field of 'Man in his working environment'. That is to say, it wished to take in the problems of industrial mental health contingent on the entry of post-adolescents into work situations, including new university graduates. David Malan's work on 'brief focal therapy' was singled out as a hopeful and very important area in which skills and training should be intensified, since it provided a workable and increasingly well-validated model of help to many properly selected cases in a short period, e.g. a dozen or so interviews. Into this area the pilot study of the clinical psychologists basing the beginnings of focal therapy on the psychological test situation seemed to fit well. This originated with a trial case by Mr John Boreham, who at the beginning of the Brief Therapy Workshop during my membership of it, reported very interesting and good therapeutic results based on his discussions with patients of their fantasies evoked by projective techniques. Such developments are in place at the Tavistock, where senior clinical psychologists and psychiatric social workers are mostly well-qualified in psychoanalysis or analytical psychology.

This chronicle must end obviously before the Tavistock's Golden Jubilee date itself, if the printed page is to appear in due time. It ends at a time of intimations of great potential changes in the National Health Service: in its structure, as expressed in the green Paper of the Ministry of Health, in its medical education, as envisaged by the Report of the Royal Commission under Lord Todd's chairmanship, and in its relations with the social and welfare services contemplated in the Report of the Seebohm Committee. At the same time, all these weighty reports are put in question by the creation of the new Department of Health and Social Security, with the departure of the Right Hon. Kenneth Robinson from the headship of a Ministry in which he had been a real friend of mental health and of the advance in psychiatric standards. Many of us will think of him with gratitude and affection, for we learnt to value his sincerity and concern for these matters during his long and committed membership of our Regional Hospital Board, before he joined the Government.

I have to conclude this account on a note of sadness. Our gracious Royal Patron, the Princess Marina, Duchess of Kent, died in September 1968. She took over in her own bereavement and was for twenty-five years an active and deeply concerned friend and supporter of the causes which unite us in mourning with many sister institutions. A moving tribute was paid to Her Royal Highness by Lord Butler, as President of the National Association for Mental Health. Confirming her real grasp and informed interest in the wide field of mental health, Lord Butler said:

> All this assiduous attention arose from an intense personal feeling for the mentally ill . . . she had a close personal relationship with the Bethlem and Maudsley Hospitals. She will be sorely missed by the Spastics Society and the British Epilepsy Association, the Tavistock Clinic and the Mental After-care Association. Those who have accompanied her on visits to . . . these bodies have been deeply impressed by Princess Marina's touching and talented care for the

sufferers, into whose lives she brought her unique way of grace and understanding. She used to say that she regarded it as a privilege for her to serve these institutions. . . .

These words are sincerely echoed in the remembrance of all those at the Tavistock who, for their part, had the privilege of meeting this charming lady and briefing her during the visits she paid us in war and peace. J. R. Rees, John Bowlby and Robert Gosling represented us at the Westminster Abbey Memorial service to this great public servant.

On 8 May 1969 we were honoured by the intimation that the Duchess's daughter, Princess Alexandra the Hon. Mrs Angus Ogilvy, had taken on her late mother's function as our Patron.

At a different level the older generations of the Tavistock were grieved to hear of the loss in 1968 of another great-hearted woman, who we were privileged to have on our staff from about 1925 until the outbreak of war. This was Dr Kathleen Todd, D.P.M., of New Zealand, who came to us already experienced in child psychiatry and psychotherapy via Oakland, California, and Boston, Mass. Our co-inhabitants at Belsize Lane will be interested to know that in 1941 Kathleen Todd was made Acting Medical Director of the Child Guidance Training Centre, then evacuated to Oxford, in which post she continued until 1946, after the Centre's return to London. Though she failed in health and never came back to what she called 'her beloved Tavi', she became for New Zealand one of the most influential figures advising on mental health and psychiatric personnel and policies. Dr Todd also endowed a fellowship for young N.Z. psychiatrists for overseas study, preferably in Europe, as well as giving money for children's homes in the Wellington area – and in South Vietnam. She published an excellent book with Lydia Jackson on child and play therapy, not listed in our index because it was a 'credit' to the C.G.T.C.

And, as already mentioned, J. R. Rees, a founder father, died in April 1969. In the preceding chapters enough is said to show what he achieved for us – the Tavistock group – his first 'baby' nearly as much as Crichton-Miller's. That this was but one phase of his strenuous life shows the breadth and creativeness of this natural, unself-conscious leader and originator. His contribution to British and international psychiatry, mental hygiene and social-welfare policies merits a volume. Many international and British honours came to him: the C.B.E. many thought an inadequate recompense for one of our most famous medical figures; the Salmon Lectureship of New York; the Clark Hall and the Maudsley Lectureships; the Lasker, Rubin and Adolph Meyer Awards – again in the U.S.A.; honorary membership of many foreign psychiatric associations as well as of our own R.M.P.A., and a special award of, first, M.R.C.P. and later Fellowship of the Royal College of Physicians. But in the hearts of those who knew J.R. well, his generosity and human warmth, lack of rancour and perennial pursuit of goodwill remain uppermost. Just as he cared less about a man's theoretical views than about what sort of person he was, so we too will remember Jack Rees for what he stood for and did rather than as a learned academic figure which is less rare in our era. We commemorated him in St Marylebone Parish Church amongst a great congregation.

In November 1969 we lost another of our most creative and admired colleagues, A. K. Rice, anthropologist and innovator, greatly mourned.

XII

Concluding Reflections

My task as a chronicler of the past would not be done if I did not attempt to draw up some sort of balance-sheet of success and failure, of national and social gain or loss from the endeavours and omissions of the Tavistock Clinic's story. Here I make a sharp break from most of what has preceded this concluding section. I have doubtless been subjective and biased in what events and personalities I have high-lighted or neglected, but at least I have mostly recorded facts of other still-living people's experience. In this section I shall be evaluative and strictly personal. No reader will be naïve enough to expect a writer of a Jubilee volume to be objective and unbiased in his summing-up when the subject of his literary portrait is his own lifelong working base, his friends and colleagues forming a living family pursuing goals in which he shared, and committing errors and misjudgements which were also his. What small measure of objectivity in this matter I may claim to have is due to my having retired from the active fray since setting out on this book and of having since had the advantage, through working on policy-forming psychiatric bodies at national level, of gaining a little more perspective of where the Tavistock and its work 'fit in' in psychological medicine past and future.

Despite Heine's pessimistic aphorism that 'the only thing we learn from history is that we do not learn from history', such a brief evaluation of a facet of British psychiatric history might be the starting-point of some reader's own reappraisal and creative thinking – not necessarily at the Tavistock or indeed in Britain.

To begin with a very broad assertion, I would hold that since its inception in 1920 the Tavistock has steadfastly represented and emphasized the psychodynamic aspects of psychiatry, and stood for 'whole-person' medicine *vis-à-vis* the trend of the times concerned increasingly with laboratory research and physico-chemical theories of health and disease. Inspired by successful applications of Freud's 'new psychology' to mass neurosis in military settings, the Tavistock was in fact favourably placed to become a mediating body between medicine and psycho-analysis in the broadest sense of that term. While from the viewpoint of orthodox Freudian theory and practice we were a body of diluters and analytic quacks, it can be said in the light of history that we made the British psychiatric world 'safe for psychoanalysis' and some of its more viable derivatives, a service which became explicitly recognized during and after the Second World War, when psychoanalysis had also matured out of its early defensive exclusiveness.

The promotion of psychoanalysis in its narrower sense however, was never a conscious aim of the founder or of the pre-war Tavistock group. H.C.M. saw in Freud's system the most coherent body of hypotheses with which to do a job which was virtually done nowhere else in Britain. This was the task of understanding and relieving the suffering of all those conditions which had also been the field of interest and study for Freud and his circle, including the deviants, like Jung and Adler: the adult neuroses, perversions, character disorders, including those manifesting chiefly at somatic levels, and – it is an important *and* – the precursor states in children as postulated by the psychogenetic theory. It can be claimed that over most of its history the Tavistock group has been patient – or task-centred rather than theory-centred, hence much more flexible and 'eclectic' (a term of mild abuse in some circles) than any orthodox 'school' could be in its choice of theoretical and heuristic approaches to concrete problems of diagnosis and therapy. It remained faithful, however, to the basic philosophy which required us to *understand* the whole person in his social and intrapsychic as well as his organismic aspects – a philosophy most clearly shown, even in 1920, by the Tavistock's multi-professional handling of psychiatric problems, setting an early pattern of interdisciplinary team work in the study of real situations which often untidily straddle abstract disciplinary boundaries. This orientation to its tasks has, I think, enabled the

Tavistock's working principles to remain remarkably consistent and continuous. Given a non-doctrinal field of interest marked only by a few cardinal points, the growth, change and sophistication in relevant fields of knowledge served to broaden and enrich rather than to threaten its position as a medico-psychological institution. This enabled it after the Second World War to welcome the newer insights and workers not only from psychoanalysis proper, but also those from the growing disciplines of the behavioural and social sciences with their methodologies for the study of human interactions and group structures. The larger Tavistock organization of the last twenty years, with its clinical and its social research wings, thus became a natural nodal point for that transdisciplinary field we may call 'community psychiatry ("sociatry") and mental health', ranging from the social development of the human infant to the dynamics of the largest human group, seen as evolutionary continuities.

It is from this basic philosophy that the Tavistock derives its design as a *clinical model*. The building of such a model was a conscious aim of Hugh Crichton-Miller. In an era still dominated by the image of 'doing good to the sick poor', this model was in many respects a revolutionary one. It fostered, many years ahead of time, an attitude to the patient which has not even today replaced the prevalent older image of our clients as a mass of ignorant inferiors to whom something good has to be done by their superiors, but whose time and anxieties are of little account. The Tavistock model of handling human beings, especially of despised neurotics, 'with nothing the matter', was based on the interest and concern of private psychotherapeutic practice. The punctually kept appointment; the courteous personal reception; the private, confidential atmosphere; the certainty of assignment to the same doctor; the unhurried *listening* to what the patient wanted to get off his chest; the cultivation rather than dismissal of the element of sympathy and participation – in short, an attempt to create a sense of security and understanding for subjective suffering – these were the main features of our clinical practice. This professional ethos, as mentioned, was an expression of H.C.M.'s philosophy, and has continued to be a cornerstone of the Tavistock's service, still evoking some astonishment and envy in people who meet it for the first time. This 'climate' or mode of professional behaviour rather than any rigid method or technique of therapy has been what we hoped to implant in our staffs and students, from receptionists to doctors.

It may be questionable whether such a *genius loci* can ever be fully transplanted or exported, either by individuals leaving to work elsewhere or in any 'daughter colonies'. Thus, I personally found it hard to maintain it in the setting of the St Bart's Hospital Psychiatric out-patient Department, where I worked as clinical assistant in 1931–2, and scarcely less hard when I established a clinic based on the Tavistock model in the Leeds teaching hospital setting in 1946–8. Perhaps H.C.M. was expecting the impossible, even if to all of us the requirements of human respect and concern for the often deep anxieties and vulnerabilities of our clientele would seem basic to medical psychology. The claim of having fashioned a new model can also apply to the pattern of staff relations and student-teacher relations within the institution. Here the original paternalism of H.C.M. had soon to give way to the establishment of a staff democracy, consistent with the interdisciplinary team structure of our clinical work and the maturity of our trainees. This also amounted, in 1931, to a revolutionary break with the tradition of consultant or medical superintendent absolutism and unquestionability. Not only election to responsibility by the staff, but voluntary mutual supervision and accountability were new and, as I see it, valuable principles. We believe that such a wide participation in managing the affairs of a professional institution has enhanced the quality of its group life. Most people I have shared this life with have been *happy* to work there, quite apart from what they might have *achieved.*

With the growth of clinical psychology and social casework as major disciplines, our staff members in these important roles have been increasingly accorded equality of status (even though it was not for us to decide their salary structures!), to the extent that what elsewhere are medical committees became in the Tavistock an inter-professional committee. This respect for other skills and surrender of medical monopoly has come near to solving a morale problem within medicine at least in *this* clinic, where our non-medical colleagues are not made to feel 'auxiliaries', implying technician status. This freedom in the history of the Clinic led to conflict and rivalry only once soon after the Second World War (see p. 189). We have much to teach both the medical and the social work professions in proper co-operation and team work without destructive rivalry, which is a latent menace in the claims of the Seebohm Committee's Report and which is alarming the medical profession.

The Tavistock, rightly or wrongly, has never attempted to go beyond the field which could be fruitfully cultivated by the originally chosen orientation. It will be recalled that this very concentration of a new and limited clinical model incurred us long hostility and obstruction from such guardians of psychiatric policy as the late Professor Mapother. He would sooner have had us as a replica of the traditional psychiatric model concerned with 'disease processes' rather than with psychodynamics of persons. This newer model, which reached its full development in the creation of the Institute of Human Relations, is well summarized in a memorandum for the Council of that body (A.913) from which I will quote significant passages:

> The Tavistock Institute grew out of the Tavistock Clinic. . . . In this lies [one of its] main features – namely, the inclusion of medical as well as non-medical social science. . . . The Clinic has specialized in the study of the psychological and social aspects of psychiatry, in the treatment of patients and of families whose disturbances can be understood in these terms, and in the prevention of such disturbances. Whilst some of its work conforms to the traditional picture of medicine, other parts do not. For example, child and adolescent psychiatry blend imperceptibly with education, child-care and criminology; whilst family psychiatry and marital counselling, by taking a family group as the object of study and assistance, break away from the medical tradition of centring attention on the individual.
>
> The Clinic . . . is expected to give priority to treatment. . . . The Institute, as an independent body, has more freedom both in the range of activities . . . and the amount of research it can do. The two bodies are complementary. It is Institute

> policy to include within its field of interest problems, such as those of psychological illness, that are traditionally . . . medical; problems such as industrial management which are not; and also problems of an intermediate sort, such as executive stress. In fact, very many problems . . . lie on the borderline; examples range from marital disturbance and socially deviant behaviour to personal tensions that arise in badly structured organizations. . . .
>
> Where the ability to draw on both the medical and the sociological parts of the spectrum [of disciplines] is of particular value is in the study of that large range of problems which require an understanding of the interplay between personality and social group. . . . Only the researcher, or project team, combining a fair grasp of sociology, social psychology and medical psychology is equipped to tackle such problems effectively.
>
> Where the Institute's work is most distinct from that of medicine is in its study of social organization and the consultative services it provides to them . . . from industrial and marketing bodies to prisons, hospitals and schools. In each case the aims are to help those concerned to clarify the objectives of their organization, to understand the social environment in which it is and will be living, to assess the extent to which the internal structure is appropriate, and to collaborate in introducing such changes as they come to recognize as desirable . . . to develop methods that will enable the organization to adapt continuously to environmental change.

Those of us who devised this model – limited only in regard to confining ourselves to the hitherto neglected part of the spectrum of 'traditional' mental disorders studied or accepted for treatment – consciously built into it this extension of a diagnostic and therapeutic intent (sociatry), equivalent to the medical model, into the apparently entirely sociological activities of controlled structural and operational change in organizations. This quasi-clinical approach arose from our experience of the indivisibility in real-life situations of biological, psychological and social factors, and of the imperative of responsible therapeutic behaviour towards any problem presented. To me this broad continuity of approach to psychodynamic and socio-dynamic problems is the chief contribution made by the Tavistock to British conceptual thinking and theory for psychological medicine, applied social science and community mental health.

It followed that our *training policy* and programmes have progressively attempted to prepare our students – both external and especially internal – for incorporating the theoretical framework and operational skills in their equipment, which are required for the range of problems in which we became interested and involved over the years. Having pioneered in the 1920s 'on-the-job' training for graduate doctors (increasingly those already trained in general psychiatry), social workers and educational psychologists in novel tasks which have slowly become, since the Second World War, a broadly recognized psychiatric activity, we set ourselves since 1946 to train also young anthropologists, sociologists, economists, etc., in the integrated skills for the practice and conceptualization of the activities just outlined. I quote again from the Council memorandum (A.913):

> Existing university departments do not equip even their post-graduate students with the range of knowledge and skills that the Institute staff must be able to apply, so that those joining . . . have to undertake further training under its auspices, and the Institute is at present able to do much less of it than is desirable.

For our clinical staffs it is not sufficient to be qualified only by their professional bodies' standards. It is not enough for a Tavistock psychiatrist to be a competent clinician and psychoanalyst. We have still to add to his equipment those techniques needed for flexibility in his family, group and community work, in individual psychopathology and institutional and social dynamics. Our clinicians participate in the training of Institute staff, and the senior members of the latter are equally engaged in sharing their skills and concepts with the clinicians, both in formal teaching and in joint projects, such as studies of executive stress or of medical institutional tensions. *Mutatis mutandis*, this holds also for the psychologists, social workers and child psychotherapists whose training is in large part the same as that for the medical members, on shared tasks and in shared seminars and case conferences. We have, by some forty years, anticipated the tardy requirements of the Royal Commission on Medical Education (Cmd. 3,569, 1968), which in its para. 132 calls psychotherapy the 'technique, which most clearly differentiates psychiatric treatment from that given in other branches of medicine' and 'has been comparatively neglected in most British medical schools'.

After advocating rather elementary experience for the aspiring 'general' psychiatrist, the Royal Commission's report admits that there 'will be a continuing need for some specialized vocational training in child psychiatry, subnormality and psychotherapy' (the latter comes last in all mentions – H.V.D.). 'The shortage of psychiatrists with advanced training in these fields is so acute that increased provision for training will have to be made, if the already pressing service needs are to be met during the next twenty years' (para. 130).

Yet there is not a single mention in that report of the achievements in this training of the Tavistock Clinic or the Cassel Hospital! One reference occurs in para. 130 to the advantages of making more use in training of *child psychiatrists* of those psychiatrists who have undergone 'formal training in psychoanalysis'. Despite our forty years of steady output of those with 'advanced training' in our field, the key posts in teaching have almost all gone to psychiatrists whose training and orientations were lacking in this, the most distinctive and essential skill for handling human beings in mental stress. I shall have occasion to recur to this aspect of psychiatric history further on.

Contributions to psychiatry by the Tavistock have not been limited to providing a new model of service and staff relations and to training a specialized kind of psychiatrist in the adult and children's fields. We have also been in the van of those pioneering new *methods* of training and study – such as the teaching group and the interdisciplinary case conference. The developments associated with the names of Michael and Enid Balint, of Kenneth Rice, Pierre Turquet and Robert Gosling (to mention only a few) in group-relations training for general practitioners, for social and marital counsellors, for family planning and public health doctors, for community and industrial managers, schoolteachers, the clergy and many others, have been instrumental in changing countless people's perceptions of their tasks in handling human relations in their own work settings.

Our contribution to the *growth of knowledge* and to the ongoing discussion about unsolved problems has been of a volume and level which stand comparison with any academic body. Its range is shown in the list of publications (which omits popular articles and re-writing) which have issued from the Tavistock since 1920 (see Appendix III). It would be a miracle if all this work had been fundamental and original. What is surprising, in view of the life lived by our institution as I have depicted it, is that so much of it has lastingly helped to shape ideas and techniques in our field. The Sutties' well-argued critique of Freud's neglect of the role of the mother in early life, and Hadfield's insistence on both an instinct of aggression and the crucial role of infantile dependence ('attachment') in psychopathology anticipated 'orthodox' psychoanalytic revisions by many years. In more formal research, the Tavistock played a major role in propagating the still novel psychosomatic method in the *nineteen-thirties* by the work of Wittkower and A. T. M. Wilson, and influenced a number of teachers in medicine towards accepting psychodynamic factors in 'organic' cardiac, gastro-intestinal and dermatological conditions. It is regrettable that after the Second World War no staff member with the necessary enthusiasm took over the interrupted psychosomatic work, from which Wilson and Wittkower had moved on to wider horizons. It is part of our tradition to leave staff members free to pursue lines of enquiry they are spontaneously interested in rather than press them into work theoretically seen to be important. This itself is worth notice.

Although it would be presumptuous to claim that the major contributions of the Army psychiatric service during the Second World War were all Tavistock achievements, it remains true that the groundwork for most of them originated in the thinking and planning of J. R. Rees and his two earliest principal aides, Ronald Hargreaves and A. T. M. Wilson. I would include in the Tavistock's achievements this trio's gift for attracting and deploying the right people recruited from elsewhere, many of whom subsequently joined the Tavistock and found there the *milieu* for their life's work. I refer here to those innovations or applications of psychodynamic theory which were translated into general psychiatry, applied personality and social psychology, and community medicine. To the former belong the concepts of group therapy evolved at Northfield Military Hospital, to which, together with the Army civil resettlement centres also, can be traced the notion of 'social reconnection' of those who have become 'alienated' (in the case of soldiers by long prisoner-of-war experiences or remote foreign service), and of a place which serves as a therapeutic 'transitional community' for this purpose – precursor of the community hostel as a halfway house in rehabilitation. I would say that the Tavistock's aim to treat people without hospitalization and loss of their social connections whenever possible is gaining ground, not only since recent legislation in the 1959 Mental Health Act, but also in the phenomenal growth of out-patient services, day hospitals, night hospitals, etc., against the sacred cow of the demand for 'beds' as the mark of psychiatric status. In the last analysis this change is an implicit, if not always explicit, recognition of the force of applying the psychodynamic theory of the human need for secure object-relations. These ideas were diffused not only by their effect on many psychiatrists who served in the Army under J.R. during the war, but also by the inception of the section of psychotherapy and social psychiatry, due to the initiative of the former Army group within the Royal Medico-Psychological Association. It is noteworthy that while these two concepts – psychotherapy and social psychiatry – were there seen as linked by the psychodynamic theory as nourished at the Tavistock and in the Army, the resistance to this theory has tended to prise 'social psychiatry' away from our concept in the direction of impersonal statistical and epidemiological studies. These can then be held to be part of 'general' psychiatry which still does not want unequivocally to own psychotherapy as a basic skill for every psychiatrist.

Another major change resulting from J.R.'s work is that relating to higher-grade mentally subnormals. The success of putting soldiers in this category into special Pioneer companies proved that they could, in their right setting, perform valuable work for their community with great benefit to their morale and human dignity. Realistic work therapy, including occupation centres and the like, in the management of psychiatric and subnormal patients was a result.

In summary, I would restate the truly outstanding and revolutionary achievements of J.R. and his team in the following way:

(*a*) The invention of the command psychiatrist as a medical-social role carrying out reconnaissance in a large structured and defined group, leading to the ascertainment and recognition of critical problems in the sphere of human relations and management.
(*b*) The invention of social psychiatry as a policy science permitting preventive technical intervention in large-scale problems.
(*c*) The fashioning of a whole series of military institutions which concretely and effectively implemented the policies advocated.
(*d*) The invention of new types of therapeutic communities.
(*e*) The invention of cultural psychiatry.

These things were possible not only because of the essentially object-relations orientation, but because of the capability nurtured in the Tavistock for the psychiatrist to work with lay personnel – in this case the military – in a collaborative partnership. In other words, the strategy of command psychiatry and the developments to which it led were psychodynamically conceived and based. At that time it would have been unlikely that psychiatrists working from a different viewpoint could have seen the importance of a free exploration of the military *milieu* and ethos as a first necessity. Even if they had, they would not have had the prior experience of our having had to win and maintain a support base for our work of the Tavistock itself. This can be illustrated by the classical anecdote, when at an inter-Service meeting a senior consultant in another Service, having heard an Army psychiatrist's description of his work in morale and training studies, exclaimed in my hearing: 'Morale – discipline? What has that to do with psychiatry?'

When other disciplines – sociologists and psychologists – came to be drawn in to implement these new psychiatric policies, they were given equality of status: it was a collaboration of equals: psychiatrist – social scientist – military officer. This brought as its long-term result a psychodynamically based philosophy of social innovation understandable and acceptable by large numbers of people, so that social and administrative change could be implemented rapidly and with consent in large and rather traditional social systems. Some of us believe this to have been a new discovery in human affairs.

These, and the steady teaching and output of those taught in the fields of family dynamics, child development, psychology and psychopathology of human relations, interaction between person and social environment, may be said to comprise our contribution to psychiatry and its related fields of community mental health.

In the field of personality and social psychology there have been notable and permanent effects on theory and practice, of which some relate directly to the Tavistock's war effort.

Most of us in the Tavistock circle would assign pride of place to Wilfred Bion's massive conceptual contribution to the theory and practice of group relations. This work laid the foundations for the therapeutic community experiment, not only at Northfield Military Hospital, already referred to, but also provided the basis for the handling of groups of severely disturbed repatriates in the civil resettlement units of the Army and the Ministry of Labour. From the creative hammering out of his views have come strong influences on the whole development of the so-called community psychiatry, as in the able hands of Maxwell Jones and of T. F. Main (the latter was at Northfield), as well as of S. H. Foulkes (likewise a Northfield staff member). The work of Bion in co-operation with Rickman influenced, I venture to say, not only the post-war clinical policy of the Tavistock Clinic itself, but was diffused widely throughout other treatment centres and hospitals for psychiatry.

Further than this, few members of the senior group of our Institute of Human Relations would deny that Bion's more sociological concepts on group structure and function gave the new venture into the study of institutions and controlled social change in them their theoretical launching platform (e.g. Elliott Jaques's work in the *Glacier project*).

It may be regrettable that the Tavistock's own staff did not have a continuing role in the development and refining of these wartime 'residential' community programmes. The Ministry of Labour did not carry on with their six C.R.U.s. But it is in any case never possible to contain all the innovations made by an institution within its own walls. None the less, the developments just stated sprang up from Bion's and similar beginnings.

The second outstanding contribution is the revolution in *personnel selection*, especially as elaborated by the War Office officer selection boards research group. 'W.O.S.B.' has become a byword, implying the replacement of hit-and-miss interviews by a more objective technique based on psychodynamic theory and professional ratings of 'test' performance in controlled social situations, done by interdisciplinary teams. The Civil Service selection boards and Unilever's central selection system for trainees are direct derivatives. In various modifications – and dilutions – this method of assessing potential leadership and executive qualities with a greatly improved degree of reliability has been applied in many spheres, including some of our Institute's own projects in industry. It is a great pity that the full publication of this piece of work has not yet occurred. The chief figures involved – Sutherland, Trist, Ben Morris, John Bowlby, W. R. Bion, Eric Wittkower – have never found the time to complete this large task. I hope that when a companion volume of the Institute's full history comes to be written in due course, W.O.S.B.s will be fully documented as one of its germinal achievements.

There is no doubt, however, that the kind of experience gathered in the Army, perhaps especially by the psychologists who joined us after the war, had an impact on the development of personality assessment techniques based on psychodynamic principles which has characterized the Tavistock's services.

Here I would cite Phillipson's Object Relations Technique, Sandler's Tavistock self-assessment inventory, Trist's work with Semeonoff on the diagnostic performance tests used in W.O.S.B. Theodora Alcock's creative use of the Rorschach is also relevant. Of later vintage is the new Interpersonal Perception Technique, related to the operational study of marital interaction, by Phillipson, Laing and Lee, for which some preliminary steps were taken in my unit. In the area of validation of hypotheses on psychodynamics by controlled clinical experiment and rigorous techniques of study, the post-war years have seen not only the work done by Bowlby and his team[1] on child development bearing on psychoanalytic and learning theory, an internationally famous and still-developing programme now including study of the effects of separation and loss also on adults.[2] We are also awaiting the full account of Ezriel's experimental study of the influence of transference interpretation on the subsequent content of patients' communications in single and group treatment – another rigorous examination of the validity of psychoanalytic theory for understanding clinical phenomena. His work, as mentioned, treats the analytic session as an experimental situation.

Combining pioneering of a new method of treating dyadic (e.g. marital) interaction with developing relevant explanatory concepts and hypotheses, the teams of the Family Discussion Bureau (now Institute of Marital Studies) and of my Marital Unit have made significant advances in an area not previously seriously studied in this country. The challenging work of Laing in analogous fields of family interaction, especially of schizophrenics, but also in marriage, has added a new dimension to the study of psychosis – in this case on the basis of contemporary work in the U.S.A. and has led to his creating a new kind of therapeutic community at Kingsley Hall, London.

Interest, however, has never been lost in individual therapy and psychopathology. There have always been 'workshops' on devising better, or at least effective, brief methods of assessment and psychotherapy on a verifiable basis, suitable for mass

[1] Notably Mary Ainsworth, Chris Heinecke, Anthony Ambrose, James Robertson, Dina Rosenbluth, H. Rudolph Schaffer and Ilse Westheimer.

[2] Especially the work of Colin Parkes.

out-patient work. Out of these efforts emerged David Malan's publications on brief psychotherapy, closely linked to problems of validation by *our* standards, not only to relief of symptoms. In this area the ongoing work by Malan, Phillipson, Gill and others promises at least some reliable measurements of therapeutic personality change.

Extra-murally, the influence of the Tavistock has always been felt in the wider spheres of voluntary mental health and human relations efforts. In the pre-war years H.C.M. and J.R. were among the direct inspirers and resource figures in the National Council for Mental Hygiene, the Child Guidance Council, the New Education Fellowship and similar movements. In the post-war years J.R. was the – yes – almost sole begetter of the World Federation for Mental Health. In a sense we can say that the Tavistock has earned its right to existence by producing this great and committed servant of human values in psychological medicine, with his genius for translating aspirations into functioning organizations, for encouraging and supporting promising workers and lines of action – not always sufficiently critically, but always generously and without seeking prestige for himself or the institution.

In all the above, I have largely omitted reference to the increasing impact of the more sociological developments in the Institute on the academic as well as institutional and industrial practice in Britain. As mentioned several times, these developments require a full history of their own by someone more competent than myself to place them in perspective. I have only attempted to sketch them in as part of the older Clinic's contribution and growth, and in their subsequent repercussions on the Clinic's own course of development. The list of published work, and noting the contribution to academic leadership of men who have obtained senior university posts on the strength of their achievements in the Institute must suffice. I cannot, however, refrain from quoting the principles of action on which our total organization was and is still founded, because these express the values which we have continuously held and which seem to me the essential basis of all adequately human medicine. The sentences come from the previously cited Institute document A.913:

> 1. The first principle of research at the Institute is that projects should spring from opportunities to collaborate in the solution of actual social problems. The second is that projects of this kind should be conducted by researchers committed in a professional role to assist those concerned.

This, my colleagues would agree, includes the whole range of aetiological research and treatment in psychiatric illness by analytic methods as well as in sociological projects.

> 2. . . . by enlisting the active co-operation of those studied, the method not only facilitates access to relevant data, but makes more probable the further testing of findings and concepts that can only be achieved in real life settings.
>
> 3. Human beings, whether individuals, families or larger groups, do not like to be intimately scrutinized . . . often, therefore, they are unwilling to provide the researcher with crucial data about themselves. When, however, they believe that he may . . . help them solve a problem that concerns them, and that he will certainly do so if he can, they are more willing to provide him with opportunities. . . . Many investigations necessary to advance physiology and pathology are permitted by the individuals investigated only because, as medical patients, they are assured of treatment. In psychological and social research the need for the subject's active collaboration is greater, since many of the relevant data concern his feelings and motives, and these are often in conflict and only partly conscious: they tend, in consequence, to be heavily guarded. Only . . . with a researcher who is . . . trusted are such feelings and motives likely to become understood and communicated.

The memorandum goes on to say that resistance to change in individuals and groups is least when an enquiry is initiated by the 'client' concerned (rather than imposed on him), and that these conditions apply whether this be a family worried about a child, an industry concerned over low productivity or a prison disturbed by staff-inmate relations:

> The tasks of the researcher are, first, to identify, as scientifically as he can, the nature of the problem; secondly, to assist the group in 'working through' to a more complete

> understanding of it, emotionally as well as intellectually, on the basis of which they may be able to fashion a new solution... by proceeding in this way ... the social scientist can come closest to exploiting methods which in the physical and biological sciences have proved a key to progress.
>
> ... Because its [i.e. the Institute's] research includes this component... a premium is placed on theory that is empirically based and of practical application and, conversely, the construction is discouraged of theoretical models remote from real life. Fields to which members of the Institute have contributed theory ... fertile in stimulating productive research in a number of centres are the behaviour of small groups, the functioning of families, the development of social relations in early childhood, the interrelatedness of work teams and the machines they use, processes of communication and persuasion, relations of organizations to their environments, and conflict resolution. [See also Appendix III.]

The clinical reader will see that in these sentences are incorporated the essential principles of that psychotherapy which is a search for better adaptation for the 'client'. It is the parent Clinic's bequest to its lusty offspring as the principles for 'searching out the secrets of institutional nature with diligence', to adapt Harvey's famous phrase. I do not know how far the other 'colonies' or half-children we helped to fashion follow these principles: the Davidson Clinic at Edinburgh, the Portman Clinic, or the Department of Psychiatry in the Leeds Medical School. That these principles are valid for the purposes of a mental health-oriented social medicine and environmental hygiene in the human sense will be difficult to gainsay.

What of the Tavistock's failures and omissions over its first half-century? Must we not admit that H.C.M.'s original dream of his model for a new norm of precept and practice in psychological medicine has been woefully slow in becoming reality? How far are all of us who laboured to make it come true responsible for this relatively modest impact on medicine in general and psychiatry in particular? In a sense, our early successes in establishing a reputation for helping neurotic patients and receiving support from influential medical and society figures contained the seeds of opposition by official psychiatry. We may have thought of ourselves as representing a 'nicer' and more 'medical' form of the New Psychology than Freud's menacing, deeply resisted original hypotheses and jargon from the godless Continent. Physicians like Farquhar Buzzard, Langdon-Brown and Arthur Hurst, involved with First World War shell-shock, by knowing the Crichton-Miller-McDougall-Rivers group, backed us. But by and large we were tarred with the Freudian brush; and who was this jumped-up G.P. Crichton-Miller, anyway, with his rich society patients and no service record in mental hospitals? We were not helped by H.C.M.'s own disdain of leading London psychiatric teachers of the day, Petrie, Armstrong-Jones, Porter Phillips or Mapother as well as of the psychoanalysts. He was too identified with his own views to be tolerant of great debate, and tended to equate opposition with personal attack. This may have made him not only overestimate the power of his model to prevail because he believed in it; it also gave one the impression that those people round him who differed were 'all out of step', from Ernest Jones to Lewis Bruce (who published a book in 1906 in which he proposed to exclude all mention of psychology from the theory of mental disorder). Thus H.C.M.s own touchy susceptibilities to deviants or critics made him think of 'his' child, the frail little 'Tavi', as a bit of a messianic centre – a feeling some readers may well detect to this day in the present chronicler's sentiments too! H.C.M.'s anomalous position between the worlds of the old mental hospital and of official psychoanalysis made for enmity and suspicion on both sides. Our emphasis on emotional and ethical compassion, closeness of the early leading figures (H.C.M., J.R., Hadfield, Browne, Bennet) to the Church, and the absence of spectacular intellectual brilliance, made for a degree of contempt or derision from the great hospitals and 'scientific' thinkers towards this 'parsons' clinic'. This stereotype lasted certainly into the Second World War, though J.R. was a more integrative thinker and a *much* more genuinely conciliatory man, to whose efforts our 'public relations' standing, such as it was, was chiefly due. It is likely that the failure to obtain major financial endowments was an accurate measure of our image.

Then, with the spectacular achievements of J.R.'s Army group, the position was rather suddenly reversed. Our ability to use creatively the new insights of mainly American work (Moreno, Kurt Lewin, Elton Mayo *et al.*) in social psychology, etc., grafted on to our own skills, made not only many 'temporary officers' from industry and the universities, but also many 'outside' psychiatrists and psychoanalysts see us as a highly successful group who should lead the revolution in British psychiatry and applied social science. And, as Enoch Powell perceived (see p. 269), we remained Crichton-Millerian or Reesian 'missionaries' ourselves.

'*Magna est veritas et prevalebit*'. Our *veritas* was, if more sophisticated and science-oriented, none the less primarily the old Tavistock one of a psychodynamic stress-relieving social action based on humanistic values. In my personal view, this model, so well expressed in the document A.913 quoted in this chapter, is the only possible one for an ethical behavioural science applied to the common weal in a free society. But we somehow did not seize the opportunity to take this lead: our financial-institutional base was still the precarious one of pre-war days, and we had brought it about that we lost our leader J.R., who might have done our public relations job for us. We alienated many who saw him as a guarantor of our continuity with the old values.

I think also that the institutional introversion which overtook us in 1946 lost us much ground. In our eagerness not to run before we could walk in the new activities, not to oversell ourselves, but first have 'the new model' established in one place – the Tavistock itself – we neglected many opportunities for making our optimal impact on the post-war psychiatric scene. We disdained to maintain our supporting base among the sanctioning 'establishment' of our society. We hoped our good works and publications would do our selling for us, but forgot that there are no universal journals, only journals and readerships for the already converted. How many British psychiatrists ever read our own *Human Relations?* We hardly even tried to publish in the *Journal of Mental Science* (now the *British Journal of Psychiatry*), in which to this day it is rare to find an article on a psychodynamic topic. For in the 'outside world', where some of the achievements of the Army group had penetrated in attenuated form – group therapy, the notion of the therapeutic community, group and interpersonal relations as the basis for psycho-social improvement etc. – the medical model of the 'disease entity', with its emphasis on biological research and drug therapy, had reasserted its older and more congenial claims in the area of its own priority, the psychoses. The successes in relieving many hitherto intractable illnesses by the physical methods and psychotropic drugs impelled the enthusiastic restatement of neurological and genetic concepts to *all* psychological ill-health, reinforced by the newly resuscitated Pavlovian-behaviourist approaches. Now psychodynamic theory and treatment was no longer shocking as between the wars; it was just irrelevant and a quaint anachronism in the new world of validated drug trials and slick factor-analysed follow-up studies. It is arguable that the ranks of psychodynamists, of which the Tavistock is the largest clinical grouping, reacted too passively to these developments – as it were, 'letting the heathen rage' not without some righteous glee, as panacea followed panacea into oblivion, from hyperthermia to cardiazol, from Rauwolfia to insulin coma, and so on.

In particular, our friendlier critics, especially those who had expected us to transform the psychiatric scene, might charge us with 'disappearing' from many areas in which Tavistock people should have been prominent. Although, for example, the programme of the N.A.M.H. and of the World Congress on Mental Health, 1948, virtually coincided with the Tavistock's interests and expertise, few of us took any prominent part in their proceedings or counsels. Also critics could say that we were slow to develop our teaching programmes, internal as well as extra-mural. And for a long period we came up with essentially the same programme as the pre-war Clinic's. It will be remembered that the Medical Planning Committee positively resolved to become a regional and not a teaching hospital, thereby foregoing the status and prerogatives of a university institution under the new N.H.S., which at one time we thought might be open to us. We saw it as an essential step to preserving our identity and our principles of work *vis-à-vis* the experience of other small institutions that opted the other way. There was only one post-graduate school and one professor of psychiatry in London, and we did not intend to become an annexe of Mapother's inheritance, as happened to the Bethlem Royal Hospital, even if that school had wanted to have us. We accepted the handicap, justifiably trusting the Ministry of Health's assurances that we would be allowed 'to be what we had been', and also to secure the link with the Tavistock Institute as a non-Governmental body. Our aim of creating a model community mental health service in a limited area never eventuated. Our position in the N.H.S. meant a diminution of our ability to develop teaching and research as our primary tasks. It could be argued that we might have succeeded by now in becoming a second teaching institution had we carried through our pre-war extension plan and created an in-patient unit, thus broadening our scope to include early and acute psychoses and necessarily the new pharmacological therapies and skills to deal with them. This aloofness from the study and use of various chemical aids to hasten recovery or to deepen insight was possibly a rigidity as great as its opposite – the neglect of psychodynamics, with which we reproached the 'hospital psychiatrists'. Precisely because we had the psychoanalytic resources, *we* should have been the people to research into the deeper effects aad reciprocal influences of drugs on personality and vice versa, even if official psychoanalysis did not do so. Such an opportunity was close to recurring around 1960, when our new building and our future were under review, and a distinguished psychopharmacological research worker explored our willingness to receive him and to provide facilities. Had he not then decided to go abroad, this marriage between the two major lines of psychiatric work might have radically altered our image and ability to attract funds and interest for the larger objectives close to our hearts.

The fact was that among the staff themselves there were not at this time people who wished or were competent to go into such biochemical or psychosomatic work, and no *fiat* from a director or a committee could have altered this, even if our internal structure had been authoritarian enough to require someone to 'volunteer'. We stuck perhaps too closely to our old last.

Equally regrettable, and perhaps more avoidable, was our failure to take the lead, under the aegis and encouragement of the Advisory Committee on Psychiatry of our Regional Hospital Board, in organizing and carrying through a remarkably advanced and comprehensive programme we devised for post-graduate education of the trainees in our region in concert with the psychiatric hospitals. We should have been ten years ahead of anything since attempted elsewhere. In the Wessex Region (which, it is true, has no medical school with a psychiatric department) the existence of a more modest scheme and its success under Dr Stephen MacKeith has called forth an adequate grant of facilities and funds by the authorities. We might also have obtained such facilities. Teachers from the abounding and diverse appropriate institutions in our Region, neurological departments and university medical schools, and in all basic sciences from genetics to cultural anthropology had shown interest. The Tavistock would have been the co-ordinating base for such a school, grafting its own wide expertise illustrated in these pages on to a first-rate course ranging from 'classical' psychiatry to sophisticated social science. The scheme died in the mid-1950s, as already recounted, for want of the necessary arduous and initially voluntary effort of administrative co-ordination. Our own teaching on what we knew and did was developed in context, but not within the broad framework of an integrative psychiatry. There might by now have been from 50 to 100 younger consultant psychiatrists all over the country trained in this school, had it eventuated.

I have also already alluded in earlier pages to our postponement of working seriously and early on adequate instruments of assessing our therapeutic results. This was always regarded as a priority. In an era which is impressed by the 'scientific', there is no criticism more damaging to psychoanalysts and therapists than their lack of validation of change in personality and of better adaptation to life of patients on which the claims for their work rest. But before such measures can be devised, adequate knowledge of the structure, growth and functioning of personality must be won. In this most elusive and complex field we have refused to over-simplify the issues like some researchers. Instead, our research strategy, and especially John Bowlby's, has been to undertake studies of personality under stress and change which can meet the canons of scientific method. If we were further on, such measuring tools would no doubt be fashioned, and the standing of dynamic psychotherapy would be higher. The absence of psychodynamically respectable measuring tools of easy application has resulted in almost total absence of follow-up work by the criteria commonly used, though universally recognized as inadequate and only useful for showing social recovery in severe psychotics, etc. This omission is perhaps counted the most typical distinguishing mark of the 'empathic', 'maternal', synaesthetic (Main's term) attitudes of the depth-therapist, in contrast to the highly rational, 'diacritical' (Main) skills and interests of the research designer. The equal development of both tendencies in doctors is rare. We can be glad that the Tavistock group has always preponderatingly contained the former, because they have given it the capacity to defend 'human' against 'theoretical' studies, which are apt to flee from the deep confrontation with differentiated persons[1] into the safer remoteness of seeing people as statistical units or bearers of classificatory labels of 'disease entities' or 'traits' abstracted for convenience. Our organization and work, in sum, has displayed the typical merits of maintaining the 'virtues' of the synaesthetic, problem-sharing and insightful approach to psychiatry *vis-à-vis* the intellectualizing epidemiologists and 'organicists'. It has also manifested the shortcomings of our genotype as viewed from the standpoint of the latter. In most ways these polarities of approach represent abiding realities in the continuing great debate within psychiatry, medicine and the human sciences, perhaps within modern man himself, which can only be resolved in the as yet unforeseeable future. Essentially it is a conflict of values which I have discussed elsewhere.[2]

[1] So much stressed, for example, by Karl Jaspers.

[2] Dicks, H. V., *Clinical Studies in Psychopathology*, 2nd Ed., London: Arnold, 1947, 221–2; 'Education for General Practice – the Psychosocial Factors', *Lancet*, ii (26 August 1950), 317–20; 'In Search of Our Proper Ethic', *Brit. J. Med. Psychol.*, 23 (1950), 1–14; 'Mental Health in the Light of Ancient Wisdom', *Ment. Hyg.*, 43 (1959), 179–93; 'The Proper Study of Mankind', *Brit J.. Psychiat.* 113 (1967), 1,333–44; 'The State of Psychotherapy in British Psychiatry', *Am. J. Psychiat.* 125 (1969), 1,232 et seq.

Prospects

If the foregoing summary was a subjective evaluation, what follows can only be described as personal speculation on the future of the Tavistock – the Clinic and the Clinic-linked activities of the Institute, perhaps all of it – in that wider prospect opened up by the fusion of health and social security in a single department of state, by the impact of the Royal Commission's Report on medical education (the Todd Report), by the proposals for restructuring our divided National Health Service into a more coherent organization (the Green Paper), and for unifying the social services (the Seebohm Report).

Even if all the assumptions on the importance of genetic inheritance in the predisposition to develop psychiatric disorders, including their specific micro-biochemical and physical accompaniments, were proven, this would not change the need for techniques of managing and preventing the complex factors of intrapsychic and social stresses in individual and group life which release or aggravate such predispositions and cause maladaptation and breakdown of personality. Thus a mental health and welfare service – indeed, a holistic medicine with its associated social and educational arms – will require in the coming half-century more of the kind of expertise, teaching and research that a place like the Tavistock has fostered. 'Nature' and 'nurture' are no longer conceivable as mutually exclusive aetiological theories, but only as interacting variables. Psychodynamic thinking and practice, distilled from psychoanalysis and the behavioural sciences, has created in the Tavistock, as at the Cassel Hospital, active reservoirs for feeding these transdisciplinary insights and hypotheses about personality in action required for community psychiatry, social casework and institutional dynamics into the helping professions involved. While the Tavistock's educational work has by the hitherto dominant psychiatric orientations always been thought of as 'highly specialized' – as it were, a post-post-graduate addition of certain narrow skills to the equipment of a few psychiatrists in the still allegedly 'marginal' areas of psychotherapy of adults and children, in social work *its central place* in the approach to *all* human stress situations from parenthood to industrial relations has been recognized much sooner. The Todd Report proposes that medical education shall see it in the same light. With the fluidity suggested by the Todd Report and by the Green Paper, the old distinctions between designated 'teaching schools' and 'regional hospitals' are likely to diminish, together with the special enclaves of the post-graduate institutes. It is clearly laid upon the Health Service (now incorporating much more of the social services) to train its personnel in the needed *vocational* skills, which is not primarily a task for universities. The Tavistock's courses, even in their present scope, are at least equivalent to post-graduate diploma level in 'human relations' for the three major professions involved. These could therefore be a basis for training the future trainers in psychotherapy and social psychiatry, social casework (in public health, child psychiatry, family and community work, probation) and clinical psychology. If university status in future is not mandatory, but a desirable linkage, then the flexibility inherent in the Tavistock Association of Governmental and non-Governmental units could be an advantage. Where in the past we strove for the hallmark of 'university recognition', we might now strive for a co-operative role in the national task of preparing the helping professions for their new co-ordinated roles in promoting mental and social health. We would expect to share with, for example, the Institute of Psychiatry that aspect of training in which we excel, without the old suspicions and fears, while benefiting from their pre-eminence in other aspects of training and research. In the emphasis the Todd Report (para. 128) has placed on adequate psychological training of future general practitioners (up to the level of specialist short of consultant rank in some cases) we would recognize an acknowledgement that what we had pioneered was becoming a desideratum for all personal medical care, hence an ongoing call on the Tavistock. Here again the early priority is for the education of the future educators. It would be no new experience for Tavistock-trained personnel to man teaching posts in our field in medical and social work departments of universities. The Todd Report, seemingly unaware of the existence of the Tavistock as such, visualizes such increased attention to psychotherapy, child psychiatry, and the elements of the social-behavioural science complex being given in university medical schools. The supply of the experts (as against those with only a purely intellectual acquaintance with our field) must for some time to come with few exceptions be drawn from where these interrelated disciplines have long been cultivated by the entire staff – as Edinburgh has recognized in inviting Sutherland to develop such work in their department of psychological medicine.

The new holistic approach to medicine advocated by the Todd Report will not be achieved under a generation or two – and then only if its recommendations are implemented for *undergraduates* (para. 199) in a balanced introduction to the psychology and sociology of human beings in trouble. The Tavistock should welcome the opportunity, if the Todd Report's proposals be accepted, of taking part in this trend-forming work. Such an opportunity might come if the likewise advocated association occurs of teaching hospitals and their schools with multi-faculty constituent institutions of London University. The Tavistock's range of research and teaching interests and experience on normal and abnormal human development, on family and social process and its stresses can offer much to the pre-clinical as well as the clinical student to counteract the at long last obvious and deplored 'dehumanization' of the future doctor under the impact of physico-chemical anatomical and physiological teaching. We would have no less to contribute to the experience of undergraduates in psychology and sociology, and would doubtless do much of our teaching in groups drawn from all these disciplines.

If, in addition to being associated in a teaching scheme, the hitherto 'extra-territorial' university hospitals were also to acquire responsibility for defined communities within their area (e.g. the U.C.H.-Royal Free combination for central north London), and if special institutions such as the Tavistock were drawn in, the latter could hope at last to implement with official blessing one of its aspirations of the last twenty years – its 'community project', offering scope to all departments of the Clinic and several units of the Institute. What a field for practical experience under socio-psychiatric guidance this could make for undergraduates and post-graduates in all the behavioural sciences, in which I include medicine. I suspect that no present teaching hospital could at present 'lay on' such a mental health service.

In the light of these potentialities for the future deployment of the Tavistock's resources, it remains to be asked what might be the effect of such moves on its structure and indeed identity. Looking outwards first, my generation have had the experience of all pioneers – of our position being first ignored, next decried and then quietly imitated without acknowledgement of sources. This form of flattery loses its charm on repetition. However faithful to Hippocrates's injunction to share our discoveries freely with our colleagues, and however aware of the mutual defence mechanisms at work, we have a right to hope that our contribution will be made in our name, and that the Tavistock will no longer take for granted that its light so shines that men will see its good works. It must acquire once again the habit of being in demand at congresses, meetings and in the counsels of our professions, correcting a lot of outdated stereotypes that serve as sticks to beat 'psychotherapy' with. Our published work will be read *after* we have made such an impact – not the other way round.

Turning inwards to look at the Tavistock's self-perception, one is sometimes struck by a dread thought. Are we like other erstwhile *avant-garde*, innovating institutions – the Daughters of the American Revolution, the Soviet Communist Party or the Progressive Schools of 1896 – set in our middle-aged ways, proclaiming the verities of yesteryear, while others have long since pushed past us? Have we perhaps our own stereotypes which we are tilting against – reactionary generals who would not have W.O.S.B.s or social psychiatry during the war or die-hard psychoanalytic bodies who could not accept group analysis or brief psychotherapy? And has the old *élan* that founded and developed the 'Tavi' on a shoestring and recreated it after the Second World War departed with the people who carried it? Has the 'security' and externally imposed framework of the N.H.S. bureaucratized us and dimmed Crichton-Miller's vision of a dedicated bunch of people who cared deeply for people in trouble and for the good doctrine? Have we –

and I mean here especially the Clinic – in fact delivered our goods and can now enter our period of senescence with the complacent sense of having been a unique, misunderstood and undervalued voice in the wilderness? Or – on the contrary – is what I have narrated in this volume just the prehistory, the heroic epic, whence we have now emerged into the national scene of 'real' history?

I cannot answer these questions. Their answer will only emerge over the next fifty years of British medical and social history. But the answer will in no small measure depend on the vision of the Tavistock's 'mission' held by the third generation of its policy-makers. I am given to extrapolating from biology. In evolution there are clearly two major vectors at work: differentiation of function (leading to specialization in organs and species) and integration (as in the adaptive behaviour of very 'simple' one-celled creatures as well as in the hierarchical regulation by the central nervous and endocrine systems of complex organisms). The total Tavistock organization, by analogy, has in the course of its evolution differentiated not only a number of units with specialized functions, but a number of skilled roles within these. The integrative function has been performed by the various structures developed for it – Council, sub-councils, committees, staff meeting, etc. – as well as by the common matrix of shared concepts and values related to the fostering of good mental health and human relations. To us, the older generation, this common matrix was the marrow of our bones; the structures evolved for sharing in it were the means, not the end. The problems of the Tavistock's future can be put in another way: if the identity, the integrated notion of us is in a name and a building, then we may not bother to maintain it. It is no good preserving cultural fossils, like some small ancient hospitals that fought the N.H.S. tooth and nail for continued separate existence though nothing original in their work or mission now justified it: this would be totemism. But if the identity, the hall-mark, is a still ongoing and distinctive integration of skills and ideas applicable to a variety of differentiated roles not duplicated elsewhere, then the preservation of the structure that permits the exchange and growth between the constituent organs is highly desirable. Not all units of the

Tavistock Institute could have survived incorporation of its mother Clinic in the Health Service. Not all units would now see any relevance to their primary chosen tasks in, for example, integrative association with the teaching hospital/multi-faculty college/special hospital mixture, as proposed by the Todd Report. They none the less see and have affirmed their interest in keeping the internal integrate or matrix of the total Tavistock organization as a corporate identity, within which their separate differentiated identities are not only preserved but positively valued, because of our having evolved a genuinely participant democratic institution. We cannot always predict when a new insight or observation made in operational research or in industrial counselling may illuminate a facet of community psychiatry, or a new finding in child psychology solve a problem in the coal-mines. But we seem to go on appreciating the potentials inherent in our peculiar mix for a 'breakthrough' in integrative studies in personal and social behaviours and dynamics.

It is this tolerant conceptual cross-fertilization for the enhancement of diagnosis and therapy on 'both sides' of our house which, if once lost, cannot easily be re-created, even if we discount all other advantages of our integrate. This is the mix which a still groping 'new psychiatry' and an applied social science in our country have scarcely begun to strive after for their own better integration. If the Tavistock now fell apart, it would have to be reinvented and retrace most of the steps – at least since the Second World War – again, and we could not then perform the new expectations from *our* mix, not simply from *our* institution. We are *de facto* just as much a special post-graduate Institute as Queen Square or the Maudsley, even if *de jure* we are in present N.H.S. ratings and in the awareness of most doctors and psychiatrists a too narrowly differentiated and rather deviant little enclave with our special mystique. I would fight hard for the preservation of such esoteric institutes, whether in tropical medicine or any other field. There *must* be such matrices embodying a guiding principle, a set of skills and a highly integrated group of people dedicated to their special 'hobbies', who together do things at a higher level of efficiency than any one of them could were he or she to represent the field elsewhere. 'Moorfields' collectively know more about eyes than their finest individual consultant working in another hospital's ophthalmic unit. Hence – though we should enter into whole-hearted co-operation with the associated hospitals and colleges which the new N.H.S. policy may soon promote – we must also remain above all ourselves. Otherwise the flow of our differentiated contribution will soon dry up – whether of men or of ideas.

I would dearly love to conclude this volume with a homily on a high ethical level addressed to my recent and future younger colleagues. I will only briefly indulge this intolerable propensity of the old to exhort their successors not to let the side down. I would once again draw their attention to our Founder's abhorrence of institutionalization and bureaucratization as a state of mind in psychological medicine. But I would also warn them against his tendency to a certain disdain and intolerance – the 'all out of step except me' syndrome of the band of devotees. This could result in selection of newcomers for congeniality rather than genius – as in ossification. Let us beware of the Devil we know – unless he has aces up his sleeve. The 'Tavi' has a long record of continuous innovation. The matrix exists to nourish the new, not to dispense the mixture as before. Without new life and creation, we would lose our place as a centre of excellence.

We have had our past. Now let us make psychiatric history!

APPENDIX I

List of Presidents, Vice-Presidents and Council Members

PRESIDENTS

H.R.H. The Duke of Kent, K.G. (1934–42)
H.R.H. The Duchess of Kent (1942–48)
(Her Royal Highness relinquished the Presidency of the Institute to become Patron of the Clinic when it joined the National Health Service, and she remained its Patron until her death in 1968.)

H.R.H. The Princess Alexandra, the Hon. Mrs Angus Ogilvy

VICE-PRESIDENTS

The Most Hon. the Marquess of Aberdeen and Temair, K.T. (1927–32)
Isabel, Marchioness of Aberdeen, G.B.E. (1927–37)
The Countess Baldwin of Bewdley, G.B.E. (1928–42)
The Right Hon. the Earl Beatty, O.M., G.C.B., G.C.V.O., D.S.O. (1927–35)
Lady Blackett (1931–3)
Sir Henry Brackenbury, LL.D., M.D. (1938–41)
Professor Sir Cyril Burt, M.A., D.SC. (1937–48)
The Lady Cynthia Colville, D.C.V.O. (1931–47)
The Marchioness of Dufferin and Ava (1927–9)
The Viscountess Erleigh (1927–8)
The Very Rev. Lionel G. B. J. Ford, M.A., PH.D., D.D. (1927–31)
Dame Katherine Furse, G.B.E., R.R.C. (1927)
H. S. Goodhart-Rendel, Esq. (1927–9)
Field Marshal Earl Haig, O.M., K.T., G.C.B. (1927)

The Right Hon. the Earl of Harewood, K.G., G.C.V.O., D.S.O. (1936–1945)
The Right Hon. the Lord Hollenden (1946–8)
The Very Rev. W. R. Inge, K.C.V.O., D.D. (1935–48)
C. W. Kimmins, Esq., M.A., D.SC. (1928–46)
The Right Hon. the Lord Leconfield, G.C.V.O., D.L. (1927–45)
Hugh Lewis, Esq. (1927–9)
The Countess of Limerick, C.B.E. (1935–47)
Miss Ishbel MacDonald (1930–6)
Professor William McDougall, LL.D., D.SC., M.B., F.R.S. (1927–38)
Lieut.-Colonel H. G. G. Mackenzie, D.S.O., M.A., M.D. (1927–45)
The Right Hon. Lord Mildmay of Flete, P.C. (1927–45)
Sir Henry Newbolt, M.A., D.LITT. (1927–38)
The Lady Margaret Nicholson (1927)
The Marchioness of Reading (1938–47)
Mrs Norman Ridgley (1937–47)
Mrs I. M. Sieff (1945–7)
Owen Hugh Smith, Esq. (1946–7)
The Most Rev William Temple, P.C., D.D. (1934–42)
The Right Hon. the Viscount Wakefield of Hythe, C.B.E., LL.D. (1935–9)
Sir Frederick Willis, K.B.E., C.B. (1933–42)

Those Vice-Presidents shown as holding office from 1927 may have been appointed earlier (between 1920 and 1926), but records are no longer available.

The office of Vice-President was discontinued in 1948 when the Tavistock Clinic became part of the National Health Service.

MEMBERS OF THE COUNCIL[1]

Harold M. Abrahams, Esq., M.A., LL.B. (1928–44)
General Sir Ronald Adam, Bart, G.C.B., D.S.O., O.B.E. (1945–53)
The Right Hon. the Lord Alness, P.C., K.C. (1938–45) (Chairman, 1938–45)
S. S. Berlanny, Esq., C.A. (1947—)
Lady Blackett (1934–44)

[1] Prior to the incorporation of the Institute in 1929 as the Tavistock Square Clinic, the governing body was known as the Executive Committee. Records of membership of the Executive Committee prior to 1927 are no longer available.

APPENDIX I

Sir Henry Brackenbury, LL.D., M.D. (1929–38) (Chairman, 1929–38)
Leonard F. Browne, Esq., M.D., J.P. (1945–60)
Professor Sir Cyril Burt, M.A., D.SC. (1932–6)
William Cash, Esq., F.C.A. (1937)
Mrs Margaret Cole (1945–8)
H. Crichton-Miller, Esq., M.D., F.R.C.P. (1929–40)
H. V. Dicks, Esq., M.D., F.R.C.P. (1947—)
H. A. Downes, Esq. (1932–3)
The Viscountess Erleigh (1929–34)
Sir Leslie Farrer, K.C.V.O. (1939–50; 1965—) (Chairman, 1946–7; 1965—)
The Right Hon. the Earl of Feversham (1933–44)
Dame Katherine Furse, G.B.E., R.R.C. (1928–41)
Professor H. R. Hamley, M.A., M.SC. (1945–7)
Douglas Hamlyn, Esq., M.C. (1937–47)
G. R. Hargreaves, Esq., O.B.E., M.R.C.S., L.R.C.P. (1946–8)
John Harvard-Watts, Esq. (1947–50)
G. D. Herbert, Esq. (1950—)
W. J. Hinton, Esq., M.A. (1945–7)
P. K. Hodgson, C.M.G., C.V.O., O.B.E. (1933–6)
J. L. Hodson, Esq. (1945–50)
The Right Hon. the Lord Hollenden (1934–45)
Miss W. E. Hollingsworth (1929–45)
R. A. Howden, Esq. (1929–50)
Rupert Hulme, Esq. (1928–36)
Christmas Humphreys, Esq., M.A., LL.B. (1939–50)
The Very Rev. W. R. Inge, K.C.V.O., D.D. (1927–34)
Sir Walter Langdon-Brown, M.D., F.R.C.P. (1938–44)
The Countess of Limerick (1927–34)
Sir Lynden Macassey, K.B.E., K.C. (1927)
Sir Dougal Malcolm, K.C.M.G. (1929–36; 1938–46)
The Very Rev. W. R. Matthews, K.C.V.O., D.D. (1935–8)
Hubert Meredith, Esq. (1935–6)
Sir William Mitchell Cotts, Bart., K.B.E. (1928–9)
Professor B. S. Morris, B.SC., ED.B. (1947—)
Conrad Ormond, Esq., B.A. (1945–8)
J. D. W. Pearce, Esq., M.D., M.B., CH.B., F.R.C.P., D.P.M. (1965—)
Bedford Pierce, Esq., M.D., F.R.C.P. (1928) (Chairman, 1928)
I. J. Pitman, Esq., M.A., M.P. (1946–50)
Colonel R. S. Rait-Kerr, C.B.E., D.S.O., M.C. (1945–8)
Neville Randall, Esq. (1934–5)
The Marchioness of Reading (1935–6)

J. R. Rees, C.B.E., M.A., M.D., F.R.C.P., D.P.H. (1946–51)
Miss Leila Rendel (1945–7)
A. K. Rice, Esq., M.A., SC.D. (1948–1969)
R. Lloyd Roberts, C.B.E. (1946)
Walter F. Roch, Esq. (1931–45)
D. Ross, Esq., B.COM., C.A. (1948—)
C. H. Scott, Esq. (1945–7)
Miss E. M. Sellar (1929–42)
Mrs I. M. Sieff (1934–44)
Professor T. S. Simey, M.A. (now Lord Simey) (1946–57)
Owen Hugh Smith, Esq. (1927–45)
J. D. Sutherland, C.B.E., PH.D., D.M.P., F.R.C.P.E. (1961—)
J. Albert Thompson, Esq., LL.D., J.P. (1938–46)
John A. F. Watson, Esq., J.P. (1945–50)
J. Douglas C. White, Esq., M.A., M.D. (1927) (Chairman, 1927)
Lady Whyte (1934—) (Chairman, 1947–65)
Sir F. J. Willis, K.B.E., C.B. (1927–32)

APPENDIX II

List of Professional Staffs and Past Trainees (Clinic), 1920–68
Bracketed year denotes last pre-War Report.

MEDICAL STAFF

		Present status (where known)
Adams, F. Shirley, M.A., M.D.	1929–(1938)	Deceased
Alcock, J. A. M.	1922–5	?
Allen, Clifford E., M.D., M.R.C.P., D.P.M.	1939[1]	Retired
Archer, B. W. Crowhurst, M.D.	1931–(1938)	?
Barton, P. F., M.A., M.B., B.CH.	1921–9	Deceased
Basden, Margaret, M.D., F.R.C.S., F.C.O.G.	1937–(1938)	
Behrman, S., M.R.C.P.	1938	In consulting practice
Bendit, L. J., M.A., M.R.C.S. L.R.C.P., D.P.M.	1929–38	Retired
Bennet, E. A., M.C., M.A., M.D., D.P.M.	1925–(1938)	In consulting practice
Berg, G. Charles, M.D., B.S., D.P.M.	1928–(1938)	Deceased
Bevan-Brown, C. M., M.A., M.B. CH.B.	1923–(1938)	In New Zealand
Bion, W. R., D.S.O., B.A., M.R.C.S., L.R.C.P.	1934–(1938)	In consulting practice, Los Angeles, Cal.
Bomford, R. R., F.R.C.P.	1938	Physician, London Hosp., Treasurer, R.C.P.
Browne, Leonard F., M.D., B.S.	1922–(1938)	Deceased
Burns, C. L. C., L.R.C.P., M.R.C.S.	1926–34	Deceased
Calver, Grace S., M.B., CH.B.	1933–(1938)	?
Clegg, E. A., M.R.C.S., L.R.C.P.	1925–37	?

[1] Assistant physician.

APPENDIX II

		Present status (where known)
Cloake, Philip C. P.	1924	Deceased
Crichton-Miller, H., M.A., M.D., M.R.C.P.	1920–(1938)	Deceased
Curnock, J. Edgley, M.R.C.S., L.R.C.P., L.D.S., R.C.S.	1938	In consulting practice
Dicks, H. V., M.A., M.D., M.R.C.P.	1928–(1938)	In consulting practice
Dodd, F. H.	1921–4	?
Duncan, A. G.	1923–4	?
Ferguson, Mary B., M.B., CH.B.	1929–(1938)	Retired
Fine, Joseph, B.SC., M.D., D.P.H., D.P.M.	1935–(1938)	In consulting appointment
Franklin, Marjorie	1923–4	Retired
Fraser, A. McLeod, M.B., CH.B.	1937–(1938)[1]	Retired
Gandy, T. H.	1921–2	?
Garrod, Marjorie, M.R.C.S., L.R.C.P.	1927–(1938)	Retired
Hadfield, J. A., M.A., M.B., CH.B.	1920–(1938)	Deceased
Hamilton Pearson, E. A., M.B., CH.B.	1920–(1938)	Deceased
Hammond, J., M.B., CH.B.	1929–31	Deceased
Hardcastle, D. N.	1923–4	Deceased
Hargreaves, G. R., M.R.C.S., L.R.C.P.	1938[1]	Deceased
Hendy, B. D., M.A., M.B., B.CH.	1931–8	Retired
Hill, T. Rowland, M.D., M.R.C.P.	1938	Deceased
Hobhouse, E. W. Neill	1920–4	?
Howe, E. Graham, M.B., B.S. D.P.M.	1926–35	Retired
Hume, J. Basil, M.S., F.R.C.S.	1934–(1938)	Retired
Hutchison, Alice M., M.D., M.R.C.P.	1923–(1938)	Retired
Hutton, Laura F., B.A., M.R.C.S., L.R.C.P.	1931–(1938)	Retired
Kitchen, M. Kathleen F., M.SC., M.B., B.S.	1935–7	?
Lander, Kathleen	1923–4	?
Lucas, R. Evelyn, M.B., CH.B.	1939[1]	Retired
Luff, Mary C., M.D., D.P.M.	1930–(1938)	Retired

[1] Assistant physician.

		Present status (where known)
Maberly, Alan, M.A., M.B., B.CH.	1939	Deceased
Miller, Emmanuel, M.A., M.R.C.P., D.P.M.	1933–(1938)	Retired
Montgomery, Eleanor A., L.R.C.P., L.R.C.S.	1922–(1938)	?
Morris, W. McGregor, F.R.C.S.(E).	1922–(1938)	?
Neame, Humphrey, F.R.C.S.	1921–(1938)	Retired
Nicolle, Grace, M.A., M.B., B.S.	1927–(1938)	Retired
Potts, W. A., M.A., M.D.	1920–35	Deceased
Redfern, A. R., M.B., CH.B.	1929–34	Retired
Rees, J. R., M.A., M.D., M.R.C.P., D.P.H.	1920–(1938)	Deceased
Rees, Mary I. Hemingway, M.B., CH.B.	1920–(1938)	Deceased
Rippon, W/Com. T. S., R.A.F. (Rtd.), O.B.E., M.R.C.S., L.R.C.P.	1934–(1938)[1]	
Rivington, Evelyn B. G.	1921–2	
Roles, F. C., M.A., B.CH., M.R.C.P.	1935–(1938)	Retired
Rowe, C. Isobel, B.M., B.CH.	1928–32	Retired
Saywell, Evelyn N., L.R.C.P. L.R.C.S.	1920–34	?
Simon, George, M.B., B.CH., D.M.R.E.	1929–(1938)	In consultant practice
Strauss, E. B., M.A., D.M., M.R.C.P.	1935–(1938)	Deceased
Suttie, Ian D., M.B., F.R.F.P.S.	1928–35	Deceased
Suttie, Jane I., M.A., M.B., CH.B.	1932–(1938)	Retired
Thoms, Amy M., M.D., M.R.C.P.	1936–(1938)	Retired
Townend, R. D. M., M.A., M.R.C.S., L.R.C.P.	1931–(1938)	?
Tremellen, Sybil E., M.R.C.S., L.R.C.P.	1928–34	Deceased
Tucker, D. L.	1920–?	?
Weber, Hilda M., B.SC., M.D., B.S., D.P.M.	1931–(1938)	Retired
Wilde, J. F., M.B., B.CH.	1932–8	Manchester
Wilson, A. T. Macbeth, M.D., B.SC.	1939	In university chair
Wilson, Henry, M.D., M.R.C.P. D.P.M.	1926–37	Deceased

[1] Assistant Physician.

		Present status (where known)
Wilson, Isabel, G. H., M.D., D.P.M.	1927–31	Retired
Wittkower, E., M.D.(Berlin), L.R.C.P.&S.	1939	In Chair, McGill Univ.
Wright, M. B., O.B.E., M.D., C.M.	1929–(1938)	Deceased
Yellowlees, D.	1920–1	In consulting practice
Young, J. C., M.C., M.D., M.S.	1926–31	Deceased

APPENDIX II

JUNIOR STAFF AND POST-GRADUATE STUDENTS

		Present status (where known)
Alford, L. B.	1921	(U.S.)
Backus, P. L., M.D., C.M.	1938	In practice
Bakewell, Helen	1926	(N.Z.)
Barber, Alice W.	1936–7	(Austr.)
Barber, G.	1921–2	
Blacker, C. P.	1928–9	
Bonnard, Augusta, M.B., B.S.	1937–(1938)	In practice
Bradley, Rosalind	1925–31	
Bridges, A. B. H.	1921	
Brook, T.	1923	
Bunbury, D. Elizabeth	1934–7	
Burbury, W. Mary	1936–7	Consultant, Lancs.
Carthew, M.	1928	(Siam)
Cheney, J.	1921	(U.S.)
Chennell, Eileen A.	1935–7	Deceased
Churchill, Stella, M.R.C.S., L.R.C.P., D.P.H.	1937–(1938)	
Closs, J. R.	1925–6	(N.Z.)
Cluver, Paul F.	1928	(S. Africa)
Cooke-Taylor, C. R.	1930–1	
Cooper, B.	1926	(Austr.)
Cowlin, Florence	1929–30	
Curran, R. D.	1930	Lord Chancellor's Visitor
Curtiss, L., M.R.C.S., L.R.C.P.	1938	
Dalby, Marjorie	1923	
Dalrymple, Leolia	1926	(U.S.)
de Peyer, Hilda, M.R.C.S., L.R.C.P.	1938	Retired
de Villiers-Pritchard, C. W.	1928	
Doherty, Winifred I., M.B., CH.B., D.P.H., D.T.M.	1925–(1938)[1]	Retired
Edelston, H., M.B., CH.B., D.P.M.	1938	Retired

[1] Appointed psychotherapist after three years' service.

APPENDIX II

		Present status (where known)
Edkins, J. E., B.SC., M.D., D.P.M.	1937–(1938)	Deceased
Edwards, F. Marjorie	1928–9	
Elias, J. P., M.B., B.S., CH.B.	1938	
Fisher, J. W.	1930	
Forbes, H. S.	1930–1	
Fordham, M. S.	1935–6	In practice
Fraser, W. H., M.B., B.S., D.P.M.	1938	(Australia)
Fraser, W. D.	1921	
Gaussen, H. S., M.R.C.S., L.R.C.P.	1938	Consultant, Exeter
Giles, Edith	1928–9	(India)
Glaister, J. Norman	1921–2	
Goitein, P. L.	1932–3	
Grace, Richard, F. T., M.D., M.R.C.P.	1937–(1938)	
Griffin, F. W. W.	1930–4	Deceased
Harris, N. G.	1926–9	Deceased
Horton, Kathleen, M.R.C.S., L.R.C.P., D.P.H.	1937–(1938)	In practice
Howard, Doris	1933–8[1]	
Iliff, Daisy G., M.R.C.S., L.R.C.P., D.P.M.	1938	
Inkster, L.	1930–2	
Ironside, A. J.	1929–30	(S. Africa)
Kapp, Dorothy M.	1933–8[1]	
Lilley, Margherita M., M.A., M.B., CH.B., D.P.H.	1932–(1938)[1]	Deceased
Mackwood, J. C., M.R.C.S., L.R.C.P.	1937–(1938)	
Macrae, Angus	1927	
Martin, Joyce, M.R.C.S., L.R.C.P.	1937–(1938)	Deceased
McGlashan, A. F., B.A., M.R.C.S., L.R.C.P.	1938	In practice
Methven, Margaret G., M.A., M.B., CH.B.	1938	Edinburgh Univ.
Millard, F. Laetitia, L.R.C.P., L.R.C.S.	1938–(1938)[1]	Retired
Mills, Hermia, M.B., B.S.	1934–(1938)[1]	In practice
Munro, Lois, M.B., B.S.	1934–(1938)[1]	In practice

[1] Appointed psychotherapist after three years' service.

APPENDIX II

		Present status (where known)
Nicolson, Caroline E., B.A., M.B.M., CH.B.	1935–(1938)[1]	
Nunan, William, M.A., M.D.	1934–(1938)[1]	
Partridge, E. Joyce	1932–7	Deceased
Parsons, Harold	1933–7[1]	
Parsons, L. D.	1923	(Ceylon)
Paterson, A. S.	1932	W. London Hosp.
Pearce, J. D., W., M.A., M.D., F.R.C.P.(E), D.P.M.	1937–(1938)	Consultant, St. Mary's H.
Pegg, George, M.A., M.R.C.S., L.R.C.P.	1937–(1938)	Deceased
Pritchard, Rosemary, B.A., M.R.C.S., L.R.C.P.	1937–(1938)	Retired
Purser, J. A., M.B., B.S., M.R.C.P.	1936–(1938)	Consultant
Reed, J. I.	1923	(U.S.)
Rosenfeld, H., M.D.(Munich), L.R.C.P.&S.	1938	In practice
Rushforth, M. Winifred	1930–1	
Scoresby-Jackson, Margaret	1929–32	
Shaw, Helen	1920–1	
Stewart, J. E. W.	1922	
Stothard, Ethel	1926–7	
Swanton, Cedric	1935	(Austr.)
Thompson, A. G., M.A., M.D., M.S., F.R.C.P.(I)	1937–(1938)	Tavi. Consultant
Thomson, Grizel, M.B., CH.B.	1934–(1938)[1]	Deceased
Thurnam, R.	1925–6	
Todd, Kathleen	1935–8	NZ. Deceased
Torrie, A., M.A., M.B., CH.B., D.P.M.	1936–(1938)	In practice
Turner, P. E.	1930–2	
Vacher, Rosalind, M.B., CH.B., D.P.M.	1936–(1938)	Retired
Vassallo, V.	1930–2	(Malta)
Wasson, Valentina P.	1932	(U.S.)
Watson, T. T. B.	1922	
Watt, A, W.	1931	Consultant, Hove

[1] Appointed psychotherapist after three years' service.

		Present status (where known)
Wentworth, M. H.	1927–8	(U.S.)
West, R. G., Ranyard, M.D., M.R.C.P., D.P.H.		
Williams, J. Harley, M.D., D.P.H.	1937–(1938)	
Wiltshire, Jessie	1930–1	
Wolfe, W. Béran	1926	Deceased (U.S.)
Wyllie, H. A.	1932–4	

APPENDIX II

SOCIAL WORKERS

		Present status (where known)
Cowles-Voysey, Mrs	1932–4	
Dickinson, Miss F. M.	1934–(1938)	
Evans, Mrs M. F.	1932–3	
Hamlyn, Mrs P. D.	1931–(1938)	
Robinson, Miss D. F., M.B.E.	1931–2	
Satow, Miss N. K.	1931–(1938)	
Sellar, Miss E. M.	1932–(1938)	
Shannon, Miss R. E.	1933–5	
Tomalin, Mrs M. R.	1933–(1938)	

EDUCATIONAL PSYCHOLOGISTS

Chesters, Miss Gwen, B.A.	1936–(1938)	
Hocart, Mrs E. G., M.A., B.SC.	1933–4	
Simmins, Miss Constance A., M.A.	1933–(1938)	Deceased

APPENDIX II

ADDITIONAL POST-WAR MEDICAL STAFF

		Present status (where known)
Balint, M., M.D.(Budapest), PH.D.(Berlin), L.R.C.P., L.R.C.S.(Ed)	1950–61	Retired, in practice.
Boenheim, C., M.D.	1938–58	Consultant, Ohio, U.S.A.
Bourne, S., M.R.C.P., M.R.C.S., D.P.M.	1959–63 and 1969-present	
Bowlby, E. J. M., M.A., M.D.	1946–present	
Bruggen, P., M.B., B.S., D.P.M.	1966–present	
Crawford, H. de L.	1939–46	Deceased.
Doyle, M., M.R.C.S., L.R.C.P.	1946–9	Deceased.
Ezriel, H., M.D.(Basle), M.R.C.S., L.R.C.P.	1945–present	
Goldblatt, T. W., M.B., B.CH., D.P.M.	1953–present	
Gosling, R. H., B.SC., M.D., D.P.M.	1956–present	Chairman of Professional Committee.
Heard, Dorothy, PH.D., M.R.C.P., M.R.C.S.	1962–present	
Holden, H., B.M., B.CH., D.OBST.R.C.O.G., D.P.M.	1964–present	
Hunter, H. D., M.B.E., M.B., CH.B., D.P.M.	1948–present	
Irwin, D. H., M.A., M.D., D.P.M.	1943–54	Consultant Psychiatrist, Essex.
Jacobs, J. J. M., F.R.C.P.E., D.P.M.	1945–63	Deceased.
Jaques, E., M.A., M.D., PH.D.	1946–8	Professor of Social Science, Brunel Univ.
Kelnar, J., M.R.C.S., L.R.C.P.	1946–present	
Mackenzie, Marion, M.R.C.S., L.R.C.P.	1950–present	Chairman, Department for Children and Parents.

APPENDIX II

		Present status (where known)
Malan, D. H., B.A., D.M., D.P.M.	1954–present	
Martin, Freda, M.D., D.P.M.	1962–present	
Mason, H. A. C., M.R.C.S., L.R.C.P., D.P.M.	1945–9	Consultant Psychiatrist Kings College and St. Thomas' Hospitals.
Miller, D. H., M.D.	1958–present	Chairman, Adolescent Department.
Miller, H. H., M.B., CH.B., D.P.M.	1947–9	Consultant Psychiatrist Herbert Hone Clinic and Brighton Probation Service.
Popper, E., M.D.	1939–55	Deceased.
Pott, M., M.R.C.S., L.R.C.P., D.P.H., D.P.M.	1936–47	Slough Child Guidance Clinic.
Shadforth, F. T., L.R.C.P., L.R.C.S.ED., D.P.M.	1937–51	Consultant Psychiatrist, University of Sussex Student Health Service.
Stein, Leopold, M.D. (Vienna)	1938–61	
Sutherland, J. D., C.B.E., F.R.C.P.E., D.P.M.	1946–68	Consultant to University of Edinburgh and Royal Edinburgh Hospital.
Soddy, K., M.D., M.R.C.S., L.R.C.P., D.P.M.	1946–8	Consultant Physician, Department of Psychological Medicine, University College Hosp.

		Present status (where known)
Turquet, P. M., M.A., M.R.C.S., L.R.C.P., D.P.M.	1952–present	Chairman, Adult Department.
MacKeith, R., M.A., F.R.C.P., D.P.H.	1946–68	
Rycroft, C. F., B.A., M.R.C.S., L.R.C.P.	1956–68	In practice.
Williams, A. Hyatt, M.D., D.P.M.	1962–present	
Wilson, J. L., M.R.C.S., L.R.C.P., D.P.M.	1959–present	
Woodhead, Barbara, M.R.C.P., D.P.M.	1955–65	In practice.
Wride, Fanny D., M.R.C.S., L.R.C.P., D.P.M., D.C.H.	1956–present	

APPENDIX II

POST-WAR MEDICAL STAFF TRAINEES

		Present status (where known)
Brenman, E., M.R.C.S., L.R.C.P., D.P.M.	1951–5	In practice.
Brough, W., M.B., B.S., D.P.M.	1962–6	Consultant Psychiatrist, London and Friern Hospitals.
Calwell, W. P. K., M.A., M.B., B.S., D.P.M.	1962–4	Director, Hoxton and Hounslow Child Guidance Clinics.
Caplan, G., M.D., D.P.M.	1947–8	Clinical Professor of Psychiatry, Harvard Medical School, Boston, U.S.A.
Craike, W. H., M.R.C.S., L.R.C.P., D.P.M.	1948–9	Consultant Psychiatrist, Paddington Clinic and Day Hospital, Earls Court Child Guidance Clinic and various Approved Schools, Homes etc.
Dare, C., B.A., M.R.C.P., D.P.M.	1968–present	
Davis, P. J. R., M.A., M.B., B.CH.	1948–50	Treasury Medical Service.

		Present status (where known)
Elder, P., M.B., B.S., D.P.M.	1963–6	Department of Psychiatry, McMaster Univ. Canada.
Evans, J., B.SC., M.R.C.P., D.P.M.	1960–3	Consultant in Child Psychiatry, Royal Hospital for Sick Children, Edinburgh.
Frazee, J., M.D.	1952–4	In practice in Canada.
Freeman, T., M.D., M.R.C.P., D.P.M.	1950–2	Consultant Psychiatrist, Holywell Hospital, Antrim.
Goodburn, J., M.B., CH.B., D.P.M.	1966–present	
Gough, D., M.A., M.B., B.CH., D.P.M.	1959–62	Consultant Child Psychiatrist, Greater London Council and Spastics Soc.
Hutchinson, D.	1958–9	Deceased.
Issroff, Judith, M.B., CH.B., D.P.M.	1966–present	
Joffe, W. G., M.B., B.CH., D.P.M.	1952–6	Senior Lecturer Academic Unit of Psychiatry, Middlesex Hospital. Hampstead Child Therapy Clinic and London Clinic of Psycho-Analysis.

		Present status (where known)
Katz, J., M.B., B.CH., D.P.M.	1948–50	Assistant Professor of Child Psychiatry, Institute of Child Health, Sydney, Australia.
Kramer, Elizabeth, M.R.C.S., L.R.C.P.	1949–51	Psycho-therapist, South London Hospital for Women and Children.
Laing, R. D., M.B., CH.B., D.P.M.	1956–60	Consultant Psychiatrist in Research in Schizophrenia.
Lewis, E., M.R.C.P., D.P.M.	1958–61	Consultant Child Psychiatrist, Charing Cross Group and Director, Psychiatric Counselling Service, University of London Institute of Education.
Lindsay, S. F., M.B., B.CH., D.P.M.	1951–5	Consultant Psychiatrist, University of Aberdeen.
Lobl, Elizabeth, M.D.	1945–51	In practice.
Maiden, A., M.R.C.S., L.R.C.P., D.C.H.	1968–present	

APPENDIX II

		Present status (where known)
Main, Agnes, M.B., B.S.	1949–52	Director, Twickenham Child Guidance Clinic.
Markillie, R. E. D., M.R.C.S., L.R.C.P., D.P.M.	1949–52	Consultant Psychiatrist and Senior Lecturer, Department of Psychiatry, Leeds Univ. Leeds R.H.B. and Wakefield Prison
Martin, K. C., M.B., B.CH., B.A.O., D.P.M.	1964–6	Lecturer Child Psychiatry, London Hosp. Medical Col., Consultant Psychiatrist to Maladjusted School.
Michell, E. P. G., M.R.C.P., D.C.H.	1957–9	Lately Physician i/c Department of Psychological Medicine, Hospital for Sick Children, Great Ormond Street. In practice.
Padel, J. H., B.A., M.B., B.S., D.P.M.	1959–64	Consultant Psychiatrist, Tavistock Institute of Human Relations. In practice.

		Present status (where known)
Pappenheim, W., B.A., M.B., B.CH., B.A.O., D.P.M.	1954–7	Consultant Child Psychiatrist, Jewish Board of Guardians, New York City.
Provis, H., M.B., CH.B., D.C.H.	1954–6	General Practice, Canada.
Pokorny, M., M.B., CH.B., D.P.M.	1968–present	
Sherrett, D., M.B., CH.B., D.P.M.	1958–62	In practice.
Smit, E., M.B., B.CH., D.P.M.	1964–7	Returned to South Africa.
Smith, T. A. L., M.A., M.B., B.CH., D.P.M.	1962–6	Consultant Psychiatrist, Surrey and Cambridgeshire Councils, Belmont and St. Helier Hospitals.
Snowdon, B. A., M.B., B.CH., D.P.M.	1967–present	
Stein, S., M.B., B.CH., D.P.M.	1955–7	Consultant Child Psychiatrist, Child Guidance Clinic, Johannesburg.
Stirrat, Jeannie, M.B., CH.B., D.P.M.	1948–50	Consultant Psychiatrist, Bournemouth and E. Dorset Hospital Group and Bournemouth Child and Family Guidance Clinic.

		Present status (where known)
Todes, C. J., M.R.C.S., L.R.C.P., D.P.M.	1965–8	Consultant Psychiatrist, Hampstead Child Therapy Clinic.
Wallbridge, D. C., M.B., B.S., D.P.M.	1964–6	Assistant Psychiatrist, Cassel Hospital.
Waterlow, Judith	1950–2	Deceased.
Wedeles, C. H. A., M.R.C.S., L.R.C.P., D.P.M.	1952–5	P.M.O. (Mental Health) London Borough of Redbridge.
Weston, Diane, M.R.C.S., L.R.C.P. D.P.M.	1966–present	
Williams, Lorna, B.SC., M.B., B.S.	1958–60	In practice.
Wilson, A. R., M.A., B.M., B.CH., D.P.M., B.OBST. R.C.O.G.	1956–60	Medical Director, Earls Court Child Guidance Clinic.
Wolf, E., M.D.(Prague)	1950–1	
Wolf, P. G., M.R.C.S., L.R.C.P., D.P.M.	1956–9	Consultant Psychiatrist, Darenth Park Hospital, Dartford.

In addition large numbers of Supernumerary Medical Trainees (including many from overseas) have undertaken periods of training of from one to four years.

APPENDIX II

POST-WAR NON-MEDICAL STAFF TRAINEES

		Present status (where known)
PSYCHOLOGISTS		
Bernstein, Mrs M.	1955–59	
Biggs, Miss J.	1950–3	In South Africa.
Blake, Mrs Y.	1951–3	
Bremner, J.	1949–51	
Bridgeman, Miss V. (now Mrs Golding)	1959–63	No appointment at present.
Buick, D.	1956–8	Hospital for Sick Children, Great Ormond Street.
Burnard, G.	1954–6	Lecturer, College of Technology.
Busfield, Miss J.	?	University of East Anglia.
Cang, S.	1960–2	Brunel University.
Cheshire, N.	?	University College of North Wales.
Cochrane, N.	?	School of Psychiatry, New South Wales, Australia.
Crockatt, P. D. N.	1969–present	
Davies, Miss D. R.	1969–present	
de Speville, Mrs	1967–8	
Dobson, Miss G.	1966–present	
Dorner, Mr S.		Hospital for Sick Children, Great Ormond Street.

APPENDIX II

		Present status (where known)
Elkan, G.	1960–3	Harperbury Hospital and Brunel University.
Foster, P. M.	1952–4	Tavistock Institute of Human Relations.
Flanders, Miss M.	1949–53	
Gaylard, Miss G. A. (now Mrs Tollenton)	1960–2	South Ockenden Hospital.
Gilbey, Miss R.	1960–4	Ingrebourne Centre and Queen Elizabeth Hospital, London.
Gleed, Miss E.	1966–present	
Harvey, Mr D.	–	Hospital Service.
Heasman, Mrs I.	1955–7	Canada.
Hildebrand, P.	1953–5	In practice as psychoanalyst.
Holland, Mrs S. D.	1968–present	
Hood, V.	1965–present	
Hooper, Miss P. (now Mrs Bishop)	1952–4	No appointment at present.
Hutton, G. J.	1951–3	Bath University.
Johnson, R. I. A.	1955–6	Deceased.
Jones, G. E.	1963–6	Shenley Hospital.
Jones, Mrs J. M.	1963–6	Shenley Hospital.
Kilcoyne, Miss A.	1969–present	
King, D.	–	Farnborough Hospital.
Lewis, J. C.	1968–present	

		Present status (where known)
Marshamn, D. M.	1967–9	
Michaels, Mrs B.	1948–50	
Miller, Miss P.	1967–8	
Mycroft, D.		Greater London Council.
Noonan, Miss E.	1967–present	
O'Kelly, Mrs E.	1953–5	
Osborne-Moss, Mrs J.	1967–present.	
Palmquist, Miss K.	1951–2	Psychotekniska Institute, Stockholm.
Pidduck, R.		Stamford House Remand Centre.
Pollock, A.	1952–3	Tavistock Institute of Human Relations.
Rakoff, V. M.	1951–2	
Rapoport, Mrs R.		Tavistock Institute of Human Relations.
Sandler, J. J.	1953–5	Institute of Psychiatry.
Sarabhai, Mrs K.		B. M. Institute, Ahmedabad, India.
Sharma, V.	1968–present	
Shepherd, R. D.		Shenley Hospital.
Slee, Miss D.		University of Surrey.
Smithells, Miss J.	1959–61	Research Unit Reading University.
Sofer, Mrs R.	1952–4	
Spensley, Mrs S.		No present appointment.

		Present status (where known)
Staunton, G.	1949–51	Park Prewett Hospital.
Toulson, Miss J. V.	1968–present	
Waddell, F. J.	1956–8	
Watson, P.	1967–8	
Whitehead, Mrs A. M.	1950–2	Educational psychologist.

SOCIAL WORKERS	*Present status (where known)*
Mrs R. Allen	New Malden Child Guidance Clinic.
Mrs Anderson	—
Mrs R. L. Arkell	—
Miss K. D. Armstrong	Deputy Children's Officer, North Riding of Yorkshire.
Miss R. Armitage	Casework Supervisor, Welfare Dept., Reading.
C. S. Bagshaw	Senior Probation Officer, City of Southampton.
Miss P. Baldock	Head Social Worker, United Oxford Hospital.
Miss P. I. Barrett	A.P.P.O., Hants.
Miss J. Baraclough	Deputy Head Medical Social Worker, Westminster Hospital.
Miss I. V. Belgrave	Assistant Children's Officer, Reading.
Mrs J. Blooman	Regional Training Officer, Probation and After-care Service.
Mrs M. Blumenau	P.S.W., Powick Mental Hospital.
Mrs Betty Booth	
Miss M. B. Boyle	Senior Caseworker, Leeds Council of Social Service.
Mrs J. Bridge	
Mrs B. Brinsdon	
Miss E. Brierley	Senior Probation Officer, Stoke on Trent.
Miss D. E. Burdis	Tutor, H.O. Northern Probation Course.

APPENDIX II

	Present status (where known)
Miss B. Butler	Lately Lecturer, Department of Social Sciences, Bedford College, London.
Miss Z. Butrym	Lecturer in Social Casework, London School of Economics.
Miss M. Chave-Jones	Casework Consultant, Camden Council of Social Service.
Mrs. U. Clarke	
Mrs F. A. Clifton	Deputy Children's Officer, Plymouth.
Mrs K. Curnock	University Teacher, School of Social Work, Leicester.
Miss B. Day	Casework Tutor, N.S.P.C.C.
Miss P. C. Deane	Assistant Principal P. O., Inner London Probation Service.
Miss B. Dickeson	P.S.W., Kilburn Child Guidance Centre.
Miss M. Dongray	Tutor, General Social Work Training, Manchester College of Commerce.
J. S. Ferguson	Lecturer in Professional Social Work, Barking Regional College of Technology.
R. J. Foren	Lecturer in Social Casework, University of Bradford.
Miss M. Goodman	Casework Supervisor, Children's Aid Society of Western Manitoba, Canada.
Miss F. Gorden	Assistant Children's Officer, London Borough of Southwark.
Miss L. Gray	Harrow Child Guidance Centre.
Mrs M. Grier	Chief Children's Officer, London Borough of Southwark.
Miss R. Hall	Area Assistant Children's Officer, Altrincham.
J. R. Halliwell	Fieldwork Organiser, Family Service Units.
Miss P. Hammond	Lecturer, Department of Sociology, University of Aberdeen.

	Present status (where known)
Mrs K. Heap	Lecturer in Social Casework, Norwegian State School of Social Work and Local Government Administration.
K. Heap	Lecturer in Social Group Work, Oslo.
Mrs F. A. Heller	
Miss J. T. Henderson	Librarian, London School of Economics.
Miss G. E. Hill	Training Officer, The Liverpool Probation Service.
P. Hughes	Children's Officer, London Borough of Greenwich.
A. W. Hunt	Principal Probation Officer, Southampton.
Mrs M. H. Johnson	Senior Probation Officer, Inner London Probation and After-care Service.
G. Jones	Principal Probation Officer, Somerset & Bath Probation Service.
Miss M. P. Keenleyside	Divisional Social Worker, Watford.
Mrs E. Kelly	
Mrs J. Kingston	Social Worker, Shenley Hospital.
Miss J. F. Knight	Principal Family Social Worker, F. W. A. Area V, London Borough of Wandsworth.
A. Lawson	Probation Officer, County of Hertford Probation Service.
Miss L. Lynch	Lecturer in Child Care, Enfield College of Technology.
G. G. Maccabee	Lecturer in Applied Social Studies, University of Nottingham.
Mrs. M. M. Martyr	Assistant Principal Probation Officer, Watford.
Miss M. T. Mayne	Senior Probation Officer, Sunderland.

	Present status (*where known*)
Mrs G. Morris	Senior Caseworker, F. W. A. Area 4.
A. B. R. MacGillivray	Principal Probation Officer, Middlesex Probation Care Services.
Miss H. McCombe	Lately Assistant Lecturer, Social Work Course, Belfast.
Mrs F. McNamee	Senior Probation Officer, Montgomery.
Miss M. McLaren	Head Social Worker, University of Newcastle-upon-Tyne.
Miss M. Morton	Caseworker, Nottingham Council of Social Service.
Miss M. M. Neal	Psychiatric Social Worker, Claybury Hospital.
G. P. Newton	Lecturer in Social Casework, National Institute of Social Work Training.
Mrs P. M. Orford	Caseworker.
Mrs M. M. Parilla	Tutor, Child Care Officer's Course, Chiswick Polytechnic.
Miss B. N. Perry	Principal Social Worker, Kingston-on-Thames.
Mrs M. Peters	P.S.W., Los Angeles, California, U.S.A.
A. F. Philp	Secretary, Family Service Units.
J. Quinn	Probation Officer, Hampshire Combined Probation and After-care Service.
Miss K. Q. Rabley	Assistant Children's Officer, Borough of Southwark.
S. Ratcliffe	Assistant Principal Probation Officer, Inner London Probation and After-care Service.
Mrs Z. Ravid	P.S.W., Halliwick Hospital.
G. A. Read	Senior Probation Officer, London Probation Service.
A. B. Robertson	Governor of Leyhill Open Prison.

	Present status (where known)
Miss S. G. Reid	Student Supervisor, Department of Medical Social Work, Dundee Royal Infirmary.
Miss B. Robinson	Area C.C.O., County of Kent.
Mrs M. Rosenbluth	Vancouver, Canada.
Miss J. Rojas	Deputy Children's Officer, London Borough of Hammersmith.
Miss M. D. Samuels	Probation Inspector, Home Office Probation and After-care Department.
Mrs J. Sarkic	Family Caseworker, London County Council.
Miss J. Shepherd	Headmistress, Knowle Hill Approved School.
J. E. Simmonds	Lecturer, University of Sussex.
Miss G. M. Stafford	Senior Probation Officer, Inner London After-care Service.
Miss O. Stevenson	Supplementary Benefits Commission, Ministry of Social Security.
Miss D. Storey	Senior Probation Officer, Gateshead.
Miss J. P. Sullivan	Senior Probation Officer, Woolwich.
Miss M. Thacker	Senior Lecturer, North West Polytechnic.
Mrs D. J. Thomas	Senior Lecturer, North West Polytechnic.
Miss M. M. Thornborough	Senior Probation Officer, London.
Mrs Y. Walczak	Tutor, South Work Certificate Course, North West Polytechnic.
Mrs M. Westland	Senior Caseworker, Chedoka Child and Family Center, Hamilton, Ontario.
N. Whittington	Senior Probation Officer, Durham.
Miss C. Woodcock	Teacher in Graduate Social Work School, Friono State College, California, U.S.A.

	Present status (where known)
Miss M. A. Yelloly	Lecturer, School of Social Work, Leicester.
Mrs D. H. Ziman	Editor, *Medical Social Work.*

CHILD PSYCHOTHERAPISTS (*NON-MEDICAL*)

		Present status (where known)
Barbour, Miss G.	1968–present	
Barnett, Miss L.	1968–present	
Blake, Mrs Y.	1950–3	Johannesburg.
Bogdanovitch, Miss S. M.	1967–present	
Boston, Mrs M.	1949–53	Paddington Green Children's Hospital and Hospital for Sick Children, Great Ormond Street.
Brenman, J.	1949–53	Hospital for Sick Children, Great Ormond Street.
Brown, Mrs F. (nee Low-Beer)	1953–7	Teaching Social Work Course, Oxford.
Crawford, G. A.	1968–present	
Daws, Mrs D. (nee Kahn)	1960–4	Paddington Green Children's Hospital.
Elkan, Mrs J. (nee Shamah)	1958–62	Paddington Green Children's Hospital and Willesden Child Guidance Clinic.
Forryan, Mrs. B. (nee Secombe)	1958–62	

		Present status (where known)
Greenhill, Miss E.	1960–2	National Association for Mental Health.
Hahn, H.	1964–8	
Hamilton, Miss V.	1968–present	
Harris, Mrs A.	1962–present	
Hilder, A.	1968–present	
Hopkins, Mrs J. (nee Phelps-Brown)	1960–6	Not at present working.
Jackson, Mrs I.	1966–9	
Langmuir-Essex, Mrs W.	1953–7	Working in a G.P. practice and teaching Social Workers.
Lush, Mrs D.	1958–64	Willesden Child Guidance Clinic.
Martin, N.	1966–present	
Miller, M.	1967–present	
Maschick, Mrs E.	1965–8	Victoria Hospital for Children, Melbourne, Austrialia.
Mykura, Miss E.	1962–6	Hospital for Sick Children, Great Ormond Street.
Orford, Mrs E.	1964–present	
O'Shaughnessy, Mrs E.	1955–9	
Pick, Mrs I.	1956–60	Practising as psychoanalyst and teaching in extramural university course for teachers.
Polke, Mrs P.	1966–present	

		Present status (where known)
Popper, Mrs Y.	1949–53	London Hospital.
Richmards, Miss E.	1966–present	
Reeves, C.	1966–present	
Roth, Mrs P.	1967–present	
Rowe, Mrs M.		Returned to U.S.A.
Ruston, Mrs M.	1967–present	
Szur, Mrs R.	1958–62	Hornsey Child Guidance Clinic.
Zadik, Mrs A.	1967–present	

In addition large numbers of clinical and educational psychologists, social workers and child psychotherapists, have undertaken training (many from abroad).

APPENDIX II

ADDITIONAL POST-WAR NON-MEDICAL PROFESSIONAL STAFF

		Present status (where known)
PSYCHOLOGISTS		
Ambrose, J. A.	1960–5	
Aston, Miss J.	1965–present	
Balfour, F.	1962–present	
Boreham, J.	1949–present	
Caspari, Miss Irene	1957–present	
Chaplin, Miss D.		
Dunne, Mrs M.	1968–present	
Gill, H. S.	1962–present	
Osborne, Mrs Elsie	1959–present	
Phillipson, H.	1946–present	
Popper, Mrs Y.	1939–63	Retired. London Hospital.
Shooter, Mrs A.	1961–present	
Upson, Mr P.	1965–present	
Williams, Mrs C.	1960–4	
Wills, Miss Doris	1947–59	
PSYCHIATRIC SOCIAL WORKERS		
Argles, Mr P.	1968–present	
Besmeres, Miss H.	1969–present	
Box, Miss S.	1969–present	
Brown, Miss D. E.	1946–present	
Chapman, Miss C.	1960–present	
Coussell, Mrs P.	1968–present	
Hunnybun, Miss N. K.	1946–55	Retired.
Irvine, Mrs E. E.	1951–66	Reader in Social Case Work, University of York.
Leared, Miss J.	1955–present	
Mainprice, Mrs J.	1967–present	
Newton, Miss J.	1961–8	

		Present status (where known)
Robertson, J.	1948–present	
Robinson, Mrs M.	1960–present	
Sinanaglou, Mrs I. O.	1968–present	
Sprince, Mrs M.	1947–51	
Stephens, Mrs J.	1956–present	
Tamplin, Miss D.	1947–60	
Templerley, Mrs J.	1968–present	
Thomson, Miss J.	1968–present	
Tod, R.	1948–51	
Watson, Miss A. M.	1960–present	
Westheimer, Miss I. J.	1955–8	
Williams, Mrs. M.	1945–present	
Woodhouse, D.	1961–present	

CHILD PSYCHOTHERAPISTS (NON-MEDICAL)

Alvarez, Mrs Anne	1962–present	
Baker, Miss S.	1968–9	
Bick, Mrs E.	1946–59	
Carr, Miss H.	1953–7 then 1963–present	
Copley, Mrs B.	1958–62 then 1967–present	
Harris, Mrs M.	1950–present	
Hoxtor, Mrs S.	1950–present	
Rosenbluth, Miss D.	1950–present	
Tustin, Mrs F.	1950–3	Aylesbury and Bletchley Child Guidance Clinics.
Wittenberg, Mrs I.	1956–60 then 1965–present	

APPENDIX III

Selected List of Major Relevant Publications by the Staffs of both Clinic and Institute, 1920–69

ABRAHAMS, Adolphe. Physical aspects of psychological disease. *Lancet* (1935) *i*, 473–6.

AINSWORTH, M. *and* BOSTON, M. Psychodiagnostic assessments of a child after prolonged separation in early childhood. *Brit. J. Med. Psychol.* (1952) *25*, 169–201.

AINSWORTH, M. *and* BOWLBY, J. Research strategy in the study of mother-child separation. *Courrier* (Centre International de l'Enfance) (1954) *4*, 105–31.

AINSWORTH, M. *see* BOWLBY, J. (1956).

ALCOCK, A. T. Conquering war strain in children. *Amer. J. Psychiat.* (1945) *102*, 372–4.

ALCOCK, A. T. Conclusions from psychiatric work among evacuated children. *Brit. J. Med. Psychol.* (1948) *21*, 181–4.

ALCOCK, A. T. Personality disturbance impairing educational ability. *Rorschach Newsletter* (Brit. Rorschach Forum) (1959) *4*, 7–12.

ALCOCK, A. T. Some personality characteristics of asthmatic children. *Brit. J. Med. Psychol.* (1960) *33*, 133–41.

ALCOCK, A. T. The reality basis of Rorschach interpretation. *Rorschach Newsletter* (Brit. Rorschach Forum) (1961) *6*, no. 2, 6–11.

ALCOCK, A. T. *The Rorschach in practice.* Tavistock Publications (1963).

ALCOCK, A. T. Some psychogenic factors in asthma. In *Transactions of the World Asthma Conference, 1965.* Chest and Heart Association (1965), pp. 85–9.

ALLEN, C. E. Some experiments in reinforcing mental analysis in cases of psychosis. *Brit. J. Med. Psychol.* (1933) *13*, 151–64.

ALLEN, C. E. The extracortical manifestations of cerebromacular degeneration. *J. Neurol. Psychopathol.* (1933) *14*, 35–44.

ALLEN, C. E. Cephalic dysotosis. *J. Neurol Psychopathol.* (1934) *14*, 640–8.

ALLEN, C. E. Introjection in schizophrenia. *Psychoanal. Rev.* (1935) *22*, 121–37.

ALLEN, C. E. The diagnosis and treatment of the early psychotic and prepsychotic. *Brit. J. Med. Psychol.* (1935) *15*, 140–52.

ALLEN, C. E. Mental disease in general practice. *Clinical J.* (1936) *65*, 199–204; 250–4.

ALLEN, C. E. Modern discoveries in medical psychology. Macmillan (1937).

ALLEN, C. E. Personality deviations in children. In MILLER, E. *The Growing Child and its problems*. Kegan Paul, Trench, Trubner & Co. (1937), pp. 109–46.

ALLEN, C. E. Adrenal dysfunction and its relation to sexuality. In BROSTER, L. R. *et al. The adrenal cortex and intersexuality*. Chapman & Hall (1938), pp. 55–136.

ALLEN, C. E. The psyche and endocrine disorders. *Proceedings of the 10th International Med. Congress for Psychotherapy*. Oxford (1938).

AMBROSE, J. A. *The smiling and related responses in early human infancy: an experimental and theoretical study of their course and significance*. Ph.D. thesis. University of London (1960).

AMBROSE, J. A. The development of the smiling response in early infancy. In FOSS, D. M. (ed.) *Determinants of Infant Behaviour*. Methuen (1961). pp. 179–204.

AMBROSE, J. A. The age of onset of ambivalence in early infancy: indications from the study of laughing. *J. Child Psychol. Psychiat.* (1963) *4*, 167–81.

AMBROSE, J. A. The concept of a critical period for the development of social responsiveness. In FOSS, B. M. (ed.) *Determinants of infant behaviour, II*. Methuen (1963), pp. 201–25.

AMBROSE, J. A. The comparative approach to early child development. In MILLER, E. (ed.) *Foundations of child psychiatry*. Pergamon Press (1968).

AMBROSE, J. A. The study of human social organisation: a review of current concepts and approaches. *Symposia of the Zoological Society of London*, no. 14 (1965).

BACAL, H. A. *see* HEATH, E. S. (1968).
see MALAN, D. H. (1968).

BALINT, M., BALINT, E., GOSLING, R. *and* HILDEBRAND, P. *A Study of doctors*. Tavistock Publications (1966).

BALINT, E. Development of Family Discussion Bureau work. *Social Casework* (1951) January, 495–500.

BALINT, E. *and* BALINT, M. Dynamics of training in groups for psychotherapy. *Brit. J. Med. Psychol.* (1955) *28*, 135–43.

BALINT, E. Training postgraduate students in social casework. *Brit. J. Med. Psychol.* (1959) *32*, 193–9.

BALINT, E. How will this marriage work ?—I. (Paper read at the Family Planning Association, London Group Conference on 'The marriage relationship', Nov. 1961). *Social Work* (1962) *19*, no. 4, 8–12.

BALINT, E. *see* BALINT, M. (1961), (1965).

BALINT, M. Training general practitioners in psychotherapy. *Brit. Med. J.* (1954) *i.* 16 Jan. 115–20. German translation: *Psyche* (1955/6) *9*, 370–89. French translation: *Psychanalyse* (1955/6) no. 2, 221–42. Abridged version: *Brit. J. Med. Psychol.* (1954) *27*, 37–41.

BALINT, M. The doctor, his patient and the illness. *Lancet* (1955) *i*, 2 Apr. 683–8.

BALINT, M. Pleasure, object and libido. Some reflection on Fairbairn's modifications of psychoanalytic theory. *Brit. J. Med. Psychol.* (1956) *29*, 162–7.

BALINT, M. *The doctor, his patient and the illness.* Pitman (1957). American edition: New York, International Universities Press, 1957. Translated into: German 1957, French 1960. Hungarian 1961. Italian 1961, Spanish 1961. 2nd Edition: Pitman Medical, 1964.

BALINT, M. Training medical students in psychotherapy. *Lancet* (1957) *ii* 23 Nov., 1015–8.

BALINT, M. The concepts of subject and object in psychoanalysis. *Brit. J. Med. Psychol.* (1958) *31*, 83–91.

BALINT, M. Training for psychosomatic medicine. In JORES, A. *and* STOKVIS, B. (eds). *Advances in psychosomatic medicine. Symposium of the Fourth European Conference on Psychosomatic Research, Hamburg 1959.* Basel (1960) pp. 167–79.

BALINT, M. *and* BALINT, E. *Psychotherapeutic techniques in medicine.* Tavistock Publications (1961). American edition: Springfield, Ill. (1962). Translated into: German 1962.

BALINT, M., BALINT, E., GOSLING, R. *and* HILDEBRAND, H. P. *A Study of Doctors.* A Mind and Medicine Monograph. Tavistock Publications (1966).

BALINT, M. *see* BALINT, E. (1955).

BAMFORTH, K. W. *see* TRIST, E. L. (1951).

BANNISTER, K. *et al. Social casework in marital problems: the development of a psychodynamic approach.* Tavistock Publications (1955). (This book was written as a co-operative effort by the staff of the Family Discussion Bureau, including K. Bannister, A. Lyons, L. Pincus, J. Robb, A. Shooter and J. Stephens.)

BANNISTER, K. Marital interaction and its impact on the family. In KING, J. F. S. (ed.) *New thinking for changing needs*. Association of Social workers (1963), pp. 6–16.

BANNISTER, K. *and* PINCUS, L. *Shared phantasy in marital problems: therapy in a four-person relationship*. Codicote Press (1965).

BANNISTER, K. *and* PINCUS, L. Seminars on marital interaction for social workers in Israel. *Social Work (1966) 23*, no. 4, 3–11.

BANNISTER, K. *see* PINCUS ,L. (1960).

BENNET, Edward A. *Heredity and environment.* In ERLEIGH, E. V. (ed.) *The mind of the growing child.* Faber & Gwyer (1928), pp. 13–25.

BENNET, Edward A. Fugue states. *Brit. J. Med. Psychol.* (1928) *8*, 143–9.

BENNET, Edward A. Treatment in the psychoneurosis. *Irish J. Med. Sci.* (1931), 6th series, 85–92.

BENNET, Edward A. Hysteria. *Probation* (1931) *1*, no. 6, 83–4.

BENNET, Edward A. Sex in relation to adolescent development. *Health and Empire* (1932) 7, 124–31.

BENNET, Edward A. Anxiety states. *Irish J. Med. Sci.* (1933), 6th series, 252–7.

BENNET, Edward A. The psychopathology of sexual perversions. *Proc. Roy. Soc. Med.* (1933) *26*, 1030–4.

BENNET, Edward A. Nullity and impotence. *Brit. J. Med. Psychol.* (1935/6) *15*, 296–304.

BENNET, Edward A. Morbid anxiety. *Med. Press and Circular* (1937) *194*, 616–19.

BENNET, Edward A. The use of dreams in psychotherapy. *Mental Hyg.* (1938) *4*, 65–9.

BENNET, Edward A. Individualism in psychotherapy. *Brit. J. Med. Psychol.* (1937/8) *17*, 293–306.

BERG, Charles. A mysterious illness. (Neurasthenia). *Med. Press and Circular* (1936) *192*, 462–5: 408–3.

BERG, Charles. The unconscious significance of hair. *Int. J. Psychoanal.* (1936) *17*, 73–78.

BEVAN-BROWN, C. M. Psychological schools—a plea for correlation. In *Individual psychology: theory and practice.* (Individual Psychology Medical Pamphlets, No. 15). C. W. Daniel (1936) pp. 9–42.

BION, W. R. *and* RICKMAN, J. Intra-group tensions in therapy. *Lancet* (1943) *ii*, 27 Nov., 678–81.

BION, W. R. The leaderless group project. *Bull. Menninger Clin.* (1946) *10*, 77–81.

BION, W. R. Advances in group and individual therapy. In FLUGEL, J. C. (ed.) *International Congress on Mental Health, Vol. 3, Proceedings of the International Conference on Medical Psychotherapy*, London 1948 (1948), H. K. Lewis, pp. 106–10.

BION, W. R. Psychiatry at a time of crisis. *Brit. J. Med. Psychol.* (1947/8) *21*, 81–9.

BION, W. R. Group Dynamics: a review. In KLEIN, M. *et al.* (eds). *New directions in psychoanalysis.* Tavistock Publications (1955), pp. 440–77.

BION, W. R. *Experiences in groups and other papers.* Tavistock Publications (1961).

BOENHEIM, C. *Practical child psychotherapy.* John Bale Medical Publications (1938).

BOENHEIM, C. *Practical Child psychotherapy.* 2nd edition. Staples (1953).

BOENHEIM, C. Group psychotherapy with adolescents. *Int. J. Group Psychother.* (1957) *7*, 398–405.

BOENHEIM, C. A follow-up study of group psychotherapy patients. *Int. J. Group Psychother. (1959) 9*, 463–4.

BOREHAM, J. L. A form of reporting projective test findings. *Rorschach Newsletter* (Brit. Rorschach Forum) (1957) 2, no. 2, 7–12.

BOREHAM, J. L. Rorschach test publication of response to psychotherapy. *Rorschach Newsletter* (1966) *11*, no. 2, 7–13.

BOREHAM, J. L. The prediction of suicide. *Rorschach Newsletter* (1967) *12*, No. 2, 5–7.

BOREHAM, J. L. The psychodynamic diagnosis and treatment of vocational problems. *Brit. J. Soc. Clin. Psychol.* (1967) *6*, 150–8.

BOREHAM, J. L. An atypical depressive record. *Brit. J. Proj. Psychol.* (1968) *13*, no. 2, 3–6.

BOREHAM, J. L. *see* WILLIAMS, C. (1961).

BOSTON, M. *see* AINSWORTH, M. (1952).
see BOWLBY, J. (1956).

BOTT, E. Urban families: conjugal roles and social networks. *Hum. Relat.* (1955) *8*, 345–84.

BOTT, E. A study of ordinary families. In *Untersuchungen Über die Familie* (Studies of the family), Vol. I. *Tubingen* (1956). pp. 29–68.

BOTT, E. Urban families: the norms of conjugal roles. *Hum. Relat.* (1956) *9*, 325–42.

BOTT, E. *Family and social network.* Tavistock Publications (1957).

BOTT, E. Family, kinship and marriage. In DOUGLAS, M. (ed). *Man in society.* Macdonald (1964), pp. 82–103.

BOWLBY, J. *Forty-four juvenile thieves; their characters and home life.* Baillière, Tindall & Cox (1946).

BOWLBY, J. Psychology and democracy. *Political Quart.* (1946) *17*, no 1, 61–76. Also in SNYDER, R. C. *and* WILSON, H. H. *Roots of political behaviour; introduction to government and politics.* New York (1946), (1949).

BOWLBY, J. Study of human relations in the child guidance clinic. *J. Social Issues* (1947) *3*, no. 2, 35–41.

BOWLBY, J. Research into the origins of delinquent behaviour. In NATIONAL ASSOCIATION FOR MENTAL HEALTH. *Why delinquency? Report of a Conference on the Scientific Study of Juvenile Delinquency. London, October 1949.* N.A.M.H. (1949) pp. 29–40. Reprinted in *Brit. Med J. i*, 11 Mar., 570–3.

BOWLBY, J. The study and reduction of group tension in the family. *Hum. Relat.* (1949) *2*, 123–8.

BOWLBY, J. *Maternal care and mental health.* (W.H.O. Monograph Series, No. 2). Geneva, World Health Organization (1951) Translated into: French 1951, Danish 1953, Yugoslav 1953, Swedish 1954, Spanish 1954, Finnish 1957, Hebrew 1957, Arabic 1960, Italian 1962, Japanese 1962, Greek 1964.
Vol. 1 Proceedings of the 1st meeting of the W.H.O. Study Group on the Psychobiological Development of the Child, Geneva 1953. Tavistock Publications, pp. 182–7.

BOWLBY, J. Presentation of a film (A two-year-old goes to hospital) by Dr Bowlby. In TANNER, J. M. *and* INHELDER, B. (eds) *Discussions on child development, Vol. 2. Proceedings of the 2nd meeting of the W.H.O. Study Group on the Psychobiological Development of the Child, London 1954.* Tavistock Publications (1956), pp. 213–34.

BOWLBY, J.; AINSWORTH, M.; BOSTON, M. *and* ROSENBLUTH, D. The effects of mother-child separation; a follow-up study. *Brit. J. Med. Psychol.* (1956) *29*, 211–47.

BOWLBY, J. An ethological approach to research in child development. *Brit. J. Med. Psychol.* (1957) *30*, 230–40.

BOWLBY, J. *Can I leave my baby?* National Association for Mental Health (1958).

BOWLBY, J. The nature of the child's tie to his mother. *Int. J. Psycho-Anal.* (1958) *39*, 350–73. German Translation: *Psyche* (1959–60) *13*, 415/56.

BOWLBY, J. A note on mother-child separation as a mental health hazard. *Brit. J. Med. Psychol.* (1958) *31*, 247–8.

BOWLBY, J. Psychoanalysis and child care. In SUTHERLAND, J. D. (ed.) *Psychoanalysis and contemporary thought.* Hogarth Press (1958), pp. 33–57. Reprinted as: The Roots of human personality. In HALMOS, P. *and* ILIFFE, A. (eds) *Readings in general psychology.* Routledge & Kegan Paul (1959), pp. 108–29.

BOWLBY, J. Comments on Professor Piaget's paper: The general problems of the psychobiological development of the child. In TANNER, J. M. *and* INHELDER, B. (eds) *Discussions on child development, Vol. 4. Proceedings of the 4th meeting of the W.H.O. Study Group on the Psychobiological Development of the Child, Geneva 1956.* Tavistock Publications (1960), 35–47.

BOWLBY, J. Separation anxiety. *Int. J. Psycho-Anal.* (1960) *41*, 89–113. German translation: *Psyche* (1961/2) *15*, 411–64.

BOWLBY, J. Grief and mourning in infancy and early childhood. *Psychoanal. Study Child.* (1960) *15*, 9–52. Reprinted in DANIELS, G. E. (ed.) *New perspectives in psychoanalysis.* New York (1965), pp. 124–69.

BOWLBY, J. Symposium on: Psychoanalysis and ethology. II. Ethology and the development of object relations. *Int. J. Psycho-Anal.* (1960) *41*, 313–17. French translation: *Rev. franc. Psychanal.* (1961) *25*, 623–31. German translation: *Psyche* (1961/2) *15*, 508–16.

BOWLBY, J. Childhood mourning and its implications for psychiatry. (Adolf Meyer Lecture). *Amer. J. Psychiat.* (1961/2) *118*, 481–98. Also published as: Childhood bereavement and psychiatric illness. In RICHTER, D. *et al.* (eds) *Aspects of psychiatric Research.* Oxford University Press (1962), pp. 262–93.

BOWLBY, J. Separation anxiety: a critical review of the literature *J. Child Psychol. Psychiat.* (1961) *1*, 251–69.

BOWLBY, J. Processes of mourning. *Int. J. Psycho-Anal.* (1961) *42*, 317–40. Reprinted in DANIELS, G. E. (ed.) *New perspectives in psychoanalysis.* New York (1965), pp. 170–217.

BOWLBY, J. Theories of psychological development in children. In MACKEITH, R. *and* SANDLER, J. (eds) *Psychosomatic aspects of paediatrics.* Pergamon Press (1961), pp. 54–66.

BOWLBY, J. Pathological mourning and childhood mourning. *J. Amer. Psychoanal. Ass.* (1963) *11*, 500–41.

BOWLBY, J. Effects on behaviour of disruption of an effectual bond. In THODAY, J. M. *and* PARKES, A. S. (eds) *Genetic and environmental influences on behaviour.* Oliver & Boyd (1968), pp. 94–108.

BOWLBY, J. *Attachment & Loss. I. Attachment.* Hogarth Press (1969).

BRACKENBURY, H. B. Address on state insurance in relation to health. *Brit. Med. J.* (1931) *i*, Supplement, 197–9.

BRIDGER, H. The Northfield Experiment. *Bull. Menninger Clin.* (1946) *10*, 71–7.

BRIDGER, H. *and* WILSON, A. T. M. Group discussion. *Mon. Rev. Brit. Counc.* (1947) *1*, 139–43.

BRIDGER, H. *and* ISDELL CARPENTER, R. Selection of management trainees. *Industr. Welf.* (1947) *29*, no. 315, 177–81.

BRIDGER, H. From school to work—a process not a procedure. *New Era* (1952) *33*, 107–11.

BRIDGER, H., Miller, E. J. *and* O'DWYER, J. J. *The doctor and sister in industry. A study of change.* Macmillan (Journals) Ltd (1964). (Reprinted from *Occup. Health* (1963) *15*.)

BROWN, D. E. The preparation of parents for treatment in a child guidance clinic. *Brit. J. Psychiatr. Soc. Work.* (1948) no. 2, 46–9.

BROWN, D. E. Interprofessional collaboration. I. An experiment in mental health consultation. In IRVINE, E. E. (ed.) *Ventures in professional co-operation.* Association of Psychiatric Social Workers (1961) pp. 1–11.

BROWNE, Leonard F. *and* HADFIELD, J. A. The psychology of spiritual healing. In MATTHEWS, W. R. *et al. Psychology and the church.* Macmillan (1925).

BROWNE, Leonard F. Child psychology. *Maternity and Child Welfare.* (1932) *16*, 74–6; 103–4; 129–31.

BROWNE, Leonard F. The psychotherapeutic treatment of tuberculous patients. *Tubercle* (1931/2) *13*, 347–52.

BROWNE, Leonard F. Personality and progress. I–IV. *Listener* (1937) *18*, 783–4; 842–3; 916; 970.

BRYANT, D. T. A survey of the development of manpower planing policies. *Brit. J. Industr. Rels.* (1965). *3*, 279–90.

BURNS, C. L. C. The psychology of the criminal. *Probation* (1930) *1*, no. 3, 38–40.

BURNS, C. L. C. Movement and types in children. *Psyche* (1930/1) *11*, no. 2, 63–6.

BURNS, C. L. C. Points in the study and treatment of the young delinquent. *Probation* (1930) *1*, no. 4, 52–3.

BURNS, C. L. C. Child guidance on the continent. *Brit. J. Educ. Psychol.* (1933) *3*, 251–68.

CALVER, G. Behaviour problems of children and their treatment. *Practitioner* (1938) *141*, 61–8.

CALVER, G. The cases at a psychological clinic attached to an infant welfare centre. *Proc. Roy. Sanit. Inst. Congress*, Southampton (1938).

CARR, H. *and* HARRIS, M. Therapeutic consultations. *J. Child Psychother.* (1966) *1*, no. 4, 13–31.

CASPARI, I. Problems of school consultation. *New Era* (1962) *43*, no. 4, 78–81.

CASPARI, I. A Rorschach record of an adolescent with severe reading difficulties and some notes on his remedial teaching. *Rorschach Newsletter* (Brit. Rorschach Forum) (1962) 7, no. 1, 3–14.

CASPARI, I. Roles and responsibilities of head teacher and teaching staff in primary schools. Tavistock Clinic (mimeog.) (1965).

CASPARI, I. *and* OSBORNE, E. L. The neighbourhood schools service of the Tavistock Clinic. School Council Working Paper, no. 15. H.M. Stationery Office (1968).

CHURCHILL, S. *On being a mother.* Gollancz (1937).

CLYNE, M. B. *Night calls; a study in general practice.* Tavistock Publications (1961).

CROOKSHANK, F. G. Organ-jargon. *Brit. J. Med. Psychol.* (1930) *10*, 295–311.

CROOKSHANK, F. G. Organ states and emotional correlates. *Psyche* (1929/30) *10*, no. 3. 65–79.

CROOKSHANK, F. G. The sexual problems of adolescence and adult life. I. *Psyche* (1929/30) *10*, no. 4, 3–21.

CROOKSHANK, F. G. The sexual problems of adolescent and adult life. II. *Psyche* (1930/1) *11*, no. 1, 21–40.

CROOKSHANK, F. G. *Individual diagnosis.* Kegan Paul, Trench, Trubner & Co. (1930).

CROOKSHANK, F. G. Individual psychology and the bases of science. *Psyche* (1930/1) *11*, no. 3, 25–44.

CROOKSHANK, F. G. *Individual sexual problems.* Kegan Paul, Trench, Trubner & Co. (1931).

CROOKSHANK, F. G. *The mongol in our midst.* 3rd edition. Kegan Paul, Trench, Trubner & Co. (1931).

CROOKSHANK, F. G. Individual psychology and general medicine. *Int. Zeit. f. Indiv.-psychol.* (1932) *10*, 35–52.

CROOKSHANK, F. G. Physical findings in psychoneurosis. In *Individual psychology and psychosomatic disorders, I.* (Individual Psychology Medical Pamphlets, no. 4). C. W. Daniel (1932), pp. 67–9.

CROOKSHANK, F. G. *Individual psychology, medicine and the bases of science.* (Individual Psychology Medical Pamphlets, no. 3a). C. W. Daniel (1932).

CROOKSHANK, F. G. Individual psychology and ill-health. In *Individual psychology and psychosomatic disorders, II.* (Individual Psychology Medical Pamphlets, no. 9). C. W. Daniel (1933), pp. 46–55.

CURLE, A. Transitional communities and social reconnection. A follow-up study of the civil resettlement of British prisoners of war. Part I. *Hum. Relat.* (1947/8) *1*, 42–68.

CURLE, A. *and* TRIST, E. L. Transitional communities and social reconnection. A follow-up study of the civil resettlement of British prisoners of war. Part II. *Hum. Relat.* (1947/8) *1*, 240–88.

CURLE, A. Incentives to work. And anthropological appraisal. *Hum. Relat.* (1949) *2*, 41–7.

DAVIS, P. J. R. Divisional psychiatry: report to the War Office. *J. Roy. Army Med. Cps.* (1946) *86*, 254–74.

DICKS, H. V. The clinical value of transduodenal biliary drainage. *St. Bartholomews Hospital Reports* (1930) *63*, 139–98.

DICKS, H. V. A clinical study of obsession. *Brit. J. Med. Psychol.* (1931/2) *11*, 234–50.

DICKS, H. V. Neurasthenia: toxic and traumatic. *Lancet* (1933) *ii*, 683–6.

DICKS, H. V. *Clinical studies in psychopathology.* Edward Arnold (1939). (2nd edition, 1947.)

DICKS, H. V. *Clinical studies in psychopathology.* 2nd edition. Arnold (1947).

DICKS, H. V. Contributor to: REES, J. R. (ed.) *The case of Rudolf Hess.* Heinemann (1948).

DICKS, H. V. Principles of mental hygiene. In HARRIS, N. G. (ed.) *Modern trends in psychological medicine.* Butterworth (1948), pp. 310–34.

DICKS, H. V. Education for general practice — the psychosocial factors. *Lancet* (1950) *ii*, 26 Aug., 317–20.

DICKS, H. V. In search of our proper ethic. (Chairman's address), *Brit. J. Med. Psychol.* (1950) *23*, 1–14.

DICKS, H. V. Personality traits and national socialist ideology. A war-time study of German prisoners of war. *Hum. Relat.* (1950) *3*, 111–54. Reprinted in LERNER, D. (ed.) *Propaganda in war and crisis.* New York (1951), pp. 100–61.

DICKS, H. V. Some psychological studies of the German character. In PEAR, T. H. (ed.) *Psychological factors of peace and war.* Hutchinson (1950), pp. 193–218.

DICKS, H. V. Observations on contemporary Russian behaviour. *Hum. Relat.* (1952) *5*, 111–75.

DICKS, H. V. Clinical studies in marriage and the family: a symposium on methods. I. Experiences with marital tensions seen in the psychological clinic. *Brit. J. Med. Psychol.* (1953) *26*, 181–96.

DICKS, H. V. The predicament of the family in the modern world. *Lancet* (1955) *i*, 5 Feb., 295–7.

DICKS, H. V. Mental hygiene in marriage. *Roy. Soc. Hlth. J.* (1957) *77*, 548–53.

DICKS, H. V. Psychological factors in prejudice. *Race* (1959) *1*, no. 1, 26–40.

DICKS, H. V. Sexual problems in marriage: a symposium. Psychodynamic aspects. *Proc. Roy. Soc. Med.* (1959) *52*, 867–72.

DICKS, H. V. *Mental health in the light of ancient wisdom. The 1st Mary Hemingway Rees Memorial Lecture of the World Federation for Mental Health, Vienna 1958.* W.F.M.H. (1959). Also in *Ment. Hyg.* (1959) *43*, 179–93.

DICKS, H. V. Some notes on Russian national society. In BLACK, C. E. (ed.) *The transformation of Russian society; aspects of social change since 1861.* Cambridge, Mass. (1960), pp. 636–52.

DICKS, H. V. National loyalty, identity and the international soldier. *International Organisation* (1963) *17*, no. 2, 425–43. Reprinted in BLOOMFIELD, L. P. (ed.) *International military forces.* Boston (1964), pp. 236–56.

DICKS, H. V. Object-relations theory and marital studies. *Brit. J. Med. Psychol.* (1963) *36*, 125–9.

DICKS, H. V. The conceptual approach to marital diagnosis and therapy, developed in the Tavistock Clinic (1964). In ABSE, D. W. *et al.* (eds) *Marriage counselling in medical practice.* Chapel Hill (1964), pp. 255–75.

DICKS, H. V. *Marital tensions.* Routledge & Kegan Paul (1967); New York (1967).

DICKS, H. V. The proper study of mankind. (Presidential Address, Royal Medico-Psychological Association, July 1967). *Brit. J. Psychiat.* (1967) *113*, 1333–44.

DICKS, H. V. The state of psychotherapy in British psychiatry. *Am. J. Psychiat.* (1969) *125*, 1232–8.

DIXON, J. J., DE MONCHAUX, C. *and* SANDLER, J. Patterns of anxiety: the phobias. *Brit. J. Med. Psychol.* (1957) *30*, 34–40.

DIXON, J. J., DE MONCHAUX, C. *and* SANDLER, J. Patterns of anxiety: an analysis of social anxieties. *Brit. J. Med. Psychol.* (1957) *30*, 107–12.

DIXON, J. J. *see* SANDLER, J. (1958).

DOYLE, M. *see* WILSON, A. T. M. (1947).

EMERY, F. E. Applied social science in British industry: a critical review. In FERRAROTTI, F. *Social research and industry in Europe — problems and perspectives*. Paris (1960), pp. 81–90.

EMERY, F. E. *and* TRIST, E. L. Socio-technical systems. In CHURCHMAN, C. W. *and* VERHULST, M. (eds) *Management sciences, models and techniques*. Vol. 2. Pergamon Press (1960), pp. 83–97.

EMERY, F. E. *and* MAREK, J. Some socio-technical aspects of automation. *Hum. Relat.* (1962) *15*, 17–25.

EMERY, F. E. *and* CHURCHMAN, C. W. On various approaches to the study of organisations. In LAWRENCE, J. R. (ed.) *Operational research and the social sciences*. Tavistock Publications (1966).

EMERY, F. E. *and* THORSRUD, E. Industrial conflict and 'industrial democracy'. In LAWRENCE, J. R. (ed.) *Operational research and the Social Sciences*. London. Tavistock Publications (1966).

EMERY, F. E. *and* TRIST, E. L. The causal texture of organisational environments. (Paper read at the 17th International Congress of Psychology, Washington 1963). *Hum. Relat.* (1965) *18*, 21–3. French translation: *Sociol. du Travail* (1964), *6e annee*, 337–50.

EMERY, F. E. *and* CASS-BEGGS, R. Food, drinks and sweets in the reduction of industrial fatigue. *Occup. Psychol.* (1965) *39*, 247–59.

[EMERY, F. E.] THORSRUD, E. *and* EMERY, F. E. Industrial conflict and 'industrial democracy'. In LAWRENCE, J. R. (ed.) *Operational research and the social sciences*. Chap. 32. Tavistock Publications (1966), pp. 439–48.

EMERY, F. E. Enterprises and their leadership. *Manpower and Applied Psychology* (1967) *1*, no. 3.

EMERY, F. E. The next thirty years: concepts, methods and anticipations. *Hum. Relat.* (1967) *20*, 199–237.

EMERY, F. E., HILGENDORF, E. Linden *and* IRVING, B. L. *The pyschological dynamics of smoking*. Tobacco Research Council (1968).

ESTERSON, A. *see* LAING, R. D. (1965).

EZRIEL, H. A psychoanalytic approach to group treatment. *Brit. J. Med. Psychol.* (1950) *23*, 59–74.

EZRIEL, H. A psychoanalytic approach to the treatment of patients in groups. *J. Ment. Sci.* (1950) *96*, 774–9.

EZRIEL, H. The psychoanalytic session as an experimental situation. *Brit. J. Med. Psychol.* (1951) *24*, 30–4.

EZRIEL, H. Notes on psychoanalytic group therapy, II. Interpretation and research. *Psychiatry* (1952) *15*, 119–26.

EZRIEL, H. Some principles of a psychoanalytic method of group treatment. In *1er Congres Mondial de Psychiatrie* (1st International Congress of Psychiatry), *Paris 1950. Comptes rendus des seances* Vol. 5. Paris (1952), pp. 239–48.

EZRIEL, H. Experimentation within the psychoanalytic session. *Brit. J. Phil. Sci.* (1956/7) *7*, 29–48; (and in continuation): Reply to Mr Spilsbury. *Brit. J. Phil. Sci.* (1956/7) *7*, 342–7.

EZRIEL, H. The role of transference in psychoanalytic and other approaches to group treatment. Proceedings of the 2nd International Congress of Group Psychotherapy, 1957. *Acta Psychother.* (*1959*) *7*, Suppl., 101–16.

FOSS, B. M. (ed.) *Determinants of infant behaviour. Proceedings of a Tavistock study group on mother-infant interaction, London, 1959.* Methuen (1961).

FOSS, B. M. (ed.) *Determinants of infant behaviour, II. Proceedings of the Second Tavistock Seminar on Mother-Infant Interaction, London 1961.* Methuen (1963).

FOSS, B. M. (ed.) *Determinants of infant behaviour, III. Proceedings of the Third Tavistock Seminar on Mother-Infant Interaction, London 1963.* Methuen (1965).

FOSTER, M. Work involvement and alienation. *Manpower and Applied Psychology* (1968) *2*, no. 1, 35–48.

FREEMAN, T. Pregnancy as a precipitant of mental illness in men. *Brit. J. Med. Psychol.* (1951) *24*, 49–54.

FRIEDMAN, L. J. *Virgin wives: a study of unconsummated marriages.* Tavistock Publications (1962).

GILL, H. S. The 'therapeutic community' as an approach to psychotherapy. *Psychotherapy* (1967) *4*, 87–91.

GORDON, R. G. Certain personality problems in relation to mental illness with special reference to suicide and homicide. *Brit. J. Med. Psychol.* (1929) *9*, 60–6.

GORDON, R. G. The physiological basis of repression and dissociation. *J. Neurol. Psychopath,* (1929) *10*, 106–13.

GORDON, R. G. The importance of psychological insight for the medical profession. *Edinburgh Med. J.* (1930) *37*, 102–8.

GORDON, R. G. *et al.* A study of the tendency towards delinquency of backward children. *Brit. Med. J.* (1930) *i*, 490–1.

GORDON, R. G. *and* THOMAS, R. S. Some observations on the mental development of feeble-minded children. *Brit. Med. J.* (1930) *i*, 1123–5.

GORDON, R. G. Paralysis in children. *Practitioner* (1930) *124*, 709–20.

[GORDON, R. G.] BERRY, R. J. A. *and* GORDON, R. G. *The mental defective; a problem in social inefficiency.* Kegan Paul, Trench, Trubner & Co. (1931).

GORDON, R. G. The problem of social adjustment. *J. Neurol. Psychopath.* (1931) *11*, 239–46.

[GORDON, R. G.] GIBSON, C. R. *and* GORDON, R. G. A case of taboparesis treated by hyperpyrexia induced by hot baths. *Brit. Med. J.* (1931) *i*, 1015–18.

GORDON, R. G. *and* NORMAN, R. M. Some psychological experiments on mental defectives in relation to the perceptual configurations which may underlie speech. Parts I and II. *Brit. J. Psychol.* (1932) *23*, 20–41; 85–113.

GOSLING, R. H. Training scheme for general practitioners. *Medical World* (1963) *99*, no. 8, 637–41.

GOSLING, R. H. *see* BALINT, M. (1965), (1966).

GOSLING, R., MILLER, D., TURQUET, P. M. *and* WOODHOUSE, D. L. *The use of small groups in training.* Tavistock Institute of Medical Psychology/Codicote Press (1967).

GOSLING, R. What is transference? In SUTHERLAND, J. D. (ed.) *The psychoanalytic approach.* Baillière, Tindall & Cassell (1968), pp. 1–10.

GOUGH, D. The visual behaviour of infants in the first few weeks of life. *Proc. Roy. Soc. Med.* (1962) *55*, 308–10.

HADFIELD, J. A. *Psychology and morals.* Methuen (1923).

HADFIELD, J. A. (ed) *Psychology and modern problems.* University of London Press (1935).

HARRIS, M. Depression and the depressive position in an adolescent boy. *J. Child Psychother.* (1965) *1*, no. 3, 33–40.

HARRIS, M. The child psychotherapist and the patient's family. *J. Child Psychother.* (1968) *2*, no. 2 50–63.

HARRIS, M. *see* CARR, H. (1966)

HEARD, Dorothy, Anxiety in nurses and teachers. *Maternal and Child Care* (1966) *2*, p. 319.

HEATH, E. S. *and* BACAL, H. A. A method of group psychotherapy at the Tavistock Clinic. *Int. J. Gp. Psychother.* (1968) *18*, 21–30.

HEATH, E. S. *see* MALAN, D. H. (1968).

HEINICKE, C. H. and WESTHEIMER, I. W. *Brief separations* Longmans Green (1966); New York (1966).

HERBERT, E. L. A case study of a group selection procedure. *Hum. Relat.* (1951) *4*, 77–94.

HERBERT, E. L. *and* TRIST, E. L. The institution of an absent leader by a students' discussion group. *Hum. Relat.* (1953) *6*, 215–48.

HERBERT, E. L. The use of group techniques in the training of teachers. *Hum. Relat.* (1961) *14*, 251–63.

HERBST, P. G. *Autonomous group functioning: an exploration in behaviour theory and measurement.* Tavistock Publications (1962).

HIGGIN, G. W. The Tavistock Institute: work in the personnel field. *Personnel Mgmt.* (1963) *45*, 148–53.

HIGGIN, G. W. *and* JESSOP, W. N. *Communications in the building industry.* National Consultative Committee of Architects, Quantity Surveyors and Builders/Tavistock Institute of Human Relations (1963). 2nd edition: Tavistock Publications (1965).

HIGGIN, G. W. *and* BRIDGER, H. The psychodynamics of an inter-group experience. *Hum. Relat.* (1964) *17*, 391–446. Reprinted as Tavistock Pamphlet No. 10, 1965.

HIGGIN, G. W. *see* TRIST, E. L. (1963).

HIGGINS, R. N. T. The concept of maladjustment: its social consequences. *Hum. Relat.* (1963) *16* 61–73.

HIGGINS, R. N. T. The perception of the body surface. *Brit. J. Med. Psychol.* (1963) *36*, 261–70.

HILL, T. R. Some neurological and psychiatric aspects of surgery. In MAINGOT, R. H. (ed.) *Postgraduate surgery, vol. 3.* Butterworth (1937).

HILL, J. M. M. *and* TRIST, E. L. A consideration of industrial accidents as a means of withdrawal from the work situation. *Hum. Relat.* (1953) *6*, 357–80.

HILL, J. M. M. *and* TRIST, E. L. Changes in accidents and other absences with length of service. *Hum. Relat.* (1955) *8*, 121–52. Reprinted together with No. 174 as *Industrial accidents, sickness, and other absences.* Tavistock Pamphlet No. 4, 1962.

HOLDEN, H. M. The Voluntary Associate Scheme. (Contribution to a Symposium on the Problem of After-Care). *Brit. J. Criminol.* (1964) *4*, 341–6.

HOLDEN, H. M. After-care and the Blackfriars Settlement. *Prison Service J.* (1965) *4*, July, p. 16.

HOLDEN, H. M. Behaviour and aversion therapy in the treatment of delinquency, III. Should aversion therapy be used in the treatment of delinquency? *Brit. J. Criminol.* (1965) *5*, 377–87.

HOLDEN, H. M. Psychotherapy of a shared syndrome in identical twins. *Brit. J. Psychiat.* (1965) *111*, 859–64.

HOLDEN, H. M. Adolescence and drugtaking. *Mental Health* (1966) Autumn issue, *25*, 33–5.

HOLDEN, H. M. Teenagers and drugs. Who are at risk? *Education* (1966) *127*, 1237–42.

HOLDEN, H. M. *and* NIVEN, B. Informal youth work in a cafe setting. *Howard J.* (1966) *12*, no. 1, 13–25.

HOLDEN, H. M. The relationship between voluntary and professional workers in the treatment of offenders. *National Association for the Care and Resettlement of Offenders, Papers & Reprints* (1968) no. 1, 17–20.

HOLDEN, H. M. Drug taking amongst young people. *Medical Digest* (1968) *13*, no. 10, 580–8.

HOOPER, Douglas *and* PADDON, Dorothy. Psychiatric roles and their meaning. *Brit. J. Soc. Clin. Psychol.* (1965) *4*, 35–8.

HOWE, E. Graham. Compulsive thinking as a castration equivalent. *Brit. J. Med. Psychol.* (1929) *9*, 159–78.

HOWE, E. Graham. *Motives and mechanisms of the mind. The Lancet* (1931).

HOWE, E. Graham. The problem adult. *Parent and Teacher* (1932) no. 2.

HOWE, E. Graham. Conflict and character. *Ment. Hyg.* (1932) no. 6, 37–41.

HOWE, E. Graham. Taking the T out of egotism. *Saturday Rev.* (1932) *153*, 558.

HOWE, E. Graham. The meaning of value. *Saturday Rev.* (1932) *153*, 608.

HOWE, E. Graham. The science of error. *Brit. J. Med. Psychol.* (1933) *13*, 1–22.

HOWE, E. Graham. The causal fallacy. *Lancet* (1934) *i*, 611–15.

HOWE, E. Graham. Sex problems of adolescence. *Ment. Hyg.* (1934) no. 9, 52–7.

HOWE, E. Graham. *I am me.* Faber & Faber (1935).

HOXTER, S. The experience of puberty. *J. Child Psychother* (1964) *1*, no. 2, 13–25.

HOXTER, S. The experience of puberty and some implications for psychotherapy. Proceedings on the 6th International Congress of Psychotherapy, London 1964. *Psychotherapy and Psychosomatics* (1965) *13*, no. 4, 30–6.

HUNNYBUN, N. K. Psychiatric social work in Great Britain. In REES, J. R. (ed.) *Modern practice in psychological medicine* Butterworth (1949), pp. 424–33.

HUNNYBUN, N. K. Psychiatric social work. In MORRIS, C. (ed.) *Social casework in Great Britain.* Faber (1950), pp. 100–26.

HUNNYBUN, N. K. The use of the relationship in casework with parents. In NATIONAL ASSOCIATION FOR MENTAL HEALTH. *11th Inter-Clinic Conference for staffs of Child Guidance Clinics.* N.A.M.H. (1955), pp. 27–45.

HUNNYBUN, N. K. Supervision, education and social casework, I. In GOLDBERG, E. M. *et al.* (eds) *The boundaries of casework. A report on a residential refresher course held by the Association of Psychiatric Social Workers. Leicester 1956.* A.P.S.W. (1956), pp. 44–9.

[HUNNYBUN, N. K.] FERARD, M. L. *and* HUNNYBUN, N. K. *The caseworker's use of relationships.* Tavistock Publications (1962).

HUNTER, D. Object-relation changes in the analysis of a fetishist. *Int. J. Psycho-Anal.* (1954) *35*, 302–12.

HUNTER, D. An approach to psychotherapeutic work with children and parents. In NATIONAL ASSOCIATION FOR MENTAL HEALTH. *11th Inter-Clinic Conference for Staffs of Child Guidance Clinics.* N.A.M.H. (1955) pp. 11–26.

HUNTER, D. Training in child psychotherapy at the Tavistock Clinic. *J. Child Psychol. Psychiat.* (1960) *1*, 87–93.

HUTCHISON, Alice M. Symptoms in children. Bad habits, sexual precocity, thieving. In *Early mental disease. The Lancet* (1926), pp. 14–19.

HUTCHISON, Alice M. Masturbation in young women. In *Modern techniques in treatment, vol. 2. The Lancet* (1926), pp. 349–52.

HUTCHISON, Alice M. The problems of the backward child. In ERLEIGH, E. V. (ed.) *The mind of the growing child.* Faber & Gwyer (1928), pp. 159–65.

HUTCHISON, Alice M. *Motives of conduct in childhood.* Jarrold (1931).

HUTTON, G. Management in a changing mental hospital. *Hum. Relat.* (1962) *15*, 283–310.

HUTTON, G. Managing systems in hospitals: the implications of a case study. *Hum. Relat.* (1962) *15*, 311–33.

HUTTON, G. *see* SOFER, C. (1958).

HUTTON, Laura F. *The single woman and her emotional problems.* Baillière, Tindall & Cox (1935).

HUTTON, Laura F. On co-education. *Brit. J. Med. Psychol.* (1936/7) *16*, 62–71.

HUTTON, Laura F. *The single woman and her emotional problems.* 2nd edition. Baillière, Tindall & Cox (1937).

HUTTON, Laura F. The adolescent girl. In MILLER, E. (ed.) *The growing child and its problems.* Kegan Paul, Trench, Trubner & Co. (1937), pp. 69–107.

INSTITUTE FOR OPERATIONAL RESEARCH. *The first four years, 1963–1967.* Tavistock Institute of Human Relations (1967).

IRVINE, E. E. Two approaches to adjustment problems among children in institutions. *Brit. J. Psychiatr. Soc. Work.* (1951) no. 5, 6–12.

IRVINE, E. E. The function and use of relationship between client and psychiatric social worker. *Brit. J. Psychiatr. Soc. Work.* (1952) no. 6, 21–6.

IRVINE, E. E. Observations on the aims and methods of child rearing in communal settlements in Israel. *Hum. Relat.* (1952) *5*, 247–75.

IRVINE, E. E. The ordeal of motherhood. *Brit. J. Psychiatr. Soc. Work.* (1952) no. 7, 3–6.

IRVINE, E. E. Research into problem families: theoretical questions arising from Dr. Blacker's investigations. *Brit. J. Psychiatr. Soc. Work.* (1954) no. 9, 24–33.

IRVINE, E. E. Opportunities for guidance in the early years. *Roy. Soc. Hlth J.* (1955) *75*, 709–14.

IRVINE, E. E. Renaissance in British casework. *Social Work* (1956) *13*, 187–94.

IRVINE, E. E. Some implications of Freudian theory for casework. *Almoner* (1956) *9*, 39–44.

IRVINE, E. E. Transference and reality in the casework relationship. *Brit. J. Psychiatr. Soc. Work.* (1956) *3*, no. 4, 15–24. Reprinted in ASSOCIATION OF PSYCHIATRIC SOCIAL WORKERS. *Relationship in casework.* A.P.S.W. (1964), pp. 55–65.

IRVINE, E. E. The use of small group discussions in the teaching of human relations and mental health. *Brit. J. Psychiatr. Soc. Work.* (1959) *5*, 26–30.

IRVINE, E. E. Commitment and objectivity. In HALMOS, P. (ed.) Moral issues in the training of teachers and social workers. *Sociological Review Monograph* (1960) no. 3, 83–7.

IRVINE, E. E. Psychosis in parents: mental illness as a problem for the family. *Brit. J. Psychiatr. Soc. Work.* (1961) *6*, 21–6.

IRVINE, E. E. (ed.) *Ventures in professional co-operation.* Association of Psychiatric Social Workers (1961) (Conclusion, pp. 97–100).

IRVINE, E. E. Mental health education in the community, the quest of sanction. *Brit. J. Psychiatr. Soc. Work.* (1964) *7*, 136–41.

IRVING, B. L. *see* EMERY, F. E. (1968).

JAQUES, E. (ed.) Social diagnosis and social therapy. *J. Social Issues* (1947) *3*, no. 2.

JAQUES, E. Social therapy: technocracy or collaboration? *J. Social Issues* (1947) *3*, no. 2, 59–66.

JAQUES, E. Some principles of organisation of a social therapeutic institution. *J. Social Issues* (1947) *3*, no. 2, 4–10.

JAQUES, E. Field theory and industrial psychology. *Occup. Psychol.* (1948) *22*, 126–33.

JAQUES, E. Interpretative group discussions as a method of facilitating social change. *Hum. Relat.* (1947/8) *1*, 533–49.

JAQUES, E. *The changing culture of a factory.* Tavistock Publications (1951).

JAQUES, E., RICE, A. K. *and* HILL, J. M. M. The social and psychological impact of a change in method of wage payment. (Glacier Project — V). *Hum. Relat.* (1951) *4*, 315–40.

JESSOP, W. N. Closing discussion. In *Manpower planning: operational research and personnel research.* (Proceedings of NATO Conference, Brussels 1965). English Universities Press Ltd (1966), pp. 289–91.

JESSOP, W. N. *see* HIGGIN, G. W. (1963).

KELNAR, J. Treatment of interpersonal relations in groups. *J. Social Issues* (1947) *3*, no. 2, 29–41.

KELNAR, J. *and* SUTHERLAND, J. D. Some current developments in psychotherapy in Great Britain. In FROMM-REICHMANN, F. *and* MORENO, J. L. (eds) *Progress in psychotherapy, 1956.* New York (1956), pp. 277–83.

KING, P. H. M. Task perception and interpersonal relations in industrial training. Development of a training project in the hosiery trade. Part I. *Hum. Relat.* (1947/8) *I*, 121–30.

KING, P. H. M. Task perception and interpersonal relations in industrial training. Part II. *Hum. Relat.* (1947/8) *1*, 373–412.

KNIGHT, J. *see* MARTIN, F. (1962).

LAING, R. D. An examination of Tillich's theory of anxiety and neurosis. *Brit. J. Med. Psychol.* (1957) *30*, 88–91.

LAING, R. D. *and* ESTERSON, A. The collusive function of pairing in analytic groups. *Brit. J. Med. Psychol.* (1958) *31*, 117–23.

LAING, R. D. *The divided self.* Tavistock Publications (1960) American edition: Chicago (1961). Translated into Spanish (1962).

LAING, R. D. *The self and others.* Tavistock Publications (1961). American edition: Chicago (1962).

LAING, R. D. Is schizophrenia a disease? *Int. J. Soc. Psychiat.* (1964) *10*, no. 3, 184–93.

LAING, R. D. *and* COOPER, D. G. *Reason and violence. A decade of Sartre's philosophy, 1950–1960.* Tavistock Publications (1964). American edition: New York (1964).

LAING, R. D. *and* ESTERSON, A. *Sanity, madness and the family. Vol. 1. Families of schizophrenics.* Tavistock Publications (1964). American edition: New York (1965).

LAING, R. D. Family and individual structure. In LOMAS, P. (ed.) *The predicament of the family.* London, Hogarth Press/Institute of Psycho-Analysis (1967).

LAING, R. D. Mystification, confusion and conflict. In BOSZORMENYI-NAGY, I. *and* FRAMO, J. L. (eds) *Intensive family therapy.* New York (1965).

LAING, R. D. Transcendental experience in relation to religion and psychosis. (Paper delivered at the International Congress of Social Psychiatry, London, August 1964). *Psychedelic Review* (1965).

LAING, R. D., COOPER, D. *and* ESTERSON, A. Results of family-oriented therapy with hospitalised schizophrenics. *Brit. Med. J.* (1965) *ii*, 1462–5.

LAING, R. D., PHILLIPSON, H. *and* LEE, A. R. *Interpersonal perception: a theory and a method of research.* Tavistock Publications/ (1966).

LAING, R. D. Religious experience and the role of organised religion. Paper for N.A.M.H. Conference, 'The role of religion in mental health'. *Guild of Health Monthly* (1966) July-August, p. 111.

LAING, R. D. Schizophrenia. In NATIONAL ASSOCIATION FOR MENTAL HEALTH. *The heart of the matter.* Report of the N.A.M.H. Annual Conference, 1966. N.A.M.H. (1966), pp. 74–8.

LUFF, Mary. A case of obsessional neurosis closely allied to schizophrenia. In *Individual psychology and sexual difficulties, I.* (Individual Psychology Medical Pamphlets, no. 3.) C. W. Daniel (1932), pp. 54–66.

LUFF, Mary. Emotional conflicts between husband and wife. *Parents and Teachers* (1934) *1*, no. 2, p. 9.

LUFF, Mary *and* GARROD, Marjorie. The after-results of psychotherapy in 500 adult cases. *Brit. Med. J.* (1935) *ii*, 54–9.

LYONS, A. *see* BANNISTER, K. (1955).
see PINCUS, L. (1960).

LYONS, A. *and* WOODHOUSE, D. L. The young and their marriages. *Mental Health* (1968) Spring issue, pp. 2–4.

MABERLY, Alan. *Commonsense and psychology.* Muller (1936).

MABERLY, Alan. After-results of child guidance. A follow-up of 500 children treated at the Tavistock Clinic 1921–1934. *Brit. Med. J.* (1939) *i*, 1130.

MACKENZIE, M. The practice of mental health in maternity and child welfare. *Medical Officer* (1956) *95*, 123–5.

MACKENZIE, M. Changing concepts in the field of child health: mental and emotional aspects. *Public Health* (1963) *77*, 107–15.

MALAN, D. H. *and* PHILLIPSON, H. The psychodynamics of diagnostic procedures. *Brit. J. Med. Psychol.* (1957) *30*, 92–8.

MALAN, D. H. On assessing the results of psychotherapy. *Brit. J. Med. Psychol.* (1959) *32*, 86–105. German translation: *Psyche* (1961–1962) *15*, 331–62.

MALAN, D. H. Symposium on psychoanalysis and validation. III. On the 'clinical' and 'objective' approaches to psychodynamic material. *Brit. J. Med. Psychol.* (1961) *34*, 15–21.

MALAN, D. H. *A study of brief psychotherapy.* Tavistock Publications (1963). American edition: Springfield, Ill. (1964). Translated into German 1965.

MALAN, D. H., HEATH, E. S. *and* BACAL, H. A. The assessment of psychodynamic change. *Proc. Roy. Soc. Med.* (1965) *58*, 522–5.

MALAN, D. H., BACAL, H.A., HEATH, E. S. *and* BALFOUR, F. H. G. A study of psychodynamic changes in untreated neurotic patients. I. Improvements that are questionable on dynamic criteria. *Brit. J. Psychiat.* (1968) *114*, 525–51.

MALAN, D. H., RAYNER, E. H., BACAL, H. A., HEATH, E. S. *and* BALFOUR, F. H. G. Psychodynamic assessment of the outcome of psychotherapy. In PORTER, R. (ed.) *The role of learning in psychotherapy.* A Ciba Foundation Symposium. J. & A. Churchill (1968), pp. 61–7.

MAREK, J. *Social and psychological responses to changing environmental demands. A study of the effects of automation in two factories.* Ph. D. thesis. University of London (1963).

MAREK, J. *see* EMERY, F. E. (1962).

MARTIN, F. *and* KNIGHT, J. Joint interviews as part of intake procedure in a child psychiatric clinic. *J. Child Psychol. Psychiat.* (1962) *3*, 17–26.

MARTIN, F. Technical problems in the treatment of adolescents beginning psychotherapy. *J. Child Psychol. Psychiat.* (1963) *4*, 109–24.

MENZIES, I. E. P. Factors affecting family breakdown in urban communities. *Hum. Relat.* (1949) *2*, 363–73.

MENZIES, I. E. P. *Technical Report. World Health Organisation: Working Conference for Public Health Nurses, Noordwijk, October, 1950.* Tavistock Institute of Human Relations (1951).

MENZIES, I. E. P. A case-study in the functioning of social systems as a defence against anxiety: a report on a study of the nursing service of a general hospital. *Hum. Relat.* (1960) *13*, 95–121. Reprinted as: Tavistock Pamphlet No. 3, 1961.

MENZIES, I. E. P. Nurses under stress. *International Nursing Review* (1960) *7*, no. 6, 9–16. Also published in *Nursing Times* (1961) *57*, 141–2; 173–4; 206–7.

MENZIES, I. E. P. *A note on driving and road accidents; (including a critical evaluation of the Ministry of Transport's Christmas 1964 poster campaign)*. British Safety Council (1965).

MENZIES, I. E. P. Some mutual interactions between organisations and their members. (Paper read at the 6th International Congress of Psychotherapy, London 1964.) *Psychother. Psychosom.* (1965) *13*, 194–200.

MENZIES, I. E. P. *see* SUTHERLAND, J. D. (1947).

MENZIES, I. E. P. *Drinking and driving. A note on drivers' reactions to the proposed Bill making it an offence to drive with a blood-alcohol concentration above a prescribed limit.* British Safety Council (1966).

MENZIES, I. E. P. *Some social and psychological aspects of road safety.* Tavistock Institute of Human Relations (1967).

MILLER, D. H. Psychosocial factors in the aetiology of disturbed behaviour. *Brit. J. Med. Psychol.* (1961) *34*, 43–52.

MILLER, D. H. *Growth to freedom.* Tavistock Publications (1964).

MILLER, D. H. Adolescence and comprehensives. *New Education* (1966) *2*, no. 5, 10–12.

MILLER, D. H. Problems of staff training in a school for delinquent adolescent boys. *Howard J. Penology* (1966) *12*, no. 1, 52–60.

MILLER, D. H. Staff training in the penal system: the use of small groups. *Hum. Relat.* (1966) *19*, 151–64.

MILLER, D. H. Adolescent psychology. In PERRY, Michael (ed.) *Crisis of confirmation.* S.C.M. Press (1967).

MILLER, D. H. Adolescence – are co-ed. schools preferable? *Where* (1967) no. 34, 15–16.

MILLER, D. H. Family interaction and adolescent therapy. In LOMAS, P. (ed.) *The predicament of the family.* Hogarth (1967) pp. 34–56.

MILLER, D. H. A model of an institution for treating delinquents. In KLARE, H. J. (ed.) *Changing concepts of crime and its treatment.* Pergamon Press (1967).

MILLER, D. H. Paying lip service to change. *Mental Health* (1967) Autumn issue, pp. 3–4.

MILLER, D. H. Uses and abuses of corporal punishment. *Mental Health* (1967) Spring issue, pp. 8–11.

MILLER, D. H. The approved school system: a critique. In CAMBRIDGE, UNIVERSITY OF, *Institute of Criminology. The residential treatment of disturbed and delinquent boys.* Cambridge, Institute of Criminology (1968), pp. 72–6.

MILLER, D. H. *see* GOSLING, R. (1967).

MILLER, Emmanuel. Child guidance and the difficult child. *J. State. Med.* (1933) *41*, 715–19.

MILLER, Emmanuel. Emotional factors in intellectual retardation. *J. Ment. Sci.* (1933) *79*, 614–25.

MILLER, Emmanuel. Sudden insanity. *Practitioner* (1933) *130*, 316–24.

MILLER, Emmanuel. Temperamental differences in the behaviour disorders of children. *Brit. J. Educ. Psychol.* (1933) *3*, 222–36.

MILLER, Emmanuel. *Insomnia and other disorders of sleep.* John Bale Sons & Danielsson (1935).

MILLER, Emmanuel. Medico-legal aspects of the aberrations of adolescence. *Medico-Legal and Criminological Rev.* (1935) *3*, 181–210.

MILLER, Emmanuel. Present discontents in psychopathology. *Brit. J. Med. Psychol.* (1935/6) *15*, 2–17.

MILLER, Emmanuel. Scientific treatment of delinquency. *Brit. Med. J.* (1936) *i*, 1112–13.

MILLER, Emmanuel. Compensation for disabilities. In *Report of the British Association Meeting, Psychological Section*, Nottingham (1937).

MILLER, Emmanuel. Education methods for children with intellectual and character abnormalities. *Report of the 1st International Congress of Child Psychiatry* (1937).

MILLER, Emmanuel. *The growing child and its problems.* Kegan Paul, Trench, Trubner & Co. (1937).

MILLER, Emmanuel. Neurosis and civilisation. In CATTELL, R. B. *et al.* (eds) *Human affairs.* Macmillan (1937).

MILLER, Emmanuel. Some psychological aspects of physiotherapy. *Brit. J. Phys. Med.* (1938) *1*, 2–6.

MILLER, Emmanuel. *The generations.* Faber & Faber (1938).

MILLER, Emmanuel. Education for parenthood. In COHEN, J. *and* TRAVERS, R. M. W. (eds) *Educating for democracy.* Macmillan (1939).

MILLER, Emmanuel. *The neuroses in war.* Macmillan (1940).
MILLER, Emmanuel. Psychiatry in children. In *British Encyclopaedia of Medical Practice*, vol. 10. 2nd edition. Butterworth (1952), pp. 289–97. (First published 1940).
MILLER, E. J. *see* BRIDGER, H. (1963).
MILLER, Hugh Crichton. The physical basis of emotional disorder. *Lancet* (1924) *i*, 378.
MILLER, Hugh Crichton. Psychology and social hygiene. *J. Soc. Hyg.* (1926) *12*, 14–24.
MILLER, Hugh Crichton. Lunacy reform. *Clin. J.* (1927) *56*, 272–6; 280–3.
MILLER, Hugh Crichton. Fear. In ERLEIGH, E. V. (ed.) *The mind of the growing child.* Faber & Gwyer (1928) pp. 147–58.
MILLER, Hugh Crichton. The real meaning of family discipline. In ERLEIGH, E. V. (ed.) *The mind of the growing child.* Faber & Gwyer (1928), pp. 179–91.
MILLER, Hugh Crichton. *Insomnia: an outline for the practitioner.* Edward Arnold (1930).
MILLER, Hugh Crichton. *Marriage, freedom and education.* SCM Press (1931).
MILLER, Hugh Crichton. Depression. *Practitioner* (1931) *126*, 130–8.
MILLER, Hugh Crichton. Discussion on the diagnosis and treatment of the milder forms of manic-depressive psychosis. *Proc. Roy. Soc. Med.* (1930) *23*, 883–6.
MILLER, Hugh Crichton. Mental health in relation to education. *Brit. Med. J.* (1932) *ii*, 234–7.
MILLER, Hugh Crichton. Primitive man and the modern patient. *Brit. Med. J.* (1932) *ii*, 430–2.
MILLER, Hugh Crichton. *Psychoanalysis and its derivatives.* Butterworth (1933).
MILLER, Hugh Crichton. Sex education. In *Conference on Mental Health, 1931. Report of the Proceedings.* Allard & Son (1931).
MILLER, Hugh Crichton. The probationer and the social contract. *Probation* (1931) *1*, no. 7, 99–100.
MILLER, Hugh Crichton. The contribution of mental hygiene to the health of school children. In *Report of Synchronised Conferences of World Educational Associations*, Oxford (1935).
MILLER, Hugh Crichton. Psychotherapeutic clinics in fact and fancy. *Brit. Med. J.* (1935) *i*, 1205–8.
MILLER, Hugh Crichton. The stewardship of mental health. *Lancet* (1935) *i*, 1292–5.

MILLER, Hugh Crichton. Educational ideals and the destinies of peoples. In HADFIELD, J. A. (ed.) *Psychology and modern problems.* University of London Press (1935), pp. 131–56.

MILLER, Hugh Crichton. Compulsion and punishment in the family. *Zeitschrift für Kinderpsychiatrie* (1935) *2*, 104–11.

MILLER, Hugh Crichton. Compulsion and punishment in the family and the school. *Ment. Hyg.* (1935) no. 11, 119–25.

MILLER, Hugh Crichton. Science and art in psychotherapy. *Nederlandsch Tijdschrift voor Psychologie* (1936) *4*, 366–74.

MILLER, Hugh Crichton. The child of tomorrow. *J. of Dutch Soc. for Ment. Hyg.* (1936).

MILLER, Hugh Crichton. Mental hygiene and preventive medicine. *Ment. Hyg.* (1936) *2*, 155–60.

MILLER, Hugh Crichton. Classification and etiology of neurosis. *Practitioner* (1936) *137*, 14–24.

MILLER, Hugh Crichton. The frontiers of psychotherapy. *Brit. J. Med. Psychol.* (1936/7) *16*, 165–83.

MILLER, Hugh Crichton. The significance of parental responsibility. *Ment. Hyg.* (1937) *21*, 8–16.

MILLER, Hugh Crichton. *Suicide: what medical psychology says about it.* National Council for Mental Hygiene (1938).

MILLER, Hugh Crichton. Sexual development of the child and adolescent. *Practitioner* (1938) *141*, 243–51.

MILLER, Hugh Crichton. The child's approach to philosophy. *Hibbert J.* (April 1938).

MILLER, Hugh Crichton. Resultant and purposive in psychiatry. *J. Ment. Sci.* (1939) *85*, 82–95.

MITCHELL, G. D. Social disintegration in a rural community. *Hum. Relat.* (1950) *3*, 279–306.

MORRIS, B. S. Education and human relations. *J. Social Issues* (1947) *3*, no. 2, 42–50.

MORRIS, B. S. Officer selection in the British Army, 1942–1945. *Occup. Psychol.* (1949) *23*, 219–34.

MURRAY, H. The sociometric stability of personal relations among retarded children. *Sociometry* (1953) *16*, 113–41. Also published as: *Sociometry Monographs* (1953), no. 28.

MURRAY, H. *An operational research study of a military training system.* Ph.D. thesis. University of London, Institute of Education (1959).

MURRAY, H. Social process in the realisation of talent. In *Proceedings of the 14th International Congress of Applied Psychology, Copenhagen 1961. Vol. 5. Industrial and business psychology.* Copenhagen (1962), pp. 80–7.

MURRAY, H. *see* TRIST, E. L. (1959), (1960), (1961), (1963).

MURRAY, J. B. *Some common psychosomatic manifestations.* 2nd edition. Oxford University Press (1951).

NICOLLE, G. Environment in the treatment of psychoneurosis. *Practitioner* (1937), p. 706.

O'KELLY, E. Some observations on relationships between delinquent girls and their parents.
Brit. J. Med. Psychol. (1955) *28*, 59–66.

O'KELLY, E. An investigation, by means of the Object Relations Test, into some of the effects of early separation from the mother on the personal relationships of adolescent delinquent girls. *J. Ment. Sci.* (1957) *103*, 381–91.

OSBORNE, E. Some problems associated with school phobia as illustrated in the Rorschach record of a six-year-old girl. *Rorschach Newsletter* (Brit. Rorschach Forum) (1963) *8*, no. 1. 3–10.

OSBORNE, E. *see* CASPARI, I. (1968).

PADDON, Dorothy *see* HOOPER, Douglas (1965).

PARKES, C. M. The effects of bereavement on physical and mental health; a study of the case records of widows. *Brit. Med. J.* (1964), *ii*, 1 Aug., 274–9.

PARKES, C. M. Recent bereavement as a cause of mental illness. *Brit. J. Psychiat.* (1964) *110*, 198–204.

PARKES, C. M. Bereavement and mental illness. Part I: A clinical study of the grief of bereaved psychiatric patients. Part II: A classification of bereavement reactions. *Brit. J. Med. Psychol* (1965) *38*, 1–12; 13–26.

PAYNE, M. A. *Oliver untwisted.* Edward Arnold (1929).

PEARSON, E. A. Hamilton. Honesty. In HOME AND SCHOOLS COUNCIL. *Advances in understanding the child.*

PHILLIPSON, H. Unconscious object relations and the techniques of the clinical psychologist. *Brit. J. Med. Psychol.* (1953) *26*, 49–57.

PHILLIPSON, H. *The Object Relations Technique.* Tavistock Publications (1955). American edition: Chicago (1960). Translated into Spanish: Buenos Aires, 1960.

PHILLIPSON, H. Directions of development in projective techniques: the projective approach in relation to diagnosis and psychotherapy *Brit. J. Med. Psychol.* (1956) *29*, 139–49.

PHILLIPSON, H. Vocational guidance as a therapeutic proc es *J. Int. Vocational Guidance Ass.* (1957/8) *1*, 125–8.

PHILLIPSON, H. The assessment of progress after at least two years of group psychotherapy. *Brit. J. Med. Psychol.* (1958) *31*, 32–42.

PHILLIPSON, H. *and* HOPKINS, J. Personality: an approach to the study of perception. *Brit. J. Med. Psychol.* (1964) *37*, 1–15.

PHILLIPSON, H. *see* LAING, R. D. (1965).
see MALAN, D. H. (1957).
see PINCUS, L. ed. (1960).

PINCUS, L. (ed.) *Marriage; studies in emotional conflict and growth.* Methuen (1960). (This book was written as a co-operative effort by the staff of the Family Discussion Bureau, including K. Bannister, V. Garden, J. Hall, A. Lyons, H. Phillipson, L. Pincus, E. Seligman and J. Stephens, with an introduction by A. G. Thompson.)

PINCUS, L. The nature of marital interaction. In YOUNG-HUSBAND, E. *comp. Social work with families.* National Institute for Social Work Training/Allen & Unwin (1965), pp. 41–55.

PINCUS, L. *Marriage problems and their implications for the family.* W.H.O. Public Health Papers no. 28. (1965), pp. 51–63,

PINCUS, L. *see* BANNISTER, K. (1966).

POTTS, W. A. Dental extractions in nervous breakdown with special reference to reactions. *Proc. Roy. Soc. Med.* (1933) *26*, 17–22.

POTTS, W. A. The diagnosis and treatment of some physical factors in nervous breakdown and incipient mental disorder. *J. Ment. Sci.* (1935) *81*, 260–4.

RAPOPORT, Rhona *see* RAPOPORT, R. N. (1967) ,(1968).

RAPOPORT, R. N., FOGARTY, M. *and* RAPOPORT, Rhona *Women and top jobs: an interim report.* Political & Economic Planning (1967).

RAPOPORT, R. N. *and* RAPOPORT, Rhona. Family transition in contemporary society. *J. Psychosom. Res.* (1968) *12*, 29–38.

RAPOPORT, R. N. The therapeutic community. In SELLS, D. (ed.) *Internat. Encyclopaedia of the Social Sciences, vol. 10.* New York (1968), pp. 207–15.

REES, J. R. Some problems in family adjustment. In ERLEIGH, E. V. (ed.) *The mind of the growing child.* Faber & Gwyer (1928), pp. 95–108.

REES, J. R. *The health of the mind.* Faber & Faber (1929).

REES, J. R. Some social psychological aspects of marriage. *Probation* (1939) *3*, 81–3.

REES, J. R. *and* ROBINSON, D. F. Modern psychiatry and social work. *Yearbook of the Hospital Almoners Association* (1931).

REES, J. R. Discussion of paper: 'Mental hygiene and the high school'. In *Proceedings of the 1st International Congress on Mental Hygiene, vol. II.* New York, International Committee for Mental Hygiene (1932), pp. 109–15.

REES, J. R. Discussion of paper: 'Organisation of special types of clinical service'. In *Proceedings of the 1st International Congress on Mental Hygiene, vol. 1.* New York, International Committee for Mental Hygiene (1932), pp. 555–60.

REES, J. R. The prophylactic treatment of mental disorders. *Practitioner* (1931) *126*, 406–14.

REES, J. R. Psychotherapeutic clinics. In CULPIN, M. *Recent advances in the study of psychoneurosis.* Churchill (1931), pp. 210–29.

REES, J. R. The healthy mind: the first five years. *Maternity and Child Welfare* (1932) *56*, 90–1.

REES, J. R. The psychology of the mother. *Maternity and Child Welfare* (1932) *56*, 61–3.

REES, J. R. The psychological causes of crime. *Probation* (1932) *1*, no. 12. 183–4.

REES, J. R. Psychological factors in the prevention and treatment of alcohol and drug addiction. *Lancet* (1932) *203*, 929–33.

REES, J. R. The causes and cure of crime: from the psychologists standpoint. *Howard J.* (1933) *3*, no. 4, 28–34.

REES, J. R. Contribution to discussion on constitutional psychopathy. *Proc. Roy. Soc. Med.* (1934) *27*, 1156–7.

REES, J. R. The neurotic. *Ment. Hyg.* (1934), no. 10, 91–4.

REES, J. R. The general practitioner and mental disorders. *Brit. Med. J.* (1935) *i*, 1303–5.

REES, J. R. The problems of outpatient clinics for psychoneurotics. *Proc. Roy. Soc. Med.* (1935) *28*, 1229–38.

REES, J. R. Prognosis in sexual neurosis. *Lancet* (1935) *i*, 948–9.

REES, J. R. Emotional disorders of adolescence. *Report of the Medical Officers of Schools Association* (1936).

REES, J. R. Neurosis: its effect on employer and employee. Speech given at Industrial Welfare Society Annual Lecture Conference (Sept. 1936) [Typescript].

REES, J. R. *The health of the mind.* 2nd edition. Faber (1936).

REES, J. R. Sexual perversions. *Practitioner* (1936) *137*, 98–107.

REES, J. R. Mental hygiene and the school. *Ment. Hyg.* (1937) *3*, 98–101.

REES, J. R. The unwilling patient. III. *Brit. J. Med. Psychol.* (1937/8) *17*, 69–70.

REES, J. R. Psychological factors in sickness and invalidism. Assurance Medical Society (1939).

REES, J. R. The magistrate and delinquency. *Ment. Hyg.* (1938) *4*, 127–32.

REES, J. R. Mental hygiene and the press. *Ment. Hyg.* (1939) *5*, 76–9.

REES, J. R. *The mental aspects of tuberculosis.* Trans. 24th Annual Conference, National Association for Prevention of Tuberculosis (1938).

REES, J. R. Strategic planning for mental health. *Ment. Hlth.* (1940) *1*, 103–6.

REES, J. R. Three years of military psychiatry in the United Kingdom. *Brit. Med. J.* (1943) *i*, 1–6.

REES, J. R. A brief impression of British military psychiatry. *Bull. Menninger Clin.* (1944) *8*, 29–35.

REES, J. R. Factors in industrial health. *Industr. Welf. and Pers. Management* (1939) *21*.

REES, J. R. 'Unfit on psychiatric grounds'. *Occup. Psychol.* (1946) *20*, 125–31.

REES, J. R. (ed.) *The case of Rudolf Hess.* Heinemann (1948).

REES, Mary I. Hemingway. The supersensitive child. In ERLEIGH, E. V. (ed.) *The mind of the growing child.* Faber & Gwyre (1928), pp. 65–80.

RICE, A. K. The role of the specialist in the community. *Hum. Relat.* (1949) *2*, 177–84.

RICE, A. K., HILL, J. M. M. *and* TRIST, E. L. The representation of labour turnover as a social process. (Glacier Project — II). *Hum. Relat.* (1950) *3*, 349–72.

RICE, A. K. The use of unrecognised cultural mechanisms in an expanding machine-shop. (Glacier Project — III). *Hum. Relat.* (1951) *4*, 143–60.

RICE, A. K. Productivity and social organisation in an Indian weaving shed. *Hum. Relat.* (1953) *6*, 297–329.

RICE, A. K. *Productivity and social organisation. The Ahmedabad Experiment.* Tavistock Publications (1958).

RICE, A. K. *The enterprise and its environment.* Tavistock Publications (1963).

RICE, A. K. *Learning for leadership.* Tavistock Publications (1965)

ROBB, M. Organ jargon. In *Individual psychology and psychosomatic disorders. I.* (Individual Medical Psychology Pamphlets, no. 4.) C. W. Daniel (1932), pp. 61–6.

ROBB, J. H. The contribution of psychopathology to sociology. *Sociol. Rev.* (1952) *44*, 53–72.

ROBB, J. H. *Working-class anti-Semite.* Tavistock Publications (1954).

ROBERTSON, J. Film: *A two-year-old goes to hospital.* 16 m.m., sound, 45 mins. English and French (1952). Tavistock Child Development Research Unit; New York, N.Y. University Film Library; Geneva, United Nations, etc. Abridged version: 16 mm., sound, 30 mins, English only.

ROBERTSON, J. *Guide to the film: A two-year-old goes to hospital.* Tavistock Publications (1953). 2nd edition 1959; 3rd edition 1965.

ROBERTSON, J. Der Verlust mütterlicher Fürsorge in früher Kindheit und einige Auswirkungen auf die Entwicklung der Persönlichkeit. *Zeitschrift für ärtzliche Fortbildung* (1957) *21–2*, 899–903.

ROBERTSON, J. Film: *Going to hospital with mother.* 16 mm., sound, 40 mins. English and French (1958) Tavistock Child Development Research Unit; New York, N.Y. University Film Library; Geneva, United Nations, etc.

ROBERTSON, J. *Guide to the film: Going to hospital with mother.* Tavistock Child Development Research Unit (1958). 2nd edition 1964.

ROBERTSON, J. Going to hospital with mother. *Proc. Roy. Soc. Med.* (1958), *52*, 381–4.

ROBERTSON, J. *Young children in hospital,* Tavistock Publications (1958). American edition: New York (1959).

ROBERTSON, J. *Hospitals and children: a parent's-eye view.* Gollancz (1962). American edition: New York (1963).

ROBERTSON, James. Effecting change in the hospitalization of children. In SHORE, M. F. (ed.) '*Red is the color of hurting*'. *Planning for children in hospital.* Bethesda, Md., National Institute of Mental Health. (1967), pp. 47–60.

ROBERTSON, James *and* BURLINGHAM, D. T. Film: *Nursery school for the blind.* Guide booklet. London, Concord Films Council/ New York, New York University Film Library (1967).

ROBERTSON, James *and* ROBERTSON, Joyce. Film: *Young children in brief separation. No. 1. Kate, aged 2 years, 5 months in fostercare for 27 days.* Guide Booklet. London, Tavistock Institute of Human Relations/New York, New York University Film Library (1968).

ROBERTSON, James *and* ROBERTSON, Joyce. Film: *Young children in brief separation. No. 3. John, aged 17 months in a residential nursery for 9 days.* London, Tavistock Institute of Human Relations/New York, New York University Film Library (1968).

ROBINSON, M. The family as the client. *Case conf.* (1968) *14*, 338–42.

ROBINSON, M. Family based therapy. Some thoughts on the family approach. *Brit. J. Psychiatr. Soc. Work.* (1968) *9*, 188–92.

ROSENBLUTH, D. *and* BOWLBY, J. The social and psychological backgrounds of tuberculous children. *Brit. Med. J.* (1955) *i*, 16 Apr., 946–9.

ROSENBLUTH, Dina. The Kleinian theory of depression. *J. Child Psychother.* (1965) *1*, no. 3, 20–5.

ROSENBLUTH, Dina. 'Insight' as an aim of treatment. *J. Child Psychother.* (1968) *2*, no. 2, 5–17.

SANDLER, J. Studies in psychopathology using a self-assessment inventory. I. The development and construction of the inventory. *Brit. J. Med. Psychol.* (1954) *27*, 142–5.

SANDLER, J. *and* POLLOCK, A. B. Studies in psychopathology using a self-assessment inventory. II. Some neurotic gastro-intestinal symptoms: functional dyspepsia in men. *Brit. J. Med. Psychol.* (1954) *27*, 146–57.

SANDLER, J. *and* POLLOCK, A. B. Studies in psychopathology using a self-assessment inventory. III. Some neurotic gastro-intestinal symptoms: functional dyspepsia in women. *Brit. J. Med. Psychol.* (1954) *27*, 235–40.

SANDLER, J. *and* POLLOCK, A. B. Studies in psychopathology using a self-assessment inventory. IV. Some neurotic gastro-intestinal symptoms: defaecatory difficulty in men and women. *Brit. J. Med. Psychol.* (1954) *27*, 241–6.

[SANDLER, J.] KANTER, V. B. *and* SANDLER, J. Studies in psychopathology using a self-assessment inventory. V. Anxiety, functional dyspepsia and duodenal ulcer; an investigation. *Brit. J. Med. Psychol.* (1955) *28*, 157–66.

SANDLER, J., DE MONCHAUX, C. *and* DIXON, J. J. Patterns of anxiety: the correlates of social anxieties. *Brit. J. Med. Psychol.* (1958) *31*, 24–31.

SANDLER, J. Psychosomatic pathology. *Brit. J. Med. Psychol.* (1958). *31*, 19–23.

SANDLER, J. The use of the Tavistock self-assessment inventory in psychosomatic research. *Proc. Roy. Soc. Med.* (1958) *51*, p. 948.

SANDLER, J. The Rorschach and the feeling of safety. *Rorschach Newsletter* (Brit. Rorschach Forum) (1959) *4*, no. 2, 2–6.

SANDLER, J. *and* HAZARI, A. The 'obsessional': on the psychological classification of obsessional character traits and symptoms. *Brit. J. Med. Psychol.* (1960) *33*, 113–22.

SANDLER, J. *see* DIXON, J. J. (1957), (1957).

SCHAFFER, H. R. Behaviour under stress: a neurophysiological hypothesis. *Psychol. Rev.* (1954) *61*, 323–33.

SELIGMAN, H. R. *see* PINCUS, L. (1960).

SEMEONOFF, B. *and* TRIST, E. L. *Diagnostic performance tests.* Tavistock Publications (1958).

SHOOTER, Antonia. The psychology of drug addiction: some literature reviewed. *Rorschach Newsletter* (1965) *10*, no. 1, 3–10.

SIMMINS, C. A. Merely dull or backward. *Ment. Welfare* (1932) *13*, 73–9.

SIMMINS, C. A. Deterioration of 'G' in psychotic patients. *J. Ment. Sci.* (1933) *79*, 704–34.

SIMMINS, C. A. The measurement of mental deterioration. *Brit. J. Med. Psychol.* (1934) *14*, 113–20.

SIMMINS, C. A. Mental incapacity: the intelligence of patients in mental hospitals. *Character and Personality* (1935/6) *4*, 25–33.

SIMMINS, C. A. Measuring the intelligence of abnormal adults. *Yearbook of Education* (1935), pp. 551–9.

SOFER, C. Reactions to administrative change. A study of staff relations in three British hospitals. *Hum. Relat.* (1955) *8*, 291–316.

SOFER, C. *The organisation from within: a comparative study of social institutions based on a sociotherapeutic approach.* Tavistock Publications (1961).

SOFER, C. The assessment of organisational change. *J. Mgmt. Studies* (1964) *1*, 128–42.

SOFER, C., JANIS, I. *and* WISHLADE, L. Social and psychological factors in changing food habits. In YUDKIN, J. *and* MACKENZIE, J. C. (eds) *Changing food habits.* MacGibbon & Kee (1964), pp. 90–108.

SOFER, C. *see* SPENCER, P. (1964).
see TRIST, E. L. (1959).

SPENCER, P. *and* SOFER, C. Organisational change and its management. *J. Mgmt. Studies* (1964) *1*, 26–47.

STEIN, L. The emotional background of stammering. *Brit. J. Med. Psychol.* (1949) *22*, 189–93.

STEIN, L. *The infancy of speech and the speech of infancy.* Methuen (1949).

STEIN, L. On talking or the communication of ideas and feelings by means of mainly audible symbols. *Brit. J. Med. Psychol.* (1951) *24*, 107–17.

STEIN, L. Stammering as a psychosomatic disorder. *Folia Phoniatr.* (1953) *5*, 12–46.

STEIN, L. The terminology of transference. *Acta Psychother.* (1955) *3*, Suppl., 674–80.
STEIN, L. What is a symbol supposed to be? *J. Anal. Psychol.* (1957) *2*, 73–84.
STEIN, L. Analytical psychology: a 'modern' science. *J. Anal. Psychol.* (1958) *3*, 43–50.
STEPHENS, J. *see* BANNISTER, K. (1955).
see PINCUS, L. (1960).
[STRAUSS, E. B.] BRAIN, W. R. *and* STRAUSS, E. B. *Recent advances in neurology.* 3rd edition. Churchill (1934).
STRAUSS, E. B. The psychogenic factor in asthma. *Guys Hosp. Reports.* (1937) *87*, 273–86.
SUTHERLAND, J. D. *and* FITZPATRICK, G. A. Some approaches to group problems in the British army. In Group psychotherapy: a symposium. *Sociometry* (1945) *8*, 443–55.
SUTHERLAND, J. D. *and* MENZIES, I. E. P. Two industrial projects. *J. Social Issues* (1947) *3*, no. 2, 51–8.
SUTHERLAND, J. D. Work and incentives in a democratic society. *Political Quart.* (1948) *19*, 117–25.
SUTHERLAND, J. D. The types of personality. In REES, J. R. (ed.) *Modern practice in psychological medicine.* Butterworth (1949) pp. 86–102.
SUTHERLAND, J. D. Clinical psychology. *Universities Quart.* (1950) *4*, Feb., 1–11.
SUTHERLAND, J. D. Notes on psychoanalytic group therapy. I. Therapy and training. *Psychiatry* (1952) *15*, 111–17.
SUTHERLAND, J. D. Psychological medicine and the National Health Service; the need for an integrated approach to research. *Brit. J. Med. Psychol.* (1952) *25*, 71–85.
SUTHERLAND, J. D. A brief reply to Dr. Eysenck and Prof. Zangwill. *Brit. J. Med. Psychol.* (1953) *26*, 313–18.
SUTHERLAND, J. D. The patient as a person. In GARLAND, H. G. *and* PHILLIPS, W. (eds) *Textbook of medicine.* Vol. I. Macmillan (1953) pp. 166–219.
SUTHERLAND, J. D. Scientific tasks for the psychological clinic. In MACE, C. A. *and* VERNON, P. E. (eds) *Current trends in British psychology* Methuen (1953), pp. 223–33.
SUTHERLAND, J. D. Psychotherapy and social casework, I. In GOLDBERG, E. M. *et al.* (eds) *The boundaries of casework. A report on a residential refresher course held by the Association of Psychiatric Social Workers, Leicester 1956.* A.P.S.W. (1956), pp. 22–35.

SUTHERLAND, J. D. Casework in a community setting. *Social Work* (1957) *14*, 265–78.

SUTHERLAND, J. D. Prevention and the treatment of psychiatric reactions to stress by psychosocial means. In TANNER, J. M. (ed.) *Stress and psychiatric disorder. Proceedings of the 2nd Oxford Conference of the Mental Health Research Fund, 1958.* Blackwell Scientific Publications (1960), pp. 104–17.

SUTHERLAND, J. D. Object-relations theory and the conceptual model of psychoanalysis. *Brit. J. Med. Psychol.* (1963) *36*, 109–20.

SUTHERLAND, J. D. Providing psychotherapeutic facilities: the changing role of the social case worker and its requirements. *Brit. J. Psychiatr. Soc. Work* (1963) *7*, 64–72.

SUTHERLAND, J. D. *and* GILL, H. S. The significance of the oneway vision screen in analytic group psychotherapy. *Brit. J. Med. Psychol.* (1964) *37*, 185–202.

SUTHERLAND, J. D. Recent advances in the understanding of small groups, their disorders and treatment. (Paper read at the 6th International Congress of Psychotherapy, London 1964). *Psychother. Psychosom.* (1965) *13*, 110–25.

SUTHERLAND, J. D. *see* KELNAR, J. (1956).

SUTHERLAND, J. D., GILL, H. S. *and* PHILLIPSON, H. Psychodiagnostic appraisal in the light of recent theoretical developments. *Brit. J. Med. Psychol.* (1967) *40*, 299–315.

SUTHERLAND, J. D. The consultant psychotherapist in the National Health Service: his role and training. *Brit. J. Psychiat.* (1968) *114*, 509–15.

SUTTIE, I. D. Some normal offenders. *Probation* (1930) *1*, no. 5, 69–70.

SUTTIE, I. D. *and* SUTTIE, Jane I. The mother: agent or object? *Brit. J. Med. Psychol.* (1932) *12*, 91–108.

SUTTIE, I. D. *and* SUTTIE, Jane I. The mother: agent or object? II. *Brit. J. Med. Psychol.* (1932) *12*, 199–233.

SUTTIE, I. D. Religion: racial character and mental and social health. *Brit. J. Med. Psychol.* (1932) *12*, 289–314.

SUTTIE, I. D. A common standpoint and foundation for psychopathology. *J. Ment. Sci.* (1933) *79*, 18–26.

SUTTIE, I. D. Is acquisitiveness an instinct? *Psyche* (1933) *13*, 154–63.

SUTTIE, I. D. Mental and social health. *Probation* (1933) *1*, no. 15, 229–30.

SUTTIE, I. D. The need for 'social' therapy. *Med. Press and Circular* (1934) *188*, 41–3.

SUTTIE, I. D. *The origins of love and hate.* Kegan Paul, Trench, Trubner & Co. (1935).

TAVISTOCK INSTITUTE OF HUMAN RELATIONS. *Social research and a national policy for science.* A paper of the Council of the Tavistock Institute of Human Relations. Tavistock Publications (Tavistock Pamphlet No. 7, 1964).

TERUEL, G. Considerations for a diagnosis in marital psychotherapy. *Brit. J. Med. Psychol.* (1966) *39*, 231–6.

THOMPSON, A. G. Abnormal psychology in relation to emotional development. In REES, J. R. (ed.) *Modern practice in psychological medicine.* Butterworth (1949), pp. 30—48.

TORRIE, A. Bromide toxicosis. In CONTROL, BOARD OF. *23rd Annual Report* (1936) Pt. 2, p. 79.

TRIST, E. L. *and* BAMFORTH, K. W. Some social and psychological consequences of the longwall method of coal-getting. *Hum. Relat.* (1951) *4*, 3–38.

TRIST, E. L. *and* SOFER, C. *Exploration in group relations.* Leicester University Press (1959).

TRIST, E. L. Social structure and psychological stress. In WALKER, C. *et al.* (eds) *Modern technology and civilisation.* New York (1962) pp. 414–18. (Expanded version of 'Work organisation at the coal face', a paper read at the 2nd Oxford Conference of the Mental Research Fund, 1958; summarized in TANNER, J. M. (ed.) *Stress and psychiatric disorder.* Blackwell Scientific Publications (1960), pp. 115–7.)

TRIST, E. L., HIGGIN, G. W., MURRAY, H. *and* POLLOCK, A. B. *Organisational choice: capabilities of groups at the coal face under changing technologies.* Tavistock Publications (1963).

TRIST, E. L. The need of the social psychiatrist to influence wider social networks and their environments. (Paper read at the 6th International Congress of Psychotherapy, London 1964.) *Psychother. Psychosom.* (1965) *13*, 229–37.

TRIST, E. L. *see* CURLE, A. (1947).
see EMERY, F. E. (1960), (1965).
see HERBERT, E. L. (1953).
see HILL, J. M. M. (1953), (1955).
see RICE, A. K. (1950), (1952).
see SEMEONOFF, B. (1958).
see WILSON, A. T. M. (1952).

TRIST, E. L. Community psychiatry: a discussion. *Int. J. Psychiat.* (1965) *1*, 574–7.

TURQUET, P. M. Aggression in nature and society, II. *Brit. J. Med. Psychol.* (1949) *22*, 156–60.

TURQUET, P. M. The criteria for a psychoanalytic interpretation, III, *Aristot. Soc. Suppl. Vol.* (1962) *36*, 121–44.

TURQUET, P. M. A seminar at work. *Medical World* (1963) *99*, no. 8, 641–8.

TURQUET, P. M. *and* THOMAE, H. Training in psychosomatic medicine: a critical review. In *Advances in psychosomatic medicine, Vol. 4.* New York (1964), pp. 167–221.

TUSTIN, F. Anorexia nervosa in an adolescent girl. *Brit. J. Med. Psychol.* (1958) *31*, 184–200.

UPSON, P. G. Some aspects of perceptual defence. *Rorschach Newsletter* (1967) *12*, no. 1, 21–34.

UPSON, P. G. The psychodynamics of reading disability on a pilot study. *Brit. J. Proj. Psychol.* (1968) *13*, no. 2, 15–21.

VAN BEINUM, H. J. J. Industrial relations on the shop floor. *Management* (1966) *13*, 130–9.

WEBER, Hilda. Hunger and appetite: a suggested correlation between physiological and psychological processes. *J. Ment. Sci.* (1930) *76*, 724–36.

WEBER, Hilda. Some points of disagreement with Freudian practice and theory. *Psyche* (1931/2) *12*, no. 1, 23–48.

WEBER, Hilda, The psychological factor in migraine. *Brit. J. Med. Psychol.* (1932) *12*, 151–73.

WEBER, Hilda. Psycho-analysis and individual psychology. *Med. Press and Circular* (1932) *184*, 366–7.

WEBER, Hilda. Parental discord in the formation of the neurotic character. In *Individual psychology and the child. II.* (Individual Psychology Medical Pamphlets, no. 8) C. W. Daniel (1933).

WEBER, Hilda. Mental disorders of the post-menopausal period. In FERGUSON, M. *et al. Awareness and the neurosis of the declining years.* C. W. Daniel (1935). (Individual Psychology Pamphlets, no. 14). pp. 31–7.

WEBER, Hilda. The post-menopausal neurosis. *Med. Press and Circular* (1935) *190*, 277–81.

WEBER, Hilda. An approach to the problem of fear in children. *J. Ment. Sci.* (1936) *82*, 136–47.

WEBER, Hilda. Fear in childhood. *Lancet* (1936) *i*, 981–4.

WEBER, Hilda. The suicidal impulse and the value of psychological treatment. *Practitioner* (1937) *139*, 168–77.

WEBER, Hilda. Suicide and the human element in therapy. *Med. Press and Circular* (1938) *196*, 115–20.

WESTHEIMER, I. *see* HEINICKE, C. M. (1965).

WHEELER, W. M. Psychodiagnostic assessments of a child after prolonged separation in early childhood. II. *Brit. J. Med. Psychol.* (1956) *29*, 248–57.

WILLIAMS, A. H. *Ehekonflikte in Psychoanalytischer Sicht in Ehekonflikte*. Stuttgart (1956).

WILLIAMS, A. H. The treatment of abnormal murderers. *Howard J. Penol.* (1965) *11*, 286–96.

WILLIAMS, A. H. Keats — La belle dame sans merci; the bad breast mother. *Amer. Imago* (1966) *23*, 63–81.

WILLIAMS, A. H. The mind of a child murderer. *Mental Health* (1967) Winter issue, pp. 7–8

WILLIAMS, C. Differential diagnosis of elderly patients showing depressive and other symptoms. *Rorschach Newsletter* (Brit. Rorschach Forum) (1957) *2*, no. 1. 14–17.

WILLIAMS, C. *and* BOREHAM, J. L. Test and re-test: before and after psychotherapy. *Rorschach Newsletter* (Brit. Rorschach Forum) (1961) *6*, no. 1, 3–15.

WILLIAMS, M. A study of hysteria in women. *J. Anal. Psychol.* (1956) *1*, 177–186.

WILLIAMS, M. Changing attitudes to death; a survey of contributions to *Psychological Abstracts* over a thirty year period. *Hum. Relat.* (1966) *19*, 405–23.

WILSON, A. T. M. *and* WRIGHT, Samson. Anti-curare action of potassium and other substances. *Quart. J. Exp. Physiol.* (1936/7) *26*, 127–39.

WILSON, A. T. M. The aetiology of the peptic ulcer. *Proceedings of the 10th International Medical Congress for Psychotherapy*. Oxford (1938).

[WILSON, A. T. M.] DAVIES, D. T. *and* WILSON, A. T. M. Observations on the life history of chronic peptic ulcer. *Lancet* (1937) *ii*, 1353–60.

WILSON, A. T. M. The psychological observations on haematemesis. *Brit. J. Med. Psychol.* (1939) *18*, 112–21.

WILSON, A. T. M. The serviceman comes home. *Pilot Papers* (1946) *1*, no. 2, 9–28.

WILSON, A. T. M. The development of a scientific basis in family casework. *Social Work* (1947) *4*, 62–9.

WILSON, A. T. M. Some implications of medical practice and social casework for action research. *J. Social Issues* (1947) *3*, no. 2, 11–28.

WILSON, A. T. M., DOYLE, M. *and* KELNAR, J. Group techniques in a transitional community. *Lancet* (1947) *i*, 21 May, 735–8.

WILSON, A. T. M. Human factors in industry. The problems of deterrents and applied social science. *Advanc. Sci.* (1947/8) *5*, 111–16.

WILSON, A. T. M. *Hospital nursing auxiliaries. Notes on a background survey and job analysis.* Tavistock Publications (1949). Shorter version in: *Hum. Relat.* (1950) *3*, 89–105.

WILSON, A. T. M. Some reflections and suggestions on the prevention and treatment of marital problems. *Hum. Relat.* (1949) *2*, 233–52.

WILSON, A. T. M. A note on some current problems of the social services. *Social Work* (1951) *8*, 504–14.

WILSON, A. T. M. Some aspects of social process. (Kurt Lewin Memorial Award Lecture). *J. Social Issues* (1951) Suppl. series no. 5.

WILSON, A. T. M., TRIST, E. L. *and* CURLE, A. Transitional communities and social reconnection. A study of the civil resettlement of British prisoners of war. In SWANSON, G. E. *et al.* (eds) *Readings in social psychology.* 2nd edition. New York (1952) pp. 561–79.

WILSON, A. T. M. Interaction between individual and culture. In TANNER, J. M. (ed.) *Prospects in psychiatric research. Proceedings of the Oxford Conference of the Mental Health Research Fund, 1952.* Blackwell Scientific Publications (1953), pp. 55–63.

WILSON, A. T. M. Social change in structured groups. In MACE, C. A. *and* VERNON, P. E. (eds) *Current trends in British psychology.* Methuen (1953), pp. 98–113.

WILSON, A. T. M. A note on social research. *Sociol. Rev.* (1955) *3*, 109–16.

WILSON, A. T. M. *see* BRIDGER, H. (1947).

WILSON, Henry. The treatment of the voluntary boarder. *J. Ment. Sci.* (1933) *79*, 102–36.

WILSON, Henry. The neurotic's physical symptoms: their early recognition. *Practitioner* (1935) *134*, 762–71.

WILSON, Henry. Psychology in relation to public health. *Public Health* (1935/6) *49*, 203–12.

WILSON, Isabel G. H. Nursing of obvious nervous illness in general hospital. *Nursing Times* (1929) *25*, 1442; 1483; 1506.

WILSON, Isabel G. H. The place of psychology in general nursing. *Nursing Times* (1929) *25*, 1366.

WILSON, Isabel G. H. Psychological help in linked symptoms of body and mind. Parts I and II. *Nursing Times* (1929) *25*, 1384; 1414.

WILSON, Isabel G. H. *Psychology in general nursing*. Arnold (1931).

WITTKOWER, Erich. *Einfluss der Gemütsbewegungen auf den Körper*. Vienna, (1936). (2nd edition, 1937.)

[WITTKOWER, Erich] DOBREFF, M., PENEFF, L. *and* WITTKOWER, Erich. Über den Einfluss von Gemütsbewegungen auf den Blutcholesteringehalt. *Zeit. fur d.ges.exp.Medizin* (1936) *98*, 428–31.

[WITTKOWER, Erich] BOURNE, G., SCOTT, R. B. *and* WITTKOWER, Erich. The psychological factor in cardiac pain. *Lancet* (1937) *ii*, 609–13.

WITTKOWER, Erich. The psychological factor in cardiac pain. *Lancet* (1937) *ii*, 665–70.

[WITTKOWER, Erich] LOWEY, A. *and* WITTKOWER, Erich. *The pathology of high altitude climate*. Oxford University Press (1937).

WITTKOWER, Erich. Some observations on the influence of emotions on bodily functions. *Proceedings of the International Congress of Psychology*, Paris (1937).

WITTKOWER, Erich. Ulcerative colitis: personality studies. *Brit. Med. J.* (1938) *ii*, 1356–60.

[WITTKOWER, Erich] KLABER, R. *and* WITTKOWER, Erich. Pathogenesis of rosacea: review with special reference to emotional factors. *Brit. J. Dermatol.* (1939) *51*, 501–24.

WITTKOWER, Erich *and* SPILLANE, J. P. Neurosis in war. *Brit. Med. J.* (1940) *i*, 223–5; 265–8; 308–10.

WITTKOWER, Erich *and* WILSON, A. T. M. Dysmenorrhoea and sterility: personality studies. *Brit. Med. J.* (1940) *ii*, 586–90.

[WITTKOWER, Erich] BOURNE, G. *and* WITTKOWER, Erich. Psychological treatment of cases with cardiac pain. *Brit. Heart J.* (1940) *2*, 25–32.

WITTKOWER, Erich, RODGER, T. F. *and* WILSON, A. T. M. Effort syndrome. *Lancet* (1946) *i*, 531–5.

WITTKOWER, E. D. The psychological aspects of venereal disease. *Brit. J. Vener. Dis.* (1948) *24*, 59.

[WITTKOWER, E. D.] TODD, G. S. *and* WITTKOWER, E. D. The psychological aspects of sanatorium management. *Lancet* (1948) *i*, 10 Jan., 49–53.

WITTKOWER, E. D. Psychiatry and the skin. *Proc. Roy. Soc. Med.* (1950) *43*, 799–801.

WITTKOWER, E. D. Acne vulgaris: a psychosomatic study. *Brit. J. Derm.* (1951) *63*, 214–23.

WITTKOWER, E. D. Eczema: a psychosomatic study. *Arch. Derm. Syph. N.Y.* (1951) *63*, 207–19.

WOODHOUSE, D. L. Casework with problem families. *Case Conf.* (1958–59) *5*, 31–9.

WOODHOUSE, D. L. Psychiatric influences in community services, II. In IRVINE, E. E. (ed.) *Ventures in professional co-operation.* Association of Psychiatric Social Workers (1961), pp. 64–76.

WOODHOUSE, D. L. How will this marriage work? — II. (Paper read at the Family Planning Association, London Group Conference on 'The marriage relationship', Nov. 1961.) *Social Work.* (1962) *19*, no. 4, 13–16.

WOODHOUSE, D. L. The marital relationship. In COUNCIL FOR TRAINING IN SOCIAL WORK. *Human growth and behaviour as a subject of study for social workers, Section II: Designing a syllabus.* C.T.S.W. (1967) pp. 21–2.

WOODHOUSE, D. L. *see* GOSLING, R. (1967).
see LYONS, A. (1968).

WRIGHT, M. B. Sociological factors which influence the suicide rate. *Psyche* (1931/2) *12*, no. 2, 52–61.

YOUNG, James. Critique of the analytical psychology of Jung. In CULPIN, M. *Recent advances in the study of psychoneuroses.* Churchill (1931), pp. 243–76.

Index

Persons included in the index are those whose policies, views or work are described in the text. A complete list of names is on pp. 328–62. Publications mentioned in the text are italicized. A complete list of publications is on pp. 363–402.

INDEX